Large Animal Orthopaedics

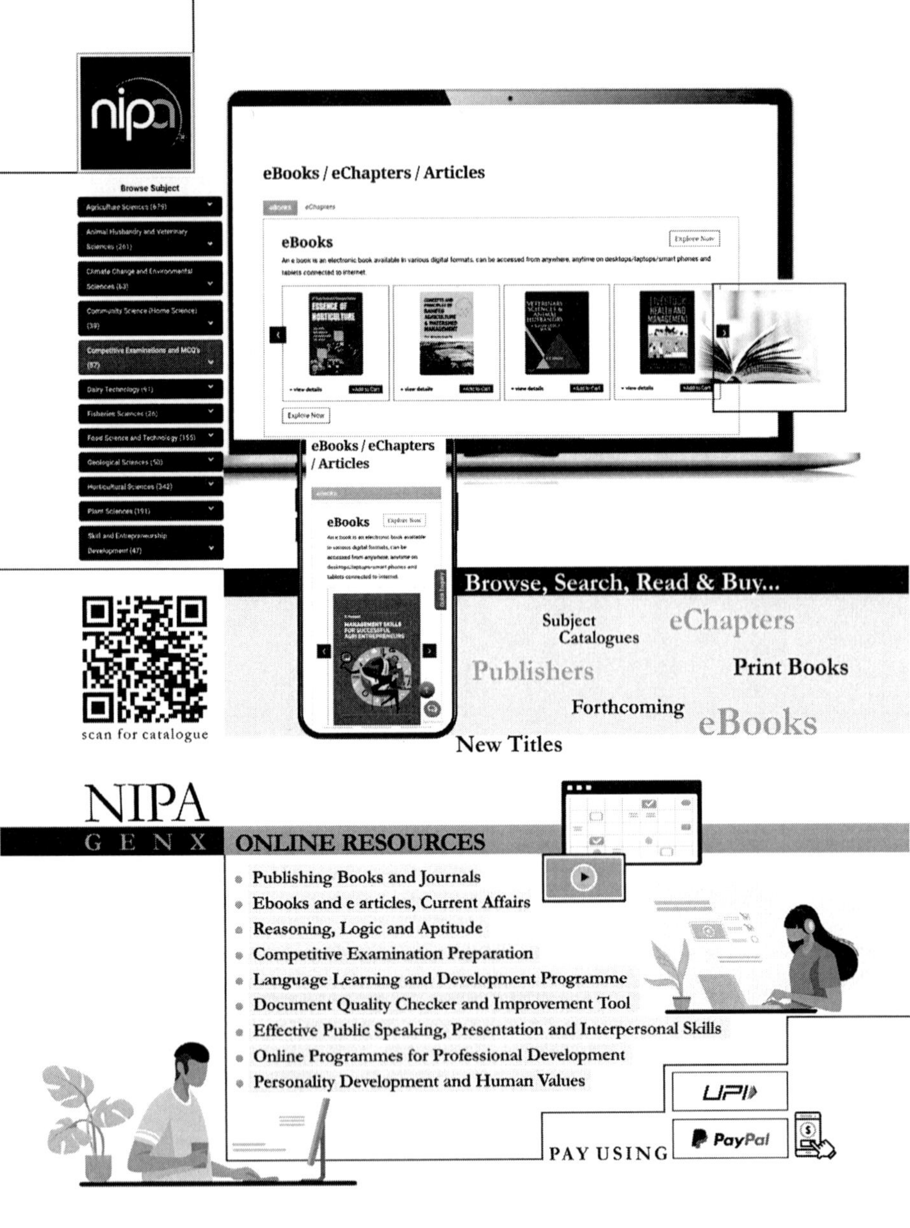

nipa
Browse Subject
eBooks / eChapters / Articles
eBooks
Explore Now
eBooks / eChapters / Articles
Browse, Search, Read & Buy...
Subject Catalogues
eChapters
Publishers
Print Books
Forthcoming
eBooks
New Titles
scan for catalogue
NIPA
GENX
ONLINE RESOURCES
Publishing Books and Journals
Ebooks and e articles, Current Affairs
Reasoning, Logic and Aptitude
Competitive Examination Preparation
Language Learning and Development Programme
Document Quality Checker and Improvement Tool
Effective Public Speaking, Presentation and Interpersonal Skills
Online Programmes for Professional Development
Personality Development and Human Values
PAY USING
UPI
PayPal

Large Animal Orthopaedics
An Illustrated Handbook on Prosthetic Fittings and Rehabilitations

Sadananda Nayak, Ph.D.
(Retired) Professor and Head
Department of Veterinary Surgery & Radiology
College of Veterinary Science & Animal Husbandary
Orissa University of Agriculture and Technology, Bhubneshwar 751 003
Orissa , Bhubaneswar

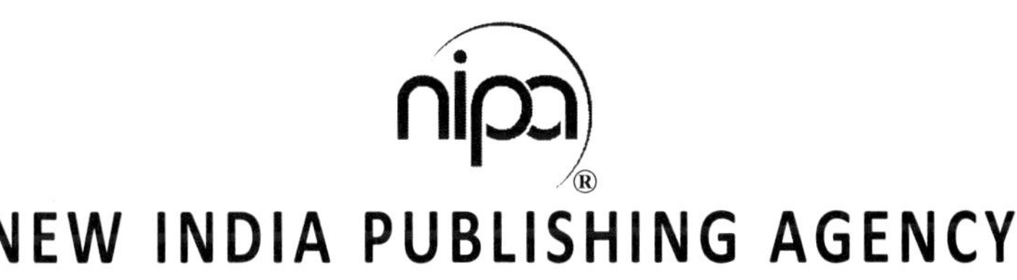

New Delhi – 110 034

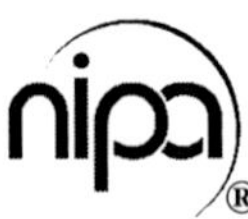

NEW INDIA PUBLISHING AGENCY
101, Vikas Surya Plaza, CU Block, LSC Market
Pitam Pura, New Delhi 110 034, India
Phone: + 91 (11)27 34 17 17 Fax: + 91(11) 27 34 16 16
Email: info@nipabooks.com
Web: www.nipabooks.com

Feedback at feedbacks@nipabooks.com

ISBN : 978-93-89130-25-6

Composed and Designed by NIPA

Dr. Jibanananda Mohanty, PhD
Professor and Head (Retd.)
Veterinary Surgery & Radiology
Ex-Dean, Faculty of Veterinary Science and Animal Husbandry
Bhubaneswar
Ex - Director
Department of Animal Husbandry and Veterinary Services, Odisha

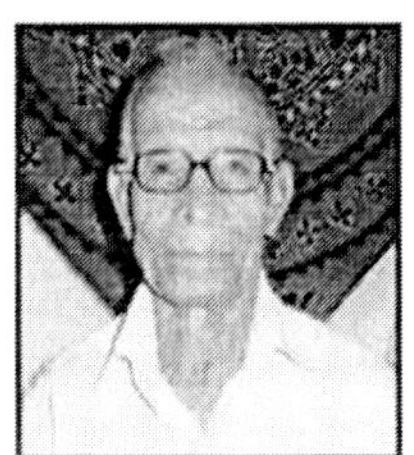

Foreword

The book "Large Animal Orthopaedics: An Illustrated Handbook on Prosthetic Fittings and Rehabilitations" is very unique because the writer Prof. (Dr.) Sadananda Nayak is himself the artist who has depicted every stage of the surgical technique as he teaches in his classes. Students need has been looked into in each presentation. Some collections have come from rare old publications of repute. Steps in modified Thomas splints fabrication, immobilization and retention of fracture and rehabilitation work has important surgical pathways for the field veterinarians as well as students In undergraduate and post graduate courses. Writer's long years of experience have been meticulously focused. The demonstrations are very nice and representative. I am sure this book will be of much use and popular among the students as well as field veterinarians.

I praise for this sincere attempt

(Dr. J.N. Mohanty)

Chintamaniswar Area, Plot No. 76, Bhubaneswar - 751 006, Odisha
Tel: 0674-2312362, Mob: +91-91787 97963

Preface

The concept of amputation, prosthetic, orthotic fitting and orthopedic rehabilitation on large animals is an innovative practice developed by the author. The author has developed several techniques of fitting of prosthetic and orthotic appliances for the large animals. Out of such practice and experience the need for publishing a book on "Large Animal Orthopaedics: An Illustrated Handbook on Prosthetic Fittings and Rehabilitations" was felt. The practical lessions and illustrations included in the book will be of very much of use for the students, teachers and researchers and practitioners in Veterinary Science in general and surgery in particular. In my 33 years of professional teaching and research experience, I feel the absence of such an illustrated book covering details of surgical techniques in teaching in a brief manner with pictorial representation. This prompted me to elaborate my experience gained in my practical fields in surgical treatment of large animals. Apart from that I have consulted a number of fellow faculty and consulted a good number of literature in the field which I wanted to reflect in the book. The basic idea behind writing this book is to publish innovative methods and new affective techniques that are easy successful and cost effective. In orthopaedic treatment in large animals fitting of articificial limbs, prosthetic and orthotic appliances, amputation and rehabilitation appear to be very rare and complicated. Large numbers of hand drawings and photographs have been incorporated in order to visualize the surgical techniques for better understanding. Fabrication of modified Thomas Splint has been demonstrated step wise using illustrations. Use of conjoined 'U' plate for better immobilization in case of lower limb fabrication in large animals is claimed as an innovative step. A sling has been fabricated for lifting of downed large animals for making them mobile to facilitate exercise of unused and paralyzed limbs using locally available materials to make it cost effective as well as availability in most rural interiors. The statement "A good surgeon is one who amputates a limb, but a better is one who save a limb". However blessings of Almighty are always behind a success.

I am extremely grateful to Dr.J.N.Mohanty, my teacher for his help and advice. I extend my gratefulness to Dr. R.K.Mahapatra, Chief Librarian, Central Library, OUAT for his encouragement for writing this book and getting this book published. I owe to my family members for their continued support and assistance in preparation of this manuscript. I convey thanks to M/S. New India Publishing

Agency, New Delhi who has taken immense interest to publish this book. Finally, I am sure this book will be a useful addition to the subject of veterinary orthopaedics providing clear understanding on surgical techniques which will be of immense benefit for the students, researchers and faculty in Veterinary Science.

Prof. Sadananda Nayak

Contents

Foreword .... *v*

Preface .... *vii*

List of Figures/Plates/Photos .... *xv*

1. Abnormal Movement of Limb 1
2. Body Symmetry of Animal in Relation to Location of Centre of Gravity 3
3. Gait of A Normal Animal, Fractured Patient and Animal with Thomas Splint 5
4. Skeletal System of Bovine 7
5. Number of Bones in Skeleton of Ox 10
6. Superficial Muscles of Fore and Hind Limbs 13
7. Skull of Ox : Dorsal View 15
8. Skull of Ox (Sinuses Opened) 17
9. Skull of Ox, without Mandible, Ventral View 18
10. Skull of Ox: Lateral Vew 21
11. Sagittal Section of Skull of Ox Without Mandible 22
12 Mandible and Hyoid Bone 23
13. Atlas 24
14. The Cervical Vertebrae 26
15. Fourth Lumbar Vertebrae and Sacrum of Ox 29
16. Scapula of Ox 32
17. Carpus and Adjacent Bones of Ox 34
18. Metacarpal and Metatarsal of Ox 36
19. Bone of Distal Part of Fore Limb of Ox 37

20. Sacrum of Ox 40

21. Bones of the Pelvic Girdle 42

22. Right Os Coxae of Ox; Lateral View 44

23. Bones of the Hind Limb 46

24. Tarsus and Adjacent Bones of Ox 50

25. Orthopaedic Instruments 52

26. First Aid in Orthopaedic Patient 54

27. Classification of Fracture 57

28. Curve Showing Degree of Inflammation and Time of Application of External Immobilisers 58

29. Bone Showing Various Level of Fracture and Their External Immobilisation Technique 60

30. Fracture Immobilizing Bandages 63

31. Various External Immobilizer for Large Animal Fracture Repair 65

32. Immobilization of Fracture by Temporary Immobilizer 66

33. Pop Bandaging Technique 67

34. Length to be Covered by P.O.P Cast for Immobilization of Fracture of Different Sites 70

35. Reinforced Pop Cast with Padded Bamboo Splints 72

36. Pop Cast With Window for Compound Fracture 74

37. Materials used for Immobilization of Fractured Limb with Gum Bandage 76

38. Arrangement of 16 Layer Padded Cloth 78

39. Fabrication of Netted Padded Bamboo Splint 80

40. Fabrication of Single U-Plate and Conjoindu-Plate Using Green Bamboo, Cane, Bread Twiser and Iron Rod 82

41. Liberal Application of GUM over the Fracture Area for Immobilisation 84

42. Application of Cotton Padded Cloth and its Retention for Immobilization of Fracture Site 86

43. Application of First Layer Padded Cloth & Its Retention with Thread 88

44. Liberal Application of Gum Over the 1st Layer Padded Cloth 90

45. Reinforcement of Gum Bandage with Padded Netted Bamboo Splint 91

46. Fixation of Protective Rubber Slipper Over Foot 93

47. Classification of Fracture & its Repair in Large Animal 95

48. Lower Level Fracture and Its Repair 97

49. Treatment of Lower Level Fracture (HINDLIMB) 101

50. Lower Level Fracture 103

51. Middle Level Fracture Repair 109

52. Middle Level Fracture 112

53. Higher Level Fracture Repair 118

54. Photo Feature of Higher Level Fracture 120

55. Highest Level Fracture (HLF) and its Management 123

56. Photo Features of Highest Level Fracture 125

57. Conjoined 'U' Plate with Ring for Immobilisation of Radius and Ulna Fracture 127

58. Hanging Pin Cast 129

59. Intramedullary Pinning of Humerus in Large Animal 131

60. Intramedullary Pinning of Femur in Large Animal 135

61. Modified Valpeau Sling for Highest Level Fore Limb Fracture 139

62. Modified Velpeau Sling for Highest Level Fracture of Hind Limb 141

63. Different Types of Thomas Splints 144

64. Thomas Splint Used in Animals (For Fore limb) 145

65. List of Requisite for Preparation of Large Animal Thomas Splint 147

66. Measurement of Ring of Thomas Splint for Large Animal 149

67. Wire Rings Required for Different Age Group of Animals 152

68. Preparation of Side Bars of Large Animal Thomas Splint 153

69. Method of Tying Ring with Bamboo Splint and Description 155

70. Padding of Thomas Splint Ring with Jute & Cotton Bandage 157

71. Medial Bending of Lower Half of Thomas Splint 159

72. Measurement of Length of Thomas Splint, Shortening of Length & Padding of Distal End 161

73. Net Fabrication in Large Animals Thomas Splint 163

74. Fitting Thomas Splint and Its Retention Over Gum Bandage 166

75. Fitting of Thomas Splint in Forelimb of Large Animal 167

76. Method of Fitting of Thomas Splint in Hind Limb of Large Animal ... 169

77. Method of Securing Thomas Splint 171

78. Method of Fixation of Hoof With the Distal End of Thomas Splint ... 172

80. Recommendation of Confinement Space and Time for Fracture Immobilised Patient 175

82. Fabrication of Durable Thomas Splint 178

84. Immobilisation of Proximal 1/3rd Metacarpal and Metatarsal Bone .. 183

85. Technique of Immobilization of Carpometacarpal and Tarsometa Tarsal or Joint Dislocation 185

86. Immobilisation Technique for Upper Third Radius-Ulna Fracture 187

87. Technique of Immobilization of Upper 3rd Tibia Fibula Fracture 189

88. Conjoined Double Thomas Splint for Both Tibia Fibula - Fracture Repair 191

89. Immobilization of Symphysial Fractured Mandible in Large Animals 193

90. Immobilization of Fracture of Ramus of Mandible 195

91. Immobilization of Limb for Flexor Tendon Repair 197

92. Digital Tendon Repair 199

93. Suturing Technique of Transected Gastrocnemious Tendon 202

94. Immobilization of Hind Limb for Tendo Achiles Repair 204

95. Hip Dislocation and It's Correction 210

96. Contracted Leg in Calves 212

97. Flushing Facility of Compound Fracture 216

98. Flushing Facility of Compound Fracture 220

99. Provision of Counter Opening and Flushing Catheter Fixation Within Infected Fracture 222

100. Classification of Tumor 223

101. Classification of Bone Tumours 224

102. Amputation of the Claw 228

103. Single Digit Amputation 232

104. Double Digit Amputation 234

105. Level of Amputation at Fore & Hind Limb by Bone Section Technique 237

106. Method of Apposing Muscle, Fascia, Skin Over Amputed Stump 241

107. Joint Disarticulation Method of Limb Amputation 244

108. Fetlock Disarticulation 247

109. Carpo-Metacarpal Joint Disarticulation 248

110. Elbow Disarticulation 249

111. Shoulder Disarticulation 250

112. Tarso-Metatarsal Joint Disarticulation Technique in Large animal 252

113. Stiffle Disarticulation 254

114. HIP Disarticulation 255

115. Figures of Various Amputees by Joint Disarticulation Method 258

116. Comparison Between Bone Section and Joint Disarticulation Method of Limb Amputation 260

117. Different Steps in Preparation of Permanent Prothesis 264

118. Different Steps in Preparation of Fore Limb Prothesis 267

119. Below Knee (B.K) Prothesis 269

120. Above Knee (A.K.) Prosthesis 270

121. Hind Foot Prosthesis-I 271

122. Below Hock (B.H.) Prosthesis -II 272

123. Above Hock (A.H.) Prosthesis – III 273

124. Amputation and Prosthetic Limb Below Carpus in Cattle 274
125. Indications for Rehabiltation of Downer's Cow Using Mobile Sling . 280
126. Requisite for Preparation of Large Animal Mobile Sling 282
127. Fabrication of Mobile Sling 284
128. Preparation of Padded Tyres for Sling Preparation 286
129. Supportive Sling 288
130. Fabrication of Mobile Sling 290
131. Method of Placing Downer Animal Within The Sling 291
132. Method of Slinging 292
133. Recommended Duration for Slinging Large Animal 294
134. Sling Rehabilitation of Calf 296
135. Importance of Rehabilitation of More Than one Limb Fractured Animal Within Mobile Sling 298
136. Rehabilitation of Large Animal in Exercise Cart 299
137. Rehabilitation of Two Limb Fractured Animal Within Mobile Sling ... 304
138. Osteology 305
139. Prosthetic Fitting 307

List of Figures/Plates/Photos

Chapter 2. Body Symmetry of Animal in Relation to Location of Centre of Gravity 3

Fig. 1: Body symmetry of animal in relation to location of centre of gravity 4

Fig. 2: Location of centre of gravity, site for measurement of length and girth of animal. 4

Chapter 3. Gait of A Normal Animal, Fractured Patient and Animal with Thomas Splint 5

Fig. 1: Gait of normal animal. Animal generally takes a lift to full extent in each step. 6

Fig. 2: Gait of normal animal (full lifting of foot) 6

Fig. 3: Gait of a fractured patient (more dragging and less lifting of foot). 6

Fig. 4: Gait of animal with light Thomas splint (less dragging and more lifting of foots). 6

Fig. 5: Gait of animal with heavy Thomas splint (more dragging and less lifting of foot) 6

Chapter 4. Skeletal System of Bovine 7

Fig. 1: Skeleton of cow. 8

Chapter 5. Number of Bones in Skeleton of Ox 10

Fig. 1: Skelton of Ox 12

Chapter 7. Skull of Ox : Dorsal View 15

Fig. 1: Skull of Ox: Dorsal View 16

Chapter 8. Skull of Ox (Sinuses Opened) 17

Fig. 1: Skull of Ox, Dorsal view, Sinuses Opened. 17

Chapter 9. Skull of Ox, without Mandible, Ventral View 18

Fig. 1. Skull of ox, without mandible, ventral view. 20

Chapter 10. Skull of Ox: Lateral Vew 21

Fig. 1: Skull of Ox: Lateral Vew 21

Chapter 11. Sagittal Section of Skull of Ox Without Mandible 22

Fig. 1: Sagittal section of Skull of Ox without mandible 22

Chapter 12. Mandible and Hyoid Bone 23

Fig. 1: Mandible 23

Fig. 2: Hyoid bone 23

Chapter 13. Atlas 24

Fig. 1: Atlas of Ox: Dorsal view. 25

Fig. 2: Atlas of Ox: Dorsal view. 25

Chapter 14. The Cervical Vertebrae 26

Fig. 1: Sixth cervical vertebra of ox: Posterior view. 28

Chapter 15. Fourth Lumbar Vertebrae and Sacrum of Ox 29

Fig. 1: Fourth Lumber Vertebrae of Ox. Posterior view 30

Fig. 2: Sacrum of Ox: Dorsal view 30

Chapter 16. Scapula of Ox 32
Fig. 1: Left scapula of ox - Lateral surface 33
Fig. 2: Glenoid angle of left scapula of horse (End view) 33
Fig. 3: Right scapula of Ox- Costal surface. 33
Chapter 17. Carpus and Adjacent Bones of Ox 34
Fig. 1: Left carpus and adjacent bones of Ox; Front view. 35
Fig. 2: Left carpus and adjacent bones of Ox; Lateral view. 35
Chapter 18. Metacarpal and Metatarsal of Ox 36
Fig. 1: Left metacarpal bone of ox: front view: the small bone has been moved laterally. 36
Fig. 2: Large metatarsal bone of ox : dorsal view 36
Chapter 19. Bone of Distal Part of Fore Limb of Ox 37
Fig. 1: Bones of distal part of fore limb of Ox: Lateral view. 38
Fig. 2: Bones of distal part of forelimb of Ox: Volar view 39
Chapter 20. Sacrum of Ox 40
Fig. 1: Sacrum of Ox; Dorsal View 40
Fig. 2: Sacrum of Ox, Ventral view 41
Chapter 21. Bones of the Pelvic Girdle 42
Fig. 1: Pelvic of cow, viewed from in front and somewhat from below. 43
Chapter 22. Right Os Coxae of Ox; Lateral View 44
Fig. 1: Right os coxae of ox; Lateral View 45
Chapter 23.Bones of the Hind Limb 46
Fig. 1: Right femur of Ox, Posterior view 48
Fig. 2: Left tibia and proximal part of fibula of ox posterior view 48
Chapter 24.Tarsus and Adjacent Bones of Ox 50
Fig. 1: Right tarsus and adjacent bones of ox- Medial view 50
Fig. 2: Right tarsus and adjacent bone of ox - Dorso -Lateral view 50
Fig. 3: Orthopaedics 51
Chapter 25.Orthopaedics Instruments 52
Fig. 1: Orthopaedics Instruments-1 52
Fig. 2: Orthopaedics Instruments-2 53
Chapter 27. Classification of Fracture 57
Fig. 1: Complete Fracture 57
Fig. 2: Green Stick Fracture 57
Fig. 3: Over riding Fracture 57
Fig. 4: Transverse Fracture 57
Fig. 5: Oblique Fracture 57
Fig. 6: Spiral Fracture 57
Fig. 7: Comminuted Fracture 57
Fig. 8: Multiple Fracture 57
Fig. 9: Avulsion Fracture 57
Fig.10: Condylar Fracture 57
Fig.11: Supra Condylar Fracture 57
Fig.12: Montegsia Fracture 57

Chapter 28.Curve Showing Degree of Inflammation and Time of Application of External Immobilisers ... 58
Fig. 1: Showing curve showing degree of inflammation and time of application of external immobilizing devices. ... 59
Chapter 29. Bone Showing Various Level of Fracture and Their External Immobilisation Technique ... 60
Fig. 1: Showing level of fractures in large animal. ... 62
Chapter 30. Fracture Immobilizing Bandages ... 63
Fig. 1: Cotton Bandage ... 63
a. Plane Cotton Bandage ... 63
b. Gamgee Bandage ... 63
Fig. 2: Adhesive Tape Bandages ... 63
a. Leukoplast ... 63
b. Micropore Tape ... 63
Fig. 3: Plaster Bandages ... 63
a. POP Bandages ... 63
b. Gypsona ... 63
Fracture Immobilizing Bandages - II ... 64
Fig. 4: Cast Bandages ... 64
a. Elastic bandages ... 64
b. Polyester cast ... 64
Fig. 5: Robert-Jones Bandages ... 64
a. Fibre glass cast ... 64
b. Crepe Bandage ... 64
Fig. 6: Fibre glass cast ... 64
a. For Horse ... 64
b. For Dog ... 64
Chapter 31.Various External Immobilizer for Large Animal Fracture Repair ... 65
Fig. 1: (a) and (b) Modified Thomas splint. ... 65
Fig. 2: (a) Caudal halfcast for forelimb ... 65
Fig. 2: (b) Caudal halfcast for hindlimb ... 65
Fig. 4: (a) Bamboo ... 65
Fig. 3: Metal conjoined U plate ... 65
Fig. 5: (b) Rope netted ... 65
Fig. 6: (c) Wire netted ... 65
Chapter 32.Immobilization of Fracture by Temporary Immobilizer ... 66
Fig. 1: Netted Bamboo splint ... 66
Fig. 2: 16-20 layer cloth padding ... 66
Fig. 3: Conjointed U-Plate ... 66
Fig. 4: Application of cloth padding over fracture site ... 66
Fig. 5: Application of bamboo splint over fracture site ... 66
Fig. 6: Application of conjoined U-Plate over fracture site ... 66
Chapter 33.Pop Bandaging Technique ... 67
Fig. 1: (a) Pop bandage roll preparation ... 69

Fig. 1: (b) Pop slint preparation 69
Fig. 2: Placement of POP splint over the fractured region at anterior & posterior surface 69
Fig. 3: (a) Metacarpal/Metatarsal - 2splints 69
Fig. 3: (b) Radius ulna / tibia fibula-4 splints 69
Fig. 4: (a) Complete POP bandage application upon limb 69
Fig. 4: (b) Cross section of POP application 69
Chapter 34. Length to be Covered by P.O.P Cast for Immobilization of Fracture of Different Sites 70
Fig. 1a: Length to be covered by POP Cast for immobilisation of Metatarsal and Tibio fibular fracture 71
FIg. lb: Above Carpus to below foot 71
Fig.lc: Above elbow to below foot 71
Fig.2a : Length to be covered for POP Cast for immobilisation of Metacarpal and Radius ulna fracture 71
Fig. 2b: Above hock to below foot 71
Fig. 2c: Above stifle to below hock 71
Chapter 35. Reinforced Pop Cast with Padded Bamboo Splints 72
Fig. 1: Application of bamboo splint over POP bandage 73
Fig. 2: Bamboo splint with soft cotton 73
Fig. 3: Cross section of limb with POP bandage and bamboo splints 73
Chapter 36.Pop Cast With Window for Compound Fracture 74
Fig. 1: Compund fracture 75
Fig. 3: Wrapping of thick padded cloth 75
Fig. 2: Fixation of flushing catheter and higher level of wound and application of soft padded absorbent cotton padding 75
Fig. 4: POP cast with window for compound fracture 75
Chapter 37.Materials used for Immobilization of Fractured Limb with Gum Bandage 76
Fig. 1: Fevicol gum-500gm. 77
Fig. 2: Green Bamboo 4-1. 77
Fig. 3: Dry bamboo 4-1 77
Fig. 4: Jute string 300-400 gm 77
Fig. 5: Bucycle tube 2'-1 77
Fig. 6: Bandage 3-4 roll 77
Fig. 7: 8-16 layer thick cloth 77
Fig. 8: Green bamboo splints -4 77
Fig. 9: Conjoined -U plate 77
Fig. 10: Netted bamboo splint 77
Fig. 11: Saw blade-2 77
Fig. 12: Double braided jute thread-10 77
Chapter 38. Arrangement of 16 Layer Padded Cloth 78
Fig 1: Making 2 equalparts of the cloth vertically 79
Fig 2: Onepiee is folded on midline and 2 layer padded cloth 79
Fig 3: 2, 4, 2 and 16 Layer cloths is further folded 79

Fig 4: The other piee of cloth from Fig. 1 is folded horzontally 79
Fig 5: 2 layer and 4 layer padded cloth 79
Chapter 39. Fabrication of Netted Padded Bamboo Splint 80
Fig 1: Marking of the bamboo splint 81
Fig 2: Grooving of the bamboo splint 81
Fig 3: Procedure for netting the bamboo splint 81
Fig 4: Netted bamboo splint (Complete) 81
Fig. 5: Padding over the bamboo splint (to avoid injury) 81
Fig 6: Width of netted padded bamboo splint ($1^1/_2$ rounding of bamboo splint over bone). 81
Chapter 40. Fabrication of Single U-Plate and Conjoindu-Plate Using Green Bamboo, Cane, Bread Twiser and Iron Rod 82
Fig. 1: U-Plate with green bamboo structure 82
Fig. 2: Bread Twiser 82
Fig. 3: U-Plate with bread twiser for fore-limb 82
Fig. 4: U-Plate with bread twiser for hindlimb 82
Fig. 5: U-Plate with cane 83
Fig. 6: Conjoint U-plate with metal of 6mm/ 8mm iron rod. 83
Chapter 41. Liberal Application of GUM over the Fracture Area for Immobilisation 84
Fig. 1: Fracture of Metacarpus 85
Fig. 2: Fracture of Radius Ulna 85
Fig. 3: Fracture of Metacarpus 85
Fig. 4: Fracture of Tibio Fibula 85
Chapter 42. Application of Cotton Padded Cloth and its Retention for Immobilization of Fracture Site 86
Fig. 1: Length of fractured limb to be covered with padding 86
Fig. 2: 16 Layer of thick sterile absorbent protective cotton padding 87
Fig. 3: Application of padded cloth over fractured site after application of traction 87
Fig. 4: Covering of padded cloth arround fractured site and its retention 87
Chapter 43. Application of First Layer Padded Cloth & Its Retention with Thread 88
Fig. 1: (a) Simple fracture of metacarpal and length of padded cloth to apply 88
Fig. 1: (b) Wrapping with padded cloth and its retention 88
Fig. 2: (a) Simple fracture of radius and ulna & length of padded cloth to be applied 89
Fig. 2: (b) Wrapping with padded cloth and its retention 89
Chapter 44. Liberal Application of Gum Over the 1st Layer Padded Cloth 90
Fig. 1: 1st layer padded cloth over the tract ured area. 90
Fig. 2: Liberal application of gum over the 1st layer padded cloth 90
Chapter 45. Reinforcement of Gum Bandage with Padded Netted Bamboo Splint 91
Fig. 1: Netted padded bamboo splint applied with adhesive gum at several places for coaptation. 92
Fig. 2: Protection of fracture site with soft bandage cotton padding with application of adhesive gum for strengthening with netted padded bamboo splint 92
Fig. 3: Strengthening of fracture site with netted padded bamboo splint wrapping with soft padding. 92

Fig. 3: (a) Wrapping of netted padded bamboo splint over the fracture site one & half round. 92
Fig. 4: Final coaptation bandage, ... 92
Chapter 46. Fixation of Protective Rubber Slipper Over Foot 93
Fig. 1: Protective Rubber tube (1 Feet long cycle tube) 94
Fig. 2: Rubber shoe protection overthe foot before thomas splint fixation 94
Fig. 3: Protective rubber shoe over netted bamboo splint 94
Fig. 4: Rubber shoe protection over 94
Chapter 47. Classification of Fracture & Its Repair in Large Animal 95
Fig. 1: Showing different levels of fracture and their appropriate method of treatment. 96
Chapter 48. Lower Level Fracture and Its Repair 97
Fig. 1: Length of limb to be coverd 99
Fig. 2: Thick cotton pad (16 layer) 99
Fig. 3: Netted bamboo splint 99
Fig. 4: Conjoint metal U plate 99
Fig. 5: Retention of cotton pad 99
Fig. 6: Bamboo splint application 99
Fig. 7: Conjoint metal U plae application 9
Immobilization of Metacarpus Compound Fracture Using Netted Bamboo Spilint and Conjoint Angular Metalic Splint (CAMS) 100
Fig. 1: Netted bamboo splint 100
Fig. 2: Conjoint angular metalic splint 100
Fig. 3: Netted bamboo splint application upon metacarpus compound fracture 100
Fig. 4: Complete immobilization of metacarpus compound fracture 100
Chapter 49. Treatment of Lower Level Fracture (HINDLIMB) 101
Fig. 1: Length of hte limb at the fracture site to be covered with coamputational bandage 102
Fig. 2: (a) Thick padded cloth 102
Fig. 2: (b) Padded netted bamboo splint 102
Fig. 2: (c) Conjoined U plate 102
Fig. 3: Protection of fracture site with thick padded cotton cloth 102
Fig. 4: Strengthening of protective cloth with padded netted bamboo splint 102
Fig. 5: Fitting of conjoined U plate at the fracture site 102
Chapter 50. Lower Level Fracture 103
Application of Bamboo Splint and Conjoint U-Plate in Lower Level Fracture 104
Management of Metacarpal Fracture by Bamboo Splint 106
Fig. 1: Unable to bear weight on the fractured limb b. 105
Fig. 2: Measurement of affected limb b (length). 105
Fig. 3: Alighment of the fractured bone fragment 105
Fig. 4: Bandaging 105
Fig. 5: Application of POP cast reinforced with bamboo splint. 105
Fig. 6: After completion of surgical procedure 105

Management of Metatarsal Fracture by Camd and Pop Cast 108
Fig. 1: Compound MC fracture 106
Fig. 2: Over riding of fracture fragment on radiograph. 106
Fig. 3: Measurement of affected limb (length). 106
Fig. 4: Alinment of the fractured bone fragment 106
Fig. 5: Temporary immobilizer application 106
Fig. 6: Weight bearing on the affected limb after healing 106
Management of Metatarsal Fracture by Camd and Pop Cast 107
Fig. 1: MT fracture in a deshi cow 107
Fig. 2. Measurement of affected limb of right MT fracture in a bull. 107
Fig. 3: Fabrication of conjoint angular metallic device (CAMD) 107
Fig. 4: Permanent immobilization with POP cast reinforced with CAMD 107
Fig. 5: After complete healing 707
Fig. 6: Left MT fracture of cow. 108
Fig. 7: Measurement of affected limb (length) 108
Fig. 8: Fabrication of conjoint angular metallic device (CAMD). 108
Fig. 9: Permanent immobilization with POP cast rein forced with CAMD. 108
Fig. 10: After complete healing 108
Chapter 51. Middle Level Fracture Repair 109
Fig. 1: Simple fracture of radius and ulna & length of padded cloth 110
Fig. 3: Padded cloth around the fracture 110
Fig. 2: Application of gum over the fracture site 110
Fig. 4: Four padded bamboo splint 110
Fig. 5: Immobilization of fracture with gum band 111
Fig. 6: Immobilization of fracture with gum bandage limb with Thomas Spli 111
Chapter 52. Middle Level Fracture 112
Application of Pop Cast and Thomas Splint in Middle Level Fracture 113
Fig. 1: Photo feature showing immobilization of radius-uina 113
Fig. 2: Photo feature showing gum bandage application of radius-ulna 113
Fig. 3: Photo feature showing thick cloth wrapping in the facture of radius-ulna ... 113
Fig. 4: Photo feature showing bamboo splint application in radius-ulna 113
Fig. 5: Photo feature showing 2nd layer gum bandage application in radius-ulna ... 113
Fig. 6: Photo feature showing limb by application of Thomas splint in radius-ulna 113
Management of Radius Ulna Fracture by Modified Thomas Splint 114
Fig. 7: Application of gum resin and covering of cloth. 114
Fig. 8: Re-strengthening of the coapted limb by application of netted bamboo splint. 114
Fig. 9: Fixation of modified Thomas splint. 114
Fig. 10: Fixation of coapted limb to the ring of modified Thomas splint. 114
Fig. 11: Fixation of MTS to hoof. 114
Fig. 12: Rehabilitation of animal within the sling. 114
Management of Radius Ulna Fracture by Modified Thomas Splint 115
Fig. 1: Casting of animal on lateral recumbency keeping the proximal level fracture limb up. 115

Fig. 2: Application of fevicol gum on the proximal level radial fracture limb. 115

Fig. 3: Application of 16 layer unsterilized clean cotton cloth over the gum. 115

Fig. 4: Application of traction. 115

Fig. 5: Application of retention knots. 115

Fig. 6: Placement of four gum impregnated bamboo splint over the cloth. 115

Tibio-Fibula Fracture Repair in Large Animal 116

Fig. 1: Correction of fracture site with traction and counter traction before immobilisation. 116

Fig. 2: Liberal application of adhesive gum over the fracture site. 116

Fig. 3: Application of soft cotton bandage strengthened with bamboo splint. 116

Fig. 4: Over padding of fracture site with gum bandage. 116

Fig. 5: Covering with netted bamboo splint and Thomas splint. 116

Fig. 6: Recovered animal. 116

Tibio-Fibula Fracture Repair in Large Animal 117

Fig. 1: Overside view of fracture site 117

Fig. 2: Liberal application of adhesive gum over the fracture site. 117

Fig. 3: Covering of fracture site with soft cotton traction and counter traction. 117

Fig. 4: Strengthening of cotton padding with bandage with green bamboo splint. .. 117

Fig. 5: Over strengthening with netted bamboo Thomas splint. 117

Fig. 6: Complete immobilisation splint 117

Chapter 53. Higher Level Fracture Repair 118

Fig.1: Left side view of cow showing immobilization technique for humerus and femur fracture with gum bandage 119

Fig. 2: Right side view of cow showing sling application for retaining the gum bandage in positition. 119

Chapter 54. Photo Feature of Higher Level Fracture 120

Modified Valpeau Sling for Management of Higher Level Fracture in Cattle 121

Fig. 1: Left side view of cow showing immobilization technique for humerus and femur fracture with gum bandage 121

Fig. 2: Right side view of cow showing sling application for retaining the gum bandage in positition. 121

Fig. 3: Photo feature showing gum bandage and sling application at femur 121

Fig. 4: Photo feature showing gum bandage and sling application at humerus 121

Humerus Fracture Repair by Modified Velpeau Sling 122

Fig. 1: Application of layer of Gum and Cotton Bandage 122

Flg. 2: Application of 2nd layer of Gum and Cotton Bandage 122

Fig. 3: Application of final layer of Gum and Cotton Bandage 122

Flg. 4: Right side view of the animal with modified Velpeu sling 122

Fig. 5: Left side view of the animal with modified Velpeau sling 122

Fig. 6: Animal after recovery 122

Chapter 55. Highest Level Fracture (HLF) and its Management 123

Fig. 1: Showing fracture of Scapula 124

Fig. 2: Showing fracture of Pelvic Girdle 124

Chapter 56. Photo Features of Highest Level Fracture 125
Fig. 1: Showing immobilization technique for highest level fracture of forelimb and hindlimb (Left side). 126
Fig. 2: Showing immobilization technique for highest level fracture, gum bandaging extending upto right sid 126
Chapter 57. Conjoined 'U' Plate with Ring for Immobilisation of Radius and Ulna Fracture 127
Fig. 1: Upper 3rd R&U fracture 128
Fig. 2a: Conjoined U plate 128
Fig. 2b: Conjoined U plate with thick cotton bandage 128
Fig. 3: Immobilise of fracture side with thick padded cloth & netted bamboo splint 128
Fig 3a: Immobilisation of Lower 3rd R&U fracture with conjoined U plate with padded ring 128
Chapter 58. Hanging Pin Cast 129
Fig. 1: Position of pin in radius ulna (Forelimb) 130
Fig. 2: Position of pin inside tibial bone (Hindlimb) 130
Chapter 59. Intramedullary Pinning of Humerus in Large Animal 131
Intramedullary Pinning of Humerus in Large Animal 133
Fig. 1: Fracture of left humerus mid shaft 133
Fig. 2: Left humerus of ox lateral view 133
Fig. 3: Intramedullary pin with drill fitter 133
Fig. 4: Close pinning of left humerus 133
Humerus Fracture Repair by Pinning and Thomas Splint 134
Fig. 1: Showing the fracture site of left humerus 134
Fig. 2: Close pinning of fractured humerus 134
Fig. 3: Close pinning completed 134
Fig. 4: Application of charge over the fracture site 134
Fig. 5: Self impregnated gum in padded netted bamboo splint 134
Fig. 6 : Application of Thomas splint 134
Chapter 60. Intramedullary Pinning of Femur in Large Animal 135
Intramedullary Pinning of Femur in Large Animal 137
Fig. 1: Mid shaft fracture of left femur 137
Fig. 2: Left femur of ox lateral view 137
Fig. 3: Intramedullary pin with drill fitter 137
Fig. 4: Close pinning of left femur 137
Femur Fracture Repair By im Pinning 138
Fig. 1: Diagnosis of fracture by palpation 138
Fig. 2: Insertion of of IM pinning by open method. 138
Fig. 3: Insertion of drainage catheter for clear out debrises. 138
Fig. 4: Closing of skin after successful reduction of fracture fragment 138
Fig. 5: Application of netted bamboo Thomas splint for immobilisation. 138
Fig. 6: Recovered animal after one month. 138
Chapter 61. Modified Valpeau Sling for Highest Level Fore Limb Fracture 139
Fig. 1: Fracture of upper 3rd humerus and scapula comes under highest level 140

Fig. 2: Covering of the fracture site as well as other healthy site of hte body with padded cloth. 140
Fig. 3: Fixation of padded cloth over the fractured site with long bandage in a fig. of 8 manner anchoring both the axila. 140
Fig. 4: A cross section of the body near the therax showing the method of wrapp cotton padding and bandage rolls. 140
Chapter 62. Modified Velpeau Sling for Highest Level Fracture of Hind Limb 141
Fig. 1: Highest level fracture (femur fracture) 142
Fig. 2: Application of cloth 142
Fig. 3: Application of cooptation bandage 142
Fig. 4: (a). Thick bandage cloth. 142
Fig. 4: (b). Figure of '8' gauze bandage 142
Fig. 5: Conjoint double Thomas splint for pelvic girdle fracture repair 143
Chapter 63. Different Types of Thomas Splints 144
Fig. 1: Fundamental structure of Thomas splint. 144
Fig. 2: Diagram of Thomas splint showing dimensions used in formula for etermining rod length. 144
Fig. 3: Simplest model of thomas splint. 144
Fig. 4: Thomas splint fashioned with No. 9 wire by J.F. Thomas (1938). 144
Fig. 5: Thomas splint prepared by W.F. Guard for a Jersey Fleifer (1953). 144
Fig. 6: Thomas splint for man (1957) Courtesy- Down Bros. Ltd.). 144
Chapter 64. Thomas Splint Used in Animals (For Fore limb) 145
Fig. 1: Thomas splint applied to a horse (Thomas, J.F. 1939) 145
Fig. 2: Thomas splint applied to a buffalo. 145
Fig. 3: Conventional method of fixation of Thomas splint using plaster of pans cast. 145
Fig. 4: Thomas splint applied to a horse (J.F., Guard 1939) 146
Fig. 5: Thomas splint applied to a buffalo 146
Fig. 6: Conventional method of fixation of Thomas splint using plaster of paris cast. 146
Chapter 65. List of Requisite for Preparation of Large Animal Thomas Splint 147
Fig. 1: Bamboo Three nicks 2" apart tying string with ring 148
Fig. 2: Selfwinding G.I. wirering. 148
Fig. 3: Jute gunny bag 148
Fig. 4: Cycle tube 1'X2 148
Fig. 5: Starting of cotton bandaging around jute bandaging 148
Fig. 6: Completion of cotton bandaging 148
Fig. 7: Complete Thomas splint net fabrication 148
Chapter 66. Measurement of Ring of Thomas Splint for Large Animal 149
Fig. 1: Showing the reference point on the bone for accurate measurement of wire 151
Fig. 2: Three and halftimes the length of humerus and femur. 151
Fig. 3: Measurement of size of ring with the help of G.I. wire 151
Fig. 4: Matching hte measurement of G.I. wire 3.5 times length of humerus or femur bone (Both measurements should be matched) 151

Chapter 67. Wire Rings Required for Different Age Group of Animals 152
Fig. 1: One round ring for young calf (Age less than 1 year) 152
Fig. 2: Two round self-winding fcadult calf (Age 2 years to 4 years) 152
Fig. 3: Three round self-winding ring for middle age cattle (Age 4 years to 6 years) 152
Fig. 4: Four round self-winding ring for old age cattle (Age above 6 years) 152
Chapter 68. Preparation of Side Bars of Large Animal Thomas Splint 153
Fig. 1: Two equal size strong bamboo 154
Fig. 2: Three nicks for tying string 154
Fig. 3: Ring type area is thinned to make an arc. 154
Fig. 4: Final bamboo splint 154
Chapter 69. Method of Tying Ring with Bamboo Splint and Description 155
Fig. 1: Fixation of ring with bamboo with clove knot. 156
Fig. 2: Upper half tying. 156
Fig. 3: Lower half tying. 156
Fig. 4: Final fixation of bamboo split with ring ring. 156
Chapter 70. Padding of Thomas Splint Ring with Jute & Cotton Bandage 157
Fig. 1: Fixation of bamboo splint with ring 158
Fig. 2: Starting of bandaging of jute on ring. 158
Fig. 3: Completion of covering of jute padding 158
Fig. 4: Starting of cotton bandaging around jute bandaging 158
Fig. 5: Completion of cotton bandaging 158
Chapter 71. Medial Bending of Lower Half of Thomas Splint 159
Fig. 1: Bending of lower half of ring of Thomas splint 160
Fig. 2: Bending of lower half of ring of Thomas splint 160
Fig. 3: Front view. 160
Fig. 4: Side view. 160
Fig. 5: Complete Thomas splint 160
Chapter 72. Measurement of Length of Thomas Splint, Shortening of Length & Padding of Distal End 161
Fig. 1: Showing correct method of taking measurement of thomas splint by positioning the leg in 90° angle to the body 162
Fig. 2: Showing incorrect method of taking measurement of thomas splint 162
Chapter 73. Net Fabrication in Large Animals Thomas Splint 163
Measurement of Length of Thomas Splint, Shortening of Length & Padding of Distal and 164
Fig. 1: Position of animal for length measurement of Thomas splint 164
Fig. 2: Shortening level or trimming of extra length. 164
Fig. 3: Soft padding to avoid pressure injury to foot. 164
Net Fabrication of Thomas Splint 165
Fig. 1: Longitudinal 165
Fig. 2: Side view 165
Fig. 3: Front view 165

Chapter 74. Fitting Thomas Splint and Its Retention Over Gum Bandage 166
Fig. 1: Immobilisation of fracture with Gum bandage 166
Fig. 2: Immobilisation of fracture with Gum 166
Chapter 75. Fitting of Thomas Splint in Forelimb of Large Animal 167
Fig. 1: Immobilization of fracture site with soft padding and netted bamboo splint. 168
Fig. 3: Thomas splint fixation over gum bandage. 168
Fig. 2: Cross section of gum bandage immobilisers. 168
Fig. 4: (a) Cross section of immobilised forelimb with thomas splint. 168
Fig. 4 (b): Cross section of immobilised hind limb with thomas splint. 168
Chapter 76. Method of Fitting of Thomas Splint in Hind Limb of Large Animal 169
Fig. 1: Immobillization of fractured hindlimb with thomas splint 170
Chapter 77.Method of Securing Thomas Splint 171
Fig. 1: Method of application of thomas splint in limbs. 171
Chapter 78. Method of Fixation of Hoof With the Distal End of Thomas Splint 172
Fig. 1: Showing direction of bandage to be winded 173
Fig. 2: 1st 2 round of bandage around hoof 173
Fig. 3: 2nd round of bandage with distal end of Thomas splint & hoof 173
Fig. 4: 3rd 2 round of bandage around front bamboo splint gap & downwards covering the foo 173
Fig. 5: 4th 2 round of bandage around posterior bamboo splint gap downwards covering the foot. 173
Fig. 6: Method of winding the bandage to include the distal end of Thomas splint with foot. Last 2 rounds covers the entire hoof. 173
Chapter 80. Recommendation of Confinement Space and Time for Fracture Immobilised Patient 175
Fig. 1: Provisionof bounded confinement space for rehabilitated immobilized patient 175
Chapter 82. Fabrication of Durable Thomas Splint 178
Fig. 1: Fabrication of Durable Thomas Splint 180
Chapter 84. Immobilisation of Proximal 1/3rd Metacarpal and Metatarsal Bone 183
Fig. 1: Metatarsal bone of Ox. 184
Chapter 85. Technique of Immobilization of Carpometacarpal and Tarsometa Tarsal or Joint Dislocation 185
Fig. 1 (a): Fracture of upper third metatarsal and dislocation of 185
Fig. 1 (b): Fracture of upper third metacarpal and dislocation of carpometacarpal joint. 185
Fig. 2: 1,2 and 3 showing fracture of upper third metacarpal and metatarsal bone and dislocation of carpometacarpal and tarsometatarsal joint. 186
Chapter 86. Immobilisation Technique for Upper Third Radius-Ulna Fracture 187
Fig. 1: Immobilisation Technique for Upper Third Radius-Ulna Fracture 188
Chapter 87. Technique of Immobilization of Upper 3rd Tibia Fibula Fracture 189
Technique of Immobilization of Upper 3rd Tibia Fibula Fracture 190
Fig. 1: Length of the limb at the fracture site to be covered with computational bandage. 190

Fig. 2: Padded netted and Conjoined bamboo splint 190
Fig. 3a : Thick padded cloth 190
Fig. 3b: Netted bamboo splint with gum 190
Fig. 3c: Modified thomas splint 190
Fig. 4: Tieing upper part of leg region with Anterior site ring of thomas splint with cotton bandage 190
Chapter 88.Conjoined Double Thomas Splint for Both Tibia Fibula - Fracture Repair 191
Fig. 1: Conjoined double Thomas splint for both tibia-fibula fracture repair 192
Fig. 2: Fitting of Thomas splint having both Tibia-fibula fracture 192
Chapter 89. Immobilization of Symphysial Fractured Mandible in Large Animals 193
Fig. 1: Bovine Skull with mandible 194
Fig. 2: Wiring technique for symphyseal fracture 194
Fig. 3: Cross-section of mandible 194
Chapter 90. Immobilisaion of Fracture of Ramus of Mandible 195
Fig. 1: Immobilisaticn of fracture of mandibie with extrnal 'U' plate and pinning. . 196
Fig. 2: 'U' plate frame with pinning device for immoblilisation of mandible fracture. 196
Fig. 3: Pinning sites, either sides of the fracture - lateral view. 196
Fig. 4: Pinning sites, either sides of the fracture - dorsal view. 196
Chapter 91. Immobilization of Limb for Flexor Tendon Repair 197
Fig. 1: Metal Frame 198
Fig. 2: Netted bamboo splint 198
Fig. 3: Thomas splint 198
Fig. 4: Immobilization of limb for flexor tendon repair 198
Chapter 92. Digital Tendon Repair 199
Fig. 1: Identification of individual tendons. 201
Fig. 2: Animal after Thomas splint application 201
Fig. 3: Fabrication of angular frame device. 201
Fig. 4: Immobilization of the limb inside the splint angular frame. 201
Chapter 93. Suturing Technique of Transected Gastrocnemious Tendon 202
Fig. 1: Transected gastrocnemius tendon. 203
Fig. 2: Suture passing technique. 203
Fig. 3: Tendon & peritendon apposition suture. 203
Fig. 4: Suturing technique of gastrocnemius 203
Chapter 94. Immobilization of Hind Limb for Tendo Achiles Repair 204
Fig. 1: Metal Frame 206
Fig. 2: Netted bamboo splint 206
Fig. 3: Thomas splint 206
Fig. 4: Immobilization of hind limb for lendo achiles repai 206
Fig. 5: a) Normal Hip joint. 208
b) Pelvic bone showing Acctabulum 208
c) Femur of ox. 208
Chapter 95. Hip Dislocation and It's Correction 210
Fig. 1: Hip dislocation in cattle 210

Fig. 2(a): Application of charge over the affected hip 210
Fig. 2(b): Extension of charge in the healthy site 210
Plate
Fig. 1: Bone showing fracture site 211
Fig. 2: Application of plaster of pahs 211
Fig. 3: Immobilisation of fracture site with cloth bandage. 211
Fig. 4: Immobilisation of fracture site with second layer of cloth padding 211
Fig. 5: Final immobilised limb with Rubber belt or suspensory bandage 211
Fig. 6: Animal kept in mobile sling for proper immobilisation 211
Chapter 96. Contracted Leg in Calves 212
Fig. 1: Calf showing bilateral contracted leg. 213
Fig. 2. (a) C.S. of fore canon at the level 214
Fig. 2. (b) L.S. of fore canon showing cutting of tendon and ligament at different levels. 214
Fig. 3: POP cast immobilisation of the contracted leg after operation. 214
Pop Bandage Technique for Contracted Leg 215
Fig. 1: Calf having contracted b: Lateral fore-limb. 215
Fig. 2: Pop cast bandage. 215
Fig. 3: Rubber shoe protection over foot. 215
Chapter 97. Flushing Facility of Compound Fracture 216
Management of Compound Fracture 216
Fig. 1: Treatment of compound fracture of radius ulna. 218
Fig. 2: Treatment of compound fracture of radius ulna. 218
Fig. 3: Treatment of compound fracture of tibio-fibula 219
Fig. 4: Treatment of compound fracture of tibio-fibula 219
Chapter 98. Flushing Facility of Compound Fracture 220
Fig. 1(a): Fixation of flushing catheter inside meta carpal compound fracture 221
Fig. 1(b): Immobilization of compound metacarpal fracture keeping the flushing .. 221
Fig. 2(a): Fixation of flushing catheter inside compound radius ulna fracture 221
Fig. 2(b): Preparation of flushing catheter 221
Fig. 2(c): Immobilization of compound radius ulna fracture keeping the flushing catheter inside 221
Chapter 102. Amputation of the Claw 228
Fig. 1: An Insentire 228
Amputation of Claw in cattle 229
Fig. 1: Exarticulation of claw (Before exarticulation) with direction of saw cut. 229
Fig. 2: Exarticulation of claw (After exarticulation). 229
Amputation of the Claw 231
Fig. 1: Course of the skin incision on the dorsal surface of the fetlock and pastern. 231
Fig. 2: The skin flap is turned up. The amputation was made thorugh the first phalanx. a. Cut surface of the 1st phalanx. 231
Fig. 3: Skin sutures after completion of hte operation. 231
Chapter 103. Single Digit Amputation 232
Fig. 1: Hoof growth with couliflower like growth in unilateral hoof 233

Fig. 2: Amputation of unilateral hoof with cancerous growth 233
Fig. 3: Hom amputation material 233
Fig. 4: After bandage cover. 233
Chapter 104. Double Digit Amputation 234
Fig. 1: Foot showing bilateral cancerous growth 236
Fig. 2: After amputation of bone the digit. 236
Fig. 3: Amputation material. 236
Fig. 4: After bandage cover. 236
Chapter 105. Level of Amputation at Fore & Hind Limb by Bone Section Technique 237
Fig. 1: Showing level of amputation at fore & hind limb. 238
Fig. 2a: Showing skin and muscle incised and reflected upward at site of incision in radius unla 239
Fig. 2b: Showing cutting of bone and suturing of muscle tendons together 239
Fig. 2c: Showing skin suturing over the top 239
Fig. 3a: Showing skin and muscle incised and reflected upward at site of incision in tibia fibula 239
Fig. 3b: Showing cutting of bone and suturing of muscle tendons together 239
Fig. 3c: Showing skin suturing over the stump 239
Various Level Amputation by Bone Section 240
Fig. 1: Forelimb amputation by bone section 240
Fig. 1(a): Below knee amputation 240
Fig. 1(b): Above knee amputation 240
Fig. 2: Hindlimb amputation by bone section 240
Fig. 2(a): Below hock amputation 240
Fig. 2(b): Above hock amputation 240
Chapter 106. Method of Apposing Muscle, Fascia, Skin Over Amputed Stump 241
Fig. 1: Left femuro tibia amputed stump showing skin flap ratio Lateral 243
Fig. 2: Closure technique of skin facia, muscle, tendon 243
Fig. 3a: Anterior group muscle united with post group and Medial group muscle united with lateral group 243
Fig. 3b: Apposition of muscle, fascia and skin over amputed stump 243
Fig. 4: Stifle amputed stump 243
Chapter 107. Joint Disarticulation Method of Limb Amputation 244
Fig. 1: B Hindlimb amputation site 246
Chapter 108. Fetlock Disarticulation 247
Fig. 1: Fetlock joint 247
Fig. 2: Skin in laceration in relation to bovine 247
Fig. 3: After both disarticulation 247
Fig. 4: Apposition of muscle and nerves 247
Fig. 5: Fircal skin closure with stem 247
Chapter 109. Carpo-Metacarpal Joint Disarticulation 248
Fig. 1: Noarmla anatomy of carpo-metacapal joint 248
Fig. 3: Skin muscle flaps 248
Fig. 2: Skin muscle flap ratio in relation to bone (1:2) 248

Fig. 4: Appositional suture of muscles and tendons 248
Fig. 5: Skin closure 248
Chapter 110. Elbow Disarticulation 249
Fig. 1: Normai anatomay of elbow joint 249
Fig. 2: Skin muscle flap ratio in relation to bon 249
Fig. 3: Skin flaps 249
Fig. 4: Appositional suture of muscle and tendons 249
Chapter 111. Shoulder Disarticulation 250
Fig. 1: Surgical anatomy for shoulder disarticulation 252
Fig. 2: Site of incision 252
Fig. 3: Blunt dissection and reflection of muscle. 252
Fig. 4: Disarticultuion and apposition of muscle 252
Fig. 5: Final colosure 252
Chapter 112. Tarso-Metatarsal Joint Disarticulation Technique in Large animal 253
Fig. 1: Anatomy of tarso meta tarso joint 253
Fig. 2: Skin flap after joint disarticulation 253
Fig. 3: Appositon of tendon & muscle (closure of skin) 253
Fig. 4: Complete closure of metatarsa joint 253
Chapter 113. Stiffle Disarticulation 254
Fig. 1: Reparable fracture of leg 254
Fig. 2: Skin flap ratio (5:1) 254
Fig. 3: Stump closure in process 254
Fig. 4: Complete closure of stiffle joint 254
Chapter 114. HIP Disarticulation 255
Fig. 1: Surgical anatomy of hip 257
Fig. 2: Reflecting muscles on the temur and their blunt dissection. 257
Fig. 3: Excision of femur and sturing 257
Chapter 115. Figures of Various Amputees by Joint Disarticulation Method 258
Fig. 1: Fetlock disarticulation. 258
Fig. 2: Fetlock disarticulation. 258
Fig. 3: Knee disarticulation. 258
Fig. 4: Hock disarticulation. 258
Fig. 5: Elbow disarticulation. 259
Fig. 6: Stifle disarticulation. 259
Chapter 116. Comparison Between Bone Section and Joint Disarticulation Method of Limb Amputation 260
Forelimb Amputees 261
Fig. 1a: Fetlock disarticulation. 261
Fig. 1b: Fetlock disarticulation. 261
Fig. 2a: Below - knee amputation 261
Fig. 2b: Below - knee amputation 261
Fig. 3a: Above - knee amputation 262
Fig. 3b: Above - knee amputation 262
Hind Limb Amputees 262

Fig. 4a: Fetlock disarticulation 262
Fig. 4b: Fetlock disarticulation 262
Fig. 5a: Below - hock amputation. 262
Fig. 5b: Below - hock amputation; 262
Fig. 6a: Above - hock amputation. 263
Fig. 6b: Above - hock amputation. 263
Chapter 117. Different Steps in Preparation of Permanent Prosthesis 264
Fig. 1: Marking on the moistened cast stokinet. 0 - Outline of sensitive area, " - Oepression+ - Prominences 1 - Border of bone U - Distal end of bone 265
Fig. 2: Negative plaster cast. 265
Fig. 3: Plaster mold or positive cast. 265
Fig. 4: Fabrication of the plastic shell. 265
Fig. 5: Alignment of duplication 265
Chapter 124. Amputation and Prosthetic Limb Below Carpus in Cattle 274
Fig. 1: The below knee stump showing free mobility of radio-carpal joint. 274
Fig. 2: The below knee stump showing semi- flexed position. 274
Fig. 3: Stance of the below knee amputee. 574
Fig. 4: Stump of the below knee amputee showing well covered and thickly padded distal end. 274
Fig. 5: Below knee amputated heifer using the stump in each step of walk. 275
Fig. 6: Application of bamboo splint bandage In case of below knee amputee during training. 275
Fig. 7: Stance of elbow disarticulated amputee showing undisturbed symmetry. ... 276
Fig. 8: Propulsion of the intact forelimb with a hopping movement, lifting the head upward. 276
Fig. 9: At walk, below elbow amputee showing propulsion of the prosthetic limb. 276
Fig. 10: At stance, below elbow amputee showing weight bearing of the prosthetic limb with canadian type 276
Fig. 11: At walk, below elbow amputee showing propulsion of the intact forelimb. 276
Fig. 12: At stance, below elbow amputee showing weight bearing of the prosthetic limb with conventional type 276
Fig. 13: Below hock prostheses (Conventional type pylon and canalian type pegleg). 277
Fig. 14: Below hock amputee at sleep, ... 277
Fig. 15: At stance below hock amputee having the prosthetic limb. 277
Fig. 17: Below hock amputee attempting to walk 277
Fig. 16: At stance below hock amputee having the prosthetic limb. 277
Fig. 18: Below hock amputee at walk. 277
Fig. 19: Above hock prostheses conventional showing type and exoskelital type. 278
Fig. 20: Walk of above hock amputee propulsion of hind leg. 278
Fig. 21: Walk of above hock amputee with conventional type prosthesis showing production of prosthetic limb. 278
Fig. 22: Stance of above hock amputee with conventional type prostheses. 278

Fig. 23: Walk of above hock amputee with exoskelital type prosthesis showing propulsion of prosthetic limb. 278
Fig. 24: Stance of above hock amputee with exoskelital type prosthesis. 278
Fig. 25. Rehabilitation 279
Chapter 126. Requisite for Preparation of Large Animal Mobile Sling 282
Fig. 1: Bicycle Motor cycle chain 283
Fig. 2: to ft. long strong bamboo 283
Fig. 3: Gunny bags 283
Fig. 6: GI. wire (6mm) 283
Fig. 4: Bicycle Tyre 283
Fig. 5: Jute string 283
Fig. 7: Saw with blade 283
Fig. 8: Axe 283
Chapter 128. Preparation of Padded Tyres for Sling Preparation 286
Fig. 1: Rope tying of tyres 286
Fig. 2: Wrapping of gunny bag over tyers 286
Fig. 3: Padded tyres for sling 286
Fig. 4: Arrangement of wrap tyres within two rods 287
Chapter 129. Supportive Sling 288
Fig. 1: Pacement of bicycle tyres over the metal frame by sliding 288
Fig. 2: Securing of bicycle tyres with strings 288
Fig. 3: Wrapping of individual bicycle tyres with gunny bags and securing in position with ropes to provide light and soft bedding 288
Chapter 130. Fabrication of Mobile Sling 290
Fig. 1: Complete sling without animal. 290
Fig. 2: Downed animal inside the mobile sling 290
Chapter 131. Method of Placing Downer Animal Within The Sling 291
Fig. 1: All the four limbs are highly lifted from ground to put the sling under the body of animal. 291
Fig. 2: Placing the animal upon the sling keeping all the four legs within the sling. 291
Chapter 132. Method of Slinging 292
Fig. 1: Method of slinging in large animal 292
Fig. 2: Method of slinging in small animal 293
Chapter 133. Recommended Duration for Slinging Large Animal 294
Fig. 1: Downed animal inside the mobile sling 294
Chapter 134. Sling Rehabilitation of Calf 296
Fig. 1: Cow with fractured tibia fibula radius ulna is rehabilitated in sling. 296
Fig. 2: A sling rehabilitated cow suckling from mother. 296
Fig. 3: A rehabilitation of a cow due to upward fixation of patella. 296
Fig. 4: Rehabilation of bilateral limb fracture of calf after immobilisation. 296
Fig. 5: Rehabilitation of metacarpal fractured buffalo under sling. 297
Fig. 6: Rehabilation of animal with both hindlimb fracture. 297

Chapter 135. Importance of Rehabilitation of More Than one Limb Fractured Animal Within Mobile Sling 298
Chapter 136. Rehabilitation of Large Animal in Exercise Cart 299
Fig. 1: Exercise cart with supporting sling for large animal with labelled path 302
Fig. 2: 302
Fig. 4: 302
Fig. 3: 302
Fig. 5: 302
Fig. 6: 303
Fig. 7: 303
Chapter 137. Rehabilitation of Two Limb Fractured Animal Within Mobile Sling 304
Fig. 1: Method of Slinging in Large Animal 304
Chapter 138. Osteology 305
Fig. 1: Lateral maleols 305
Fig. 2: Gait of normal animal. Animal generally takes a lift to full extent in each step 306
Fig. 3: Gait of normal animal (full lifting of foot) 306
Fig. 4: Gait of a fractured patient (more dragging and less lifting of foot). 306
Fig. 5: Gait of animal with light Thomas splint (less dragging and more lifting of foots) 306
Fig. 6: Gait of animal with heavy Thomas splint (more dragging and less lifting of foot) 306
Chapter 139. Prosthetic Fitting 307
Forelimb Amputees 308
Fig. 1a: Fetlock disarticulation. 308
Fig. 2a: Meta carpal amputation 308
Fig. 3a: Radius ulna amputation 308
Fig. 1b: Fetlock disarticulation. 308
Fig. 2b: Carpo-metacarpal disarticulation 308
Fig. 3b: Elbow disarticulation 308
Hind Limb Amputees 309
Fig. 4a: Fetlock disarticulation 309
Fig. 4b: Fetlock disarticulation 309
Fig. 5a: Meta tarsal amputation. 309
Fig. 5b: Transometa tarsal disarticulation 309
Fig. 6a: Tibiofibula 309
Fig. 6b: Stifle disarticulation 309

1

Abnormal Movement of Limb

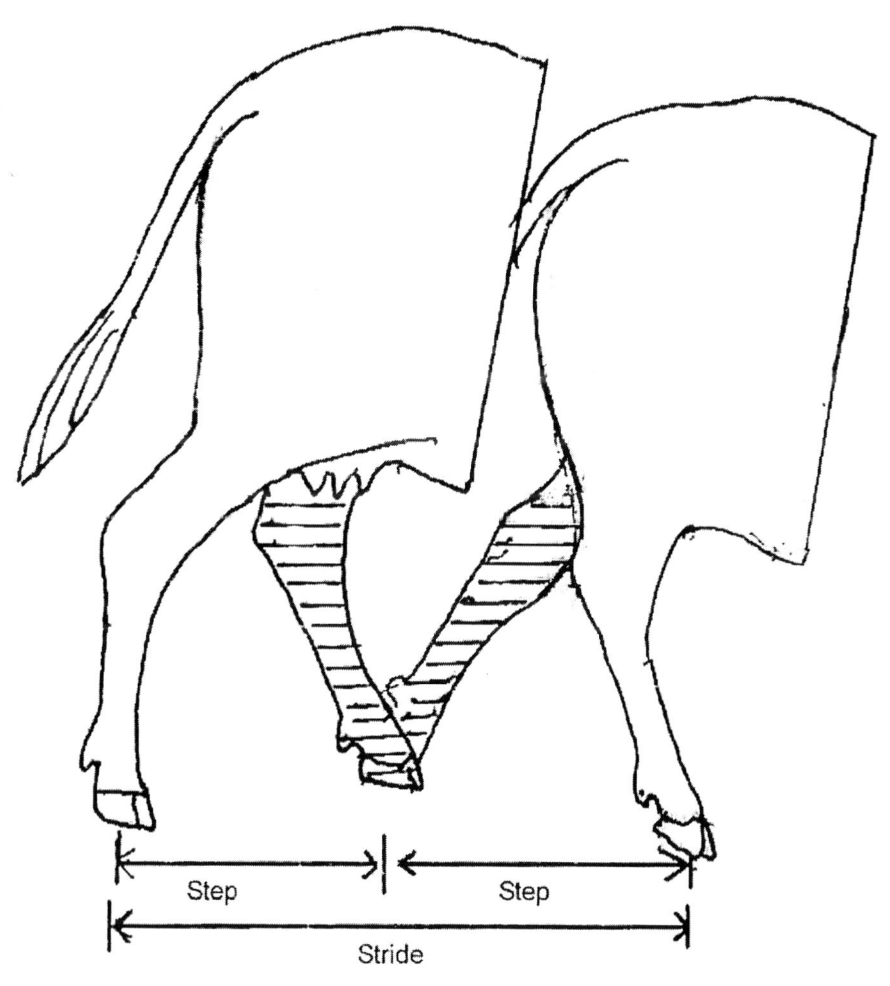

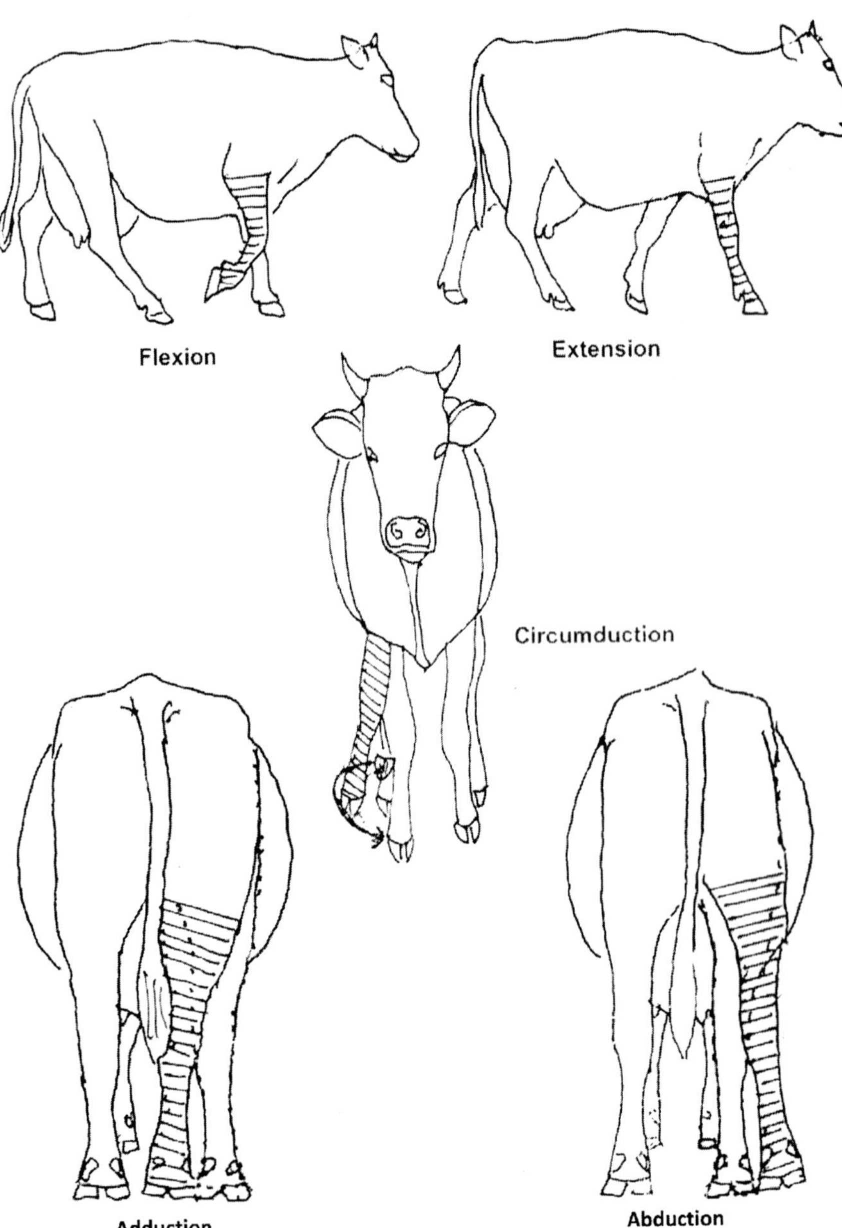
Flexion
Extension
Circumduction
Adduction
Abduction

2

Body Symmetry of Animal in Relation to Location of Centre of Gravity

Centre of gravity

It is most commonly located is the middle of the rib cage, just caudal to the line separating the cranial and middle third of the body because the CG & located more cranially. The forelimbs bear 60-65% of body weight. This causes an increased stress of forelimb and increase incidence of lameness. The horse that is taller over the group than the wither has an additional disadvantage, because PTS CG is shifted further forwards.

1. Long backed horses may develop a swing in the gait that alters the movement of their limbs. Such horses are prone to speedy cutting. Cross firing & back problem due to muscle ligament strain.
2. Short backed horses may develop a swing in the gait that alters the movement of these limbs. Such horses are prone to speedy cutting, cross firing & back problem due to muscle and ligament strain.
3. Hence body should be pleasing, in balance with limbs and well proportioned. Body conformation is not common cause of lameness.

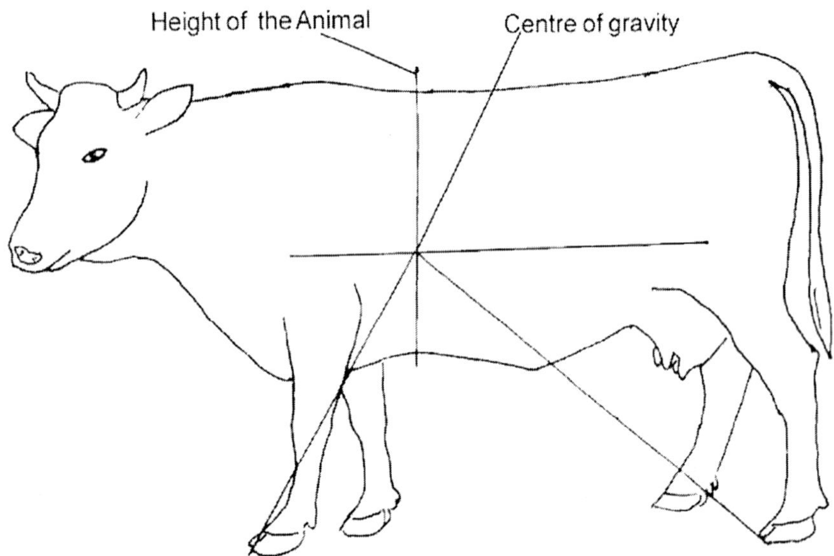

Fig. 1: Body symmetry of animal in relation to location of centre of gravity

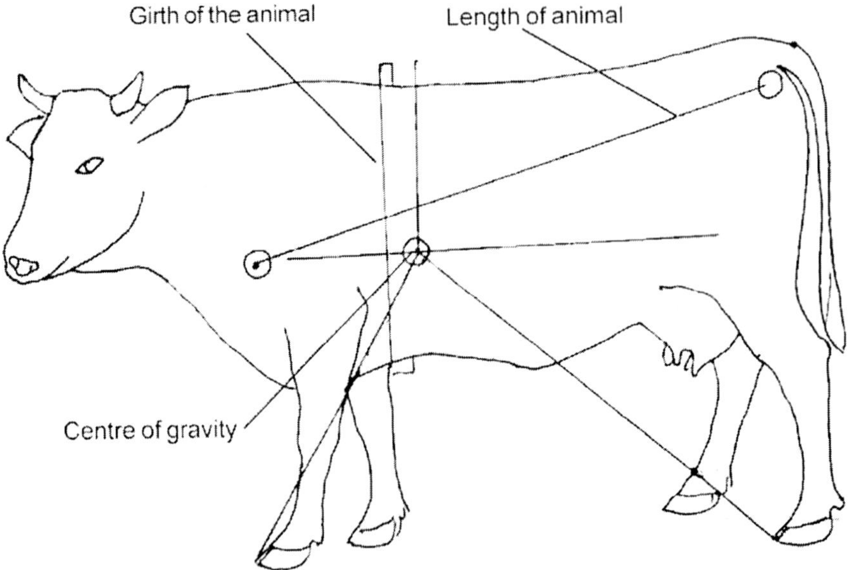

Fig. 2: Location of centre of gravity, site for measurement of length and girth of animal.

3

Gait of A Normal Animal, Fractured Patient and Animal with Thomas Splint

Gait of A Normal Animal

- This is a four - beat gait. Walking can be of various forms, but regardless of the form, it must be an even four beat gait.
- When a regular sequence is lost, identified by four hoof beats at precise interyals, the cattle is no longer walking.
- The walking sequence is lateral because both feet of one side hit the ground before the two feet of opposite side strike.
- Propulsion primarily results from the hindlimbs, and the forelimbs simply follow.
- The length of stride in the walk will usually vary between 5 1/2 and 6 ft. This distance is measured between successive imprints of the same foot.
- The step will vary between 33 and 39 inches and is the measurement made between the imprints made by a pair of forefeet or the imprints made by a pair of hind feet.
- The sequence of the hoof beats can be described according to this pattern: (1) near - hind, (2) near - fore, (3) off - hind, (4) off - fore.
- This gait is sometimes described as beginning with a forelirnb as ; (1) off — fore, (2) near - hind, (3) near - fore, and (4) off - hind.
- This description is not proper according to the way the cattle starts, but it is proper after it is in motion.

In the walk there is never a moment at which fewer than two feet are in contact with the ground. There is no period of suspension or no moment when only one foot is in contact with the ground.

GAIT OF A NORMAL ANIMAL, FRACTURED PATIENT AND ANIMAL WITH THOMAS SPLINT

Gait it is the pattern of movement of the limbs of animal during locomotinover a solid substrate

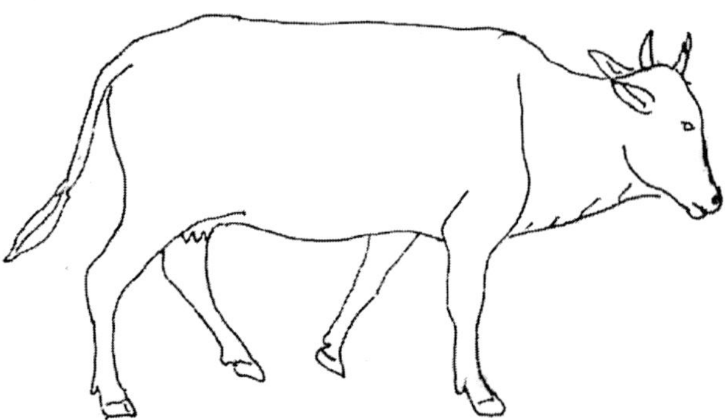

Fig. 1: Gait of normal animal. Animal generally takes a lift to full extent in each step.

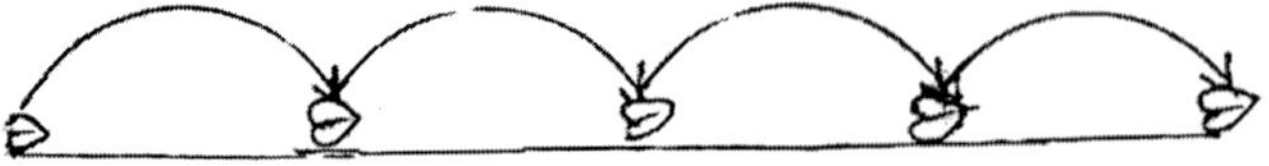

Fig. 2: Gait of normal animal (full lifting of foot)

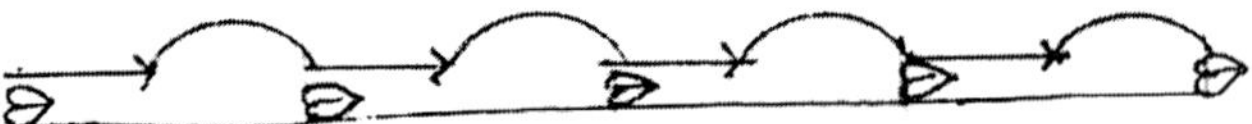

Fig. 3: Gait of a fractured patient (more dragging and less lifting of foot).

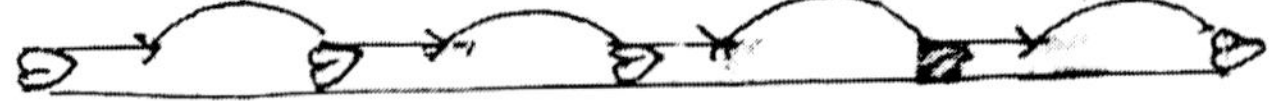

Fig. 4: Gait of animal with light Thomas splint (less dragging and more lifting of foots). s).

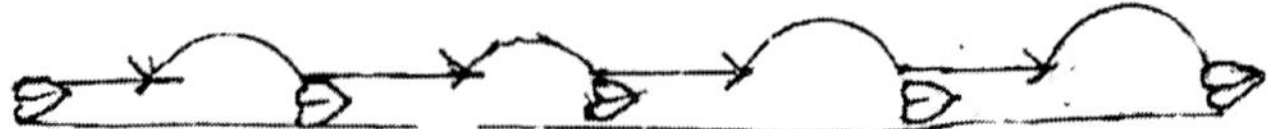

Fig. 5: Gait of animal with heavy Thomas splint (more dragging and less lifting of foot)

4

Skeletal System of Bovine

1. Tubercoxae
2. Twelth thoracic vertebra
3. First lumbar vertebra
4. Last rib
5. First coccygeal vertebra
6. Sacrum
7. Tuber ischii
8. T rochanter major
9. Femur
10. Lateral condyle of Tibia
11. Tibia
12. Distal end of fibula
13. Tuber calcis
14. Tarsus
15. Metatarsus
16. Phalanges
17. Patella
18. Ilium
19. Tuber sacrale
20. Last lumbar vertebra
21. Atlas
22. Seventh cervical vertebra
23. First thoracic vertebra
24. Cartilage of scapula
25. Scapula
26. Spine of scapula
27. Acromian
28. Lateral tuberosity of humerus
29. Deltoid tuberosity
30. Humerus
31. Sixth rib
32. Sixth costal cartilage
33. Manubrium
34. Sternum
35. Olecranon
36. Radius
37. Ulna
38. Carpus
39. Accessory carpal bone
40. Meta carpus
41. Phalanges.

Skeletal System of Bovine

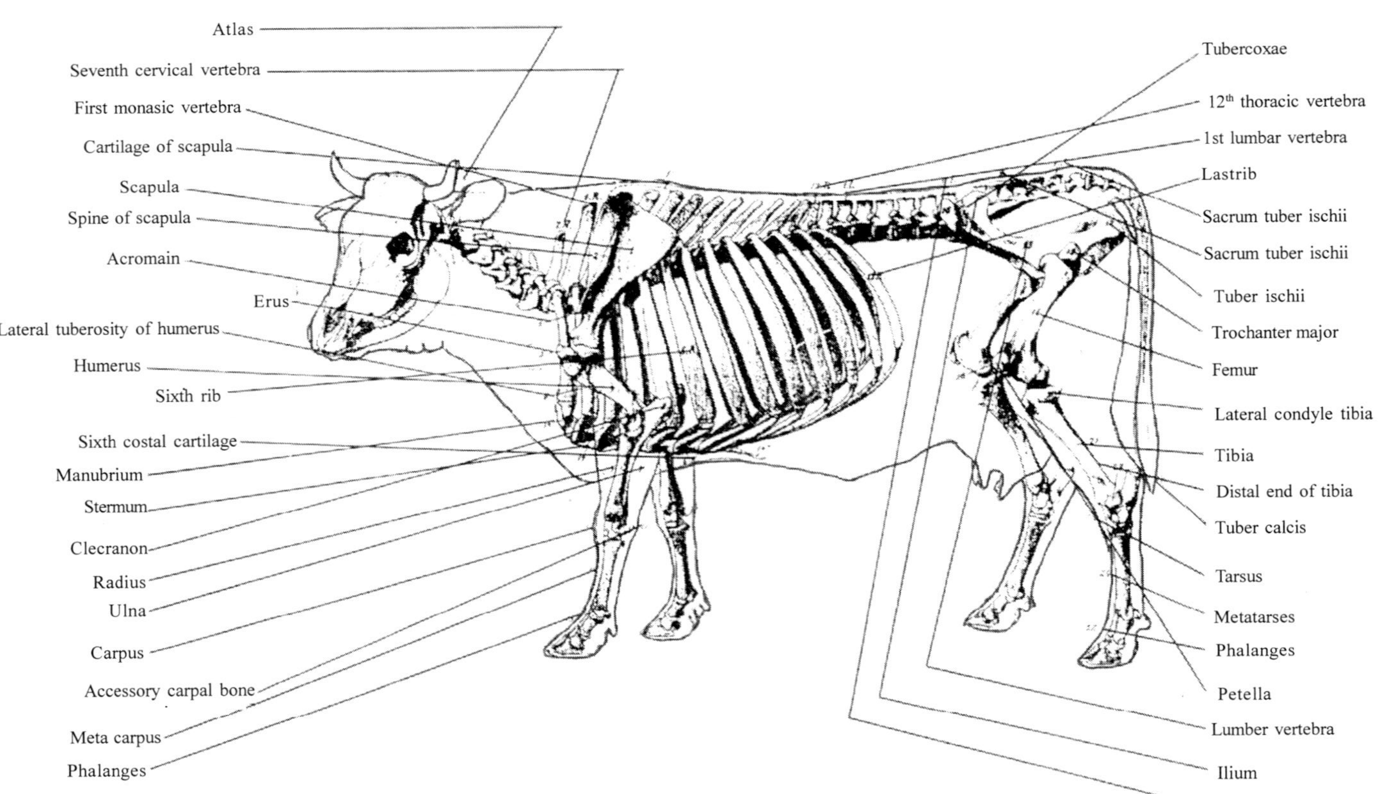

Fig. 1: Skeleton of cow.

Number of Bones in Skeleton of ox

SKULL (including hyoid and mandible) Total = 32	Vertebral column (approximately) Total = 51 (apprx)	Ribs+Sternum (26 + 1) Total = 27	Forelimb (24x2) Total = 48	Hindlimb (24x2) Total = 48	Visceral bones Total = 2
CRANIAL BONES (11) 1. Occipital (1) 2. Interparietal (2) 3. Parietal (2) 4. Sphenoid (1) 5. Ethmoid (T) 6. Frontal (2) 7. Temporal (2) FACIAL BONES(17) 1. Lacrimal (2) 2. Malar (2) 3. Maxilla (2) 4. Pre maxi!la(2) 5. Palatine (2) 6. Nasal (2) 7. Ptery'goid (2) 8. Turbinate (2) 9 Vomer (1) Cornua! process (2) Hyoid (1) Mandible (1)	Cervical (7) Thoracic (13) Lumbar (6) Sacral (5) Coccygeal(15-25)	Ribs =13 pairs (26) Sternum =1	Each forelimb has : 1. Scapula (1) 2. Humerus (1) 3. Radius (1) 4. Ulna(1) 5. Carpals(6) 6. Metacarpals(2) 7. Pha!anges(6) 8. Sesamoid ; (6) Proximal (4) Distal(2) Total bones in one fore limb=24 Total bones in 2 fore!imb=24x2=48	Each hindlimb has ; 1.Os coxae(l) 2. Femur (1) 3. Patella (1) 4. Tibia (1) 5. Fibula (1) 6. Tarsal (5) 7. Metatarsal(2) 8. Phalanges (6) 9. Sesamoid (6) Proximal (4) Distal(2) Total bones in one hind limb=24 Total bones In 2 hind!imb=24x2=48	Os cordis (2)

TOTAL NUMBER OF BONES IN SKELETON OF OX =208

References: Page 126, Sisson S.& Grossman, J.D. (1953). The Anatomy of the Domestic animals W.B. Saunders Co. Philadelphia.

5*

Number of Bones in Skeleton of Ox

*Table starts from next page

SKULL (including hyoid and mandible) Total = 32	Vertebral column (approximately) Total = 51 (apprx)	Ribs+Sternum (26 + 1) Total = 27	Forelimb (24x2) Total = 48	Hindlimb (24x2) Total = 48	Visceral bones Total = 2
CRANIAL BONES (11)	Cervical (7)	Ribs =13 pairs	Each forelimb has :	Each hindlimb has ;	Os cordis
1. Occipital (1)	Thoracic (13)	(26)	1. Scapula (1)	1.Os coxae(l)	(2)
2. Interparietal (2)	Lumbar (6)	Sternum =1	2. Humerus (1)	2. Femur (1)	
3. Parietal (2)	Sacral (5)		3. Radius (1)	3. Patella (1)	
4. Sphenoid (1)	Coccygeal(15-25)		4. Ulna(1)	4. Tibia (1)	
5. Ethmoid (T)			5. Carpals(6)	5. Fibula (1)	
6. Frontal (2)			6. Metacarpals(2)	6. Tarsal (5)	
7. Temporal (2)			7. Pha!anges(6)	7. Metatarsal(2)	
FACIAL BONES(17)			8. Sesamoid ; (6)	8. Phalanges (6)	
			Proximal (4)	9. Sesamoid (6)	
1. Lacrimal (2)			Distal(2)	Proximal (4)	
2. Malar (2)				Distal(2)	
3. Maxilla (2)					
4. Pre maxi!la(2)			Total bones in one	Total bones in one	
5. Palatine (2)			fore limb=24	hind limb=24	
6. Nasal (2)			Total bones in 2	Total bones In 2	
7. Ptery'goid (2)			fore!imb=24*2=48	hind!imb=24*2=48	
8. Turbinate (2)					
9 Vomer (1)					
Cornua! process (2)					
Hyoid (1)					
Mandible (1)					

TOTAL NUMBER OF BONES IN SKELETON OF OX =208

References: Page 126, Sisson S.& Grossman, J.D. (1953). The Anatomy of the Domestic animals W.B. Saunders Co. Philadelphia.

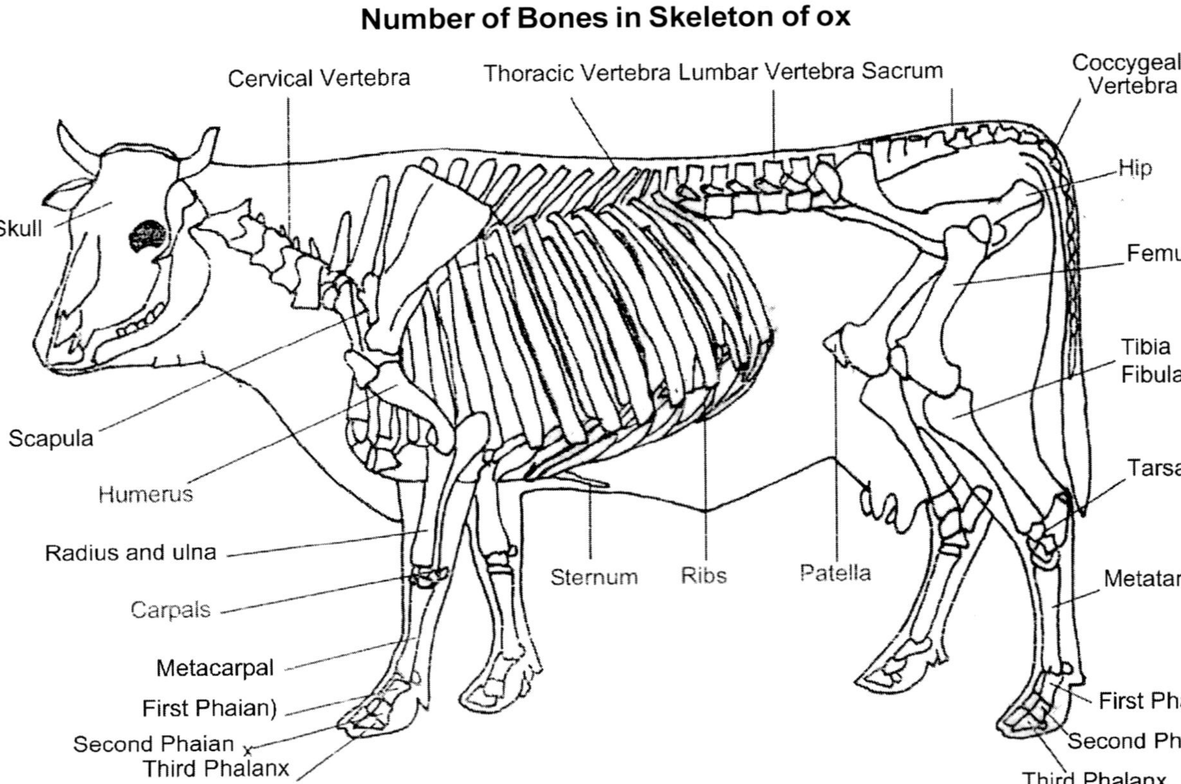

Fig. 1: Skelton of Ox

References: Page 126, Sisson S.& Grossman, J.D. (1953). The Anatomy of the Domestic animals W.B. Saunders Co. Philadelphia. p. 126

6

Superficial Muscles of Fore and Hind Limbs

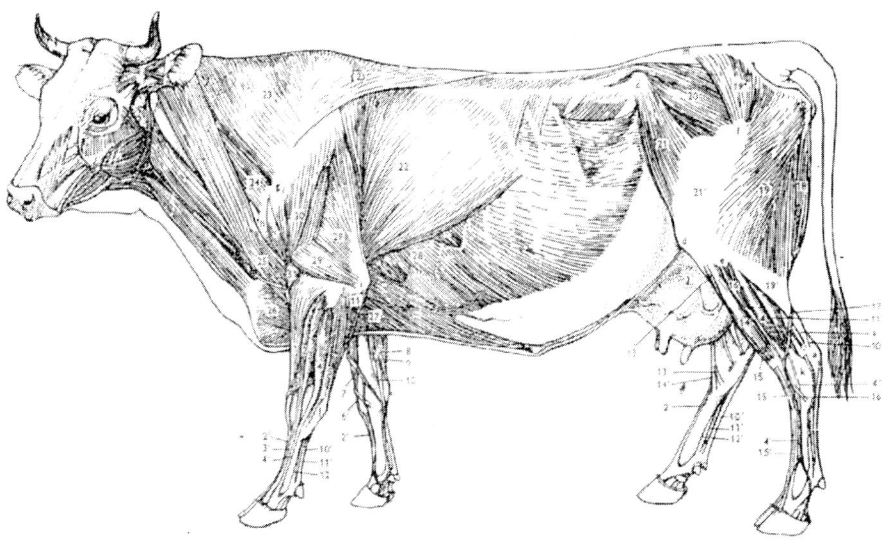

1: extensor carpi radialis
2: m. extensor digiti III propr.
2: its tendon
3: m. extensor digiti communis
3: its tendon
4: m. extensor digiti IV. propr.
4': its tendon :
5: m. ulnaris lateralis
6: m. extensor carpi obliquus
6: its tendon
7: cephalic vein
8: m. flexor carpi radialis
9: m. flexor carpi ulnaris
10: superficial part of m. flexor digiti supf.
10: superficial flexor tendon
19: superficial gluteal part of biceps
20: gluteus medius (middle gluteal)

11: ulnar head of m. flexor digiti prof.
11: deep flexor tendon
12: suspensory ligament
13: m. tibialis cranialis
13: its medial tendon of insertion
14: m. peroneus tertius
14: its tendon
15: m. extensor digiti pedis longus
15: its tendon
16: m. peroneus longus
16': its tendon
17: lateral saphenous vein
18: m. semitendinosus
19: m. biceps femoris
19: its aponeurosis (cut)

21: m. tensor fasciae latae
21. its aponeurosis
22 m. latissimus dorsi
23 m. trapezius
24 m. omotransversarius
25 m. brachiocephalicus
26 m. pectoralis supf.
27 m, pectoralis prof.
28 m. serratus ventralis
29: long and lateral heads of m. brachii
30 m. deltoideus
31 m. brachialis

a: tuber calcanei
a': common calcanean tendon (mainly tendoAchillis)
b: tuber ischii
c: tuber coxae
d: patella
e: lateral condyle of tibia and head of fibula
f: greater trochanter of femur
g: spine of scapula
h: major tuberosity of humerus
i: olecranon tuber of ulna
j: accessory carpal bone
k: lateral malleolus
m: tuber sacrale

7

Skull of Ox : Dorsal View

The condition in the young subject is as follows:

The two parietals are united with each other and also with the interparietal and supraoccipital. The resulting mass is somewhat horse shoe shaped. Its occipital part (planum occipitale) forms the greater part of the posterior wall of the cranium and bears about its centre the tubersity for the attachment of the ligamentum nuche. From either side of this a line curves outward and divide the surface into an upper smooth area and a lower area which is rough for muscular technique. The upper borderjoins the frontal bone and concurs In the formation of the frontal eminence. The temperal part (Plana temporalla) are much smaller and are concave externally; they join the frontal above and the squamous temporal below. A median occipital crest extends ventrally from the external occipital protuberance.

Skull of Ox : Dorsal View

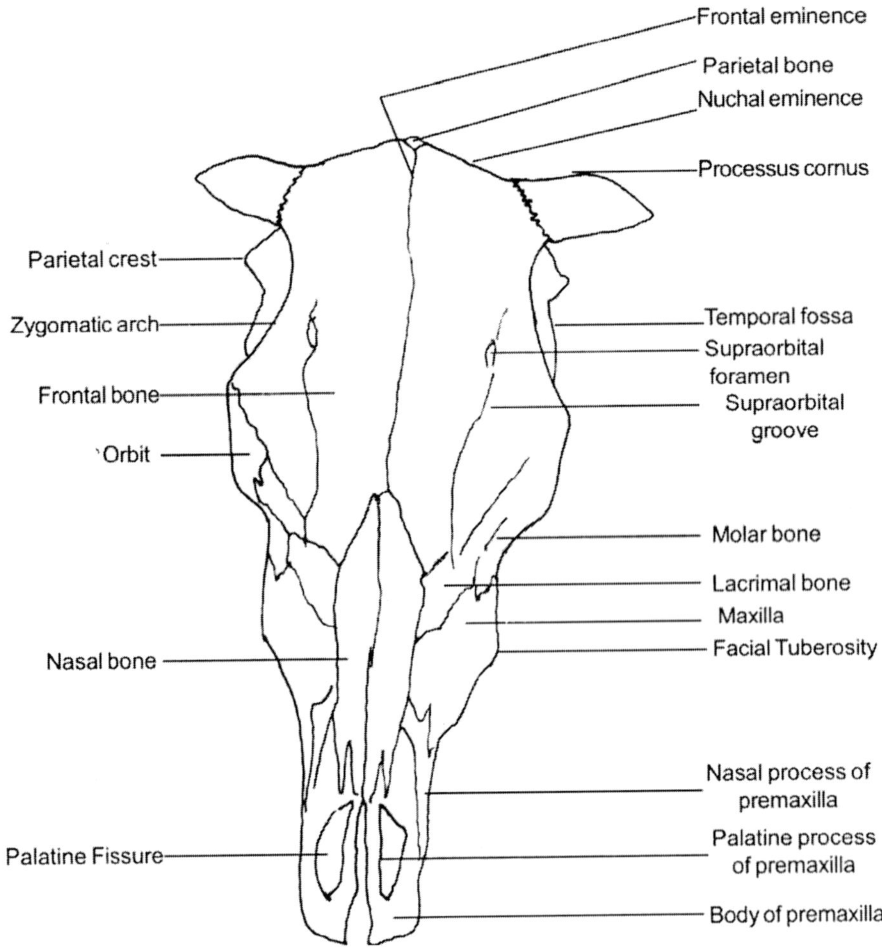

Fig. 1: Skull of Ox: Dorsal View

8

Skull of Ox (Sinuses Opened)

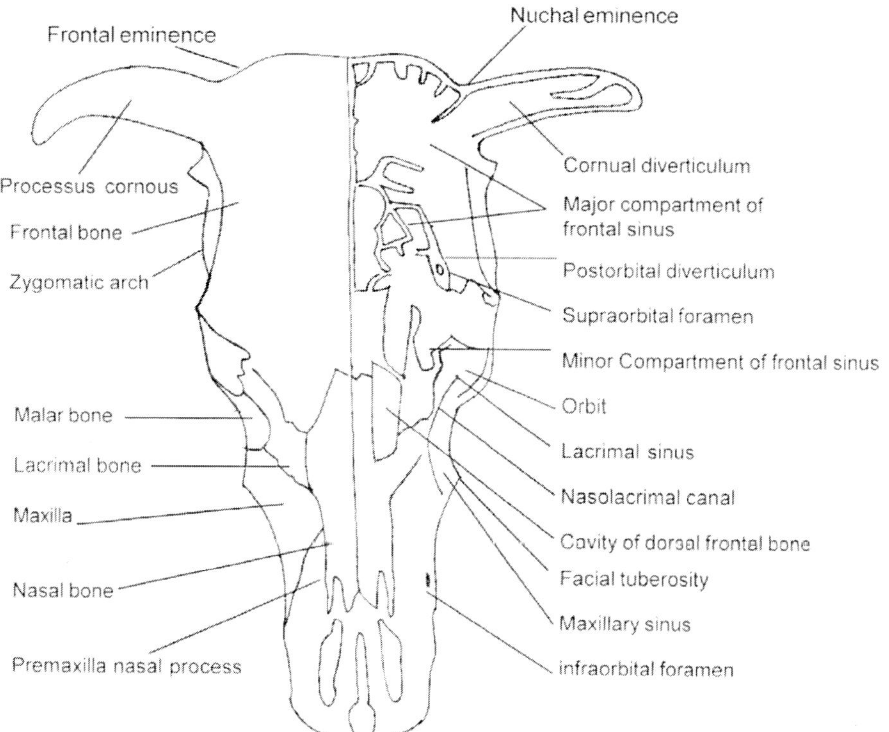

Fig. 1: Skull of Ox, Dorsal view, Sinuses Opened.

9

Skull of Ox, without Mandible, Ventral View

1. Foramen magnum
2. Occipital condyle
3. Paramastoid process
4. Condyloid foramen
5. Foramen lacerum
6. Basilar part of occipital condyle
7. Basilar tubercles
8. Bulla tympanica
9. Foramen ovale(concealed by muscular process)
10. Meatus acusticus externus
11. Zygomatic process of temporal bone
12. Condyle of same
13. External opening of temporal canal
14. Processus cornus
15. Muscular process of temporal bone
16. Pterygoid crest
17. Orbital opening of supraorbital canal
18. Choanae or posterior nbares
19. Hamulus of pterygoid bone
20. Cest formed by pterygoid processes of sphenoid and palatine bones
21. Horizontal part of palatine bone

22. Anterior palatine foramen
23. Lacrimal bulla
24. Maxillary tuberosity
25. Palatine process of maxilla
26. Zygomatic process of malar bone
27. Facial tubersoty
28. Body of pemaxilla
29. Palatine process of same
30. Palatine fissure
31. Incisive fissure
32. Premolars
33. Molars

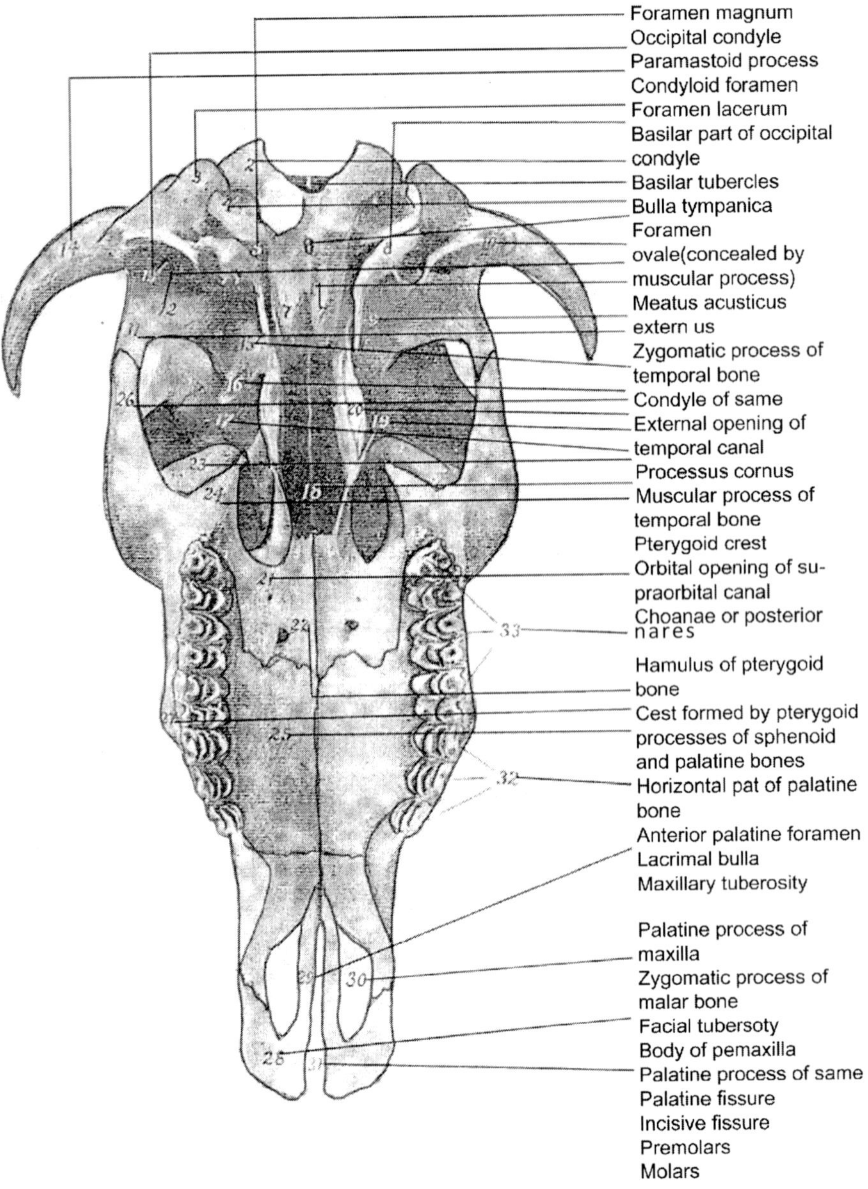

Fig. 1. Skull of ox, without mandible, ventral view.

10

Skull of Ox: Lateral View

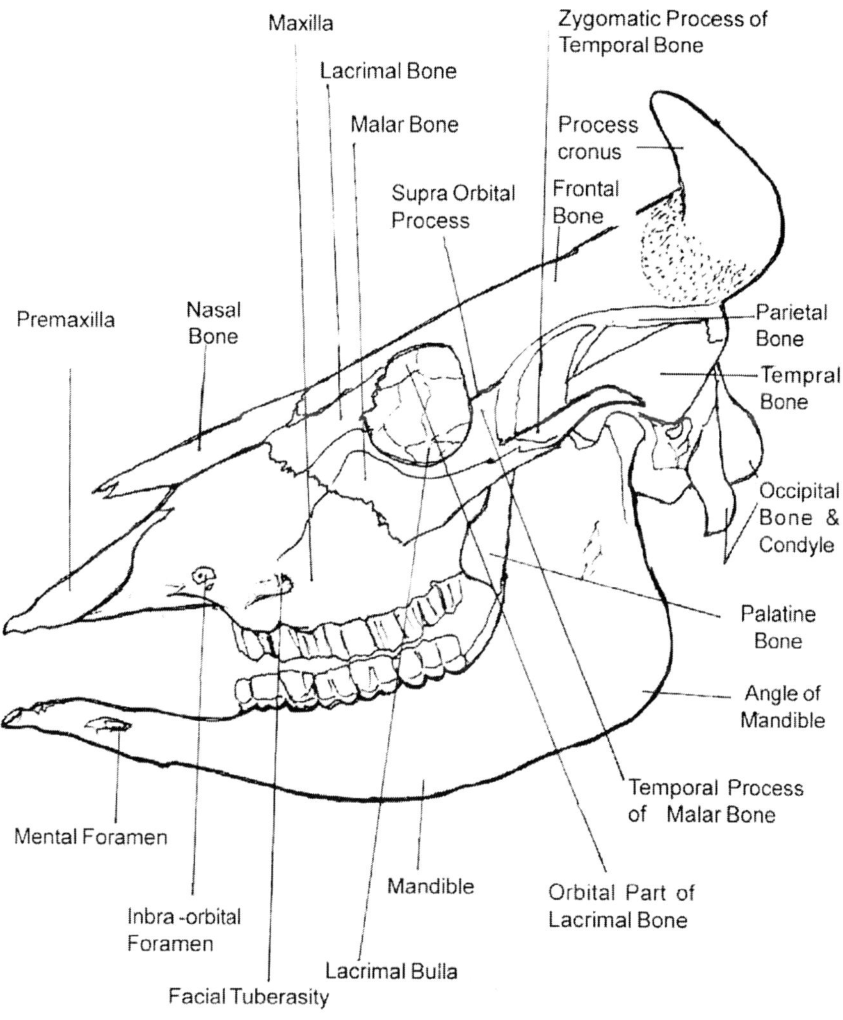

Fig. 1: Skull of Ox: Lateral Vew

References: Sisson and Grossman J.D. (1953). The Anatomy of the Domestic Animals 4th Edh. W.B Saunders Co. Philadelphia., P.138.

11

Sagittal Section of Skull of Ox Without Mandible

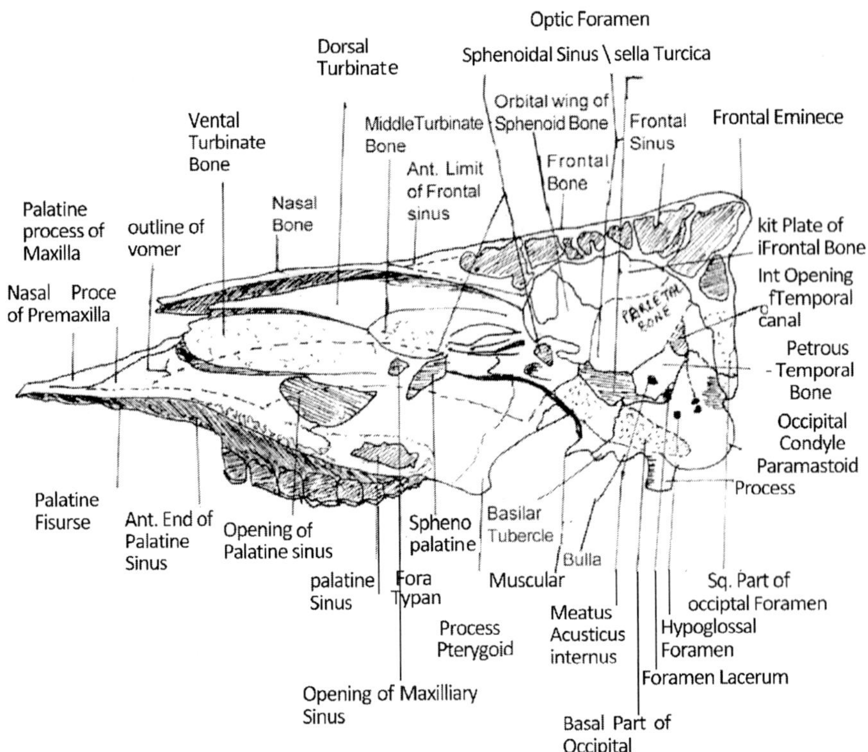

Fig. 1: Sagittal section of Skull of Ox without mandible

Reference: Sisson and Grossman, J.D. (1953). The Anatomy of the Domestic Animals. 4th Edn. W.B. Saunders Co. Philadelphia., P. 133.

12

Mandible and Hyoid Bone

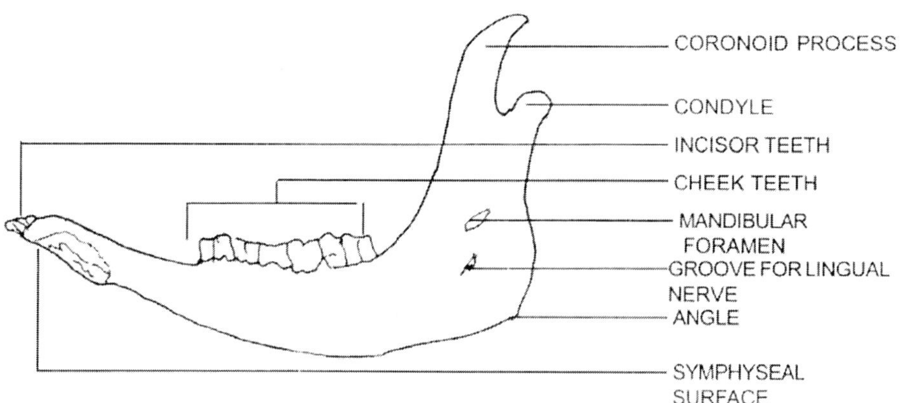

Fig. 1: Mandible

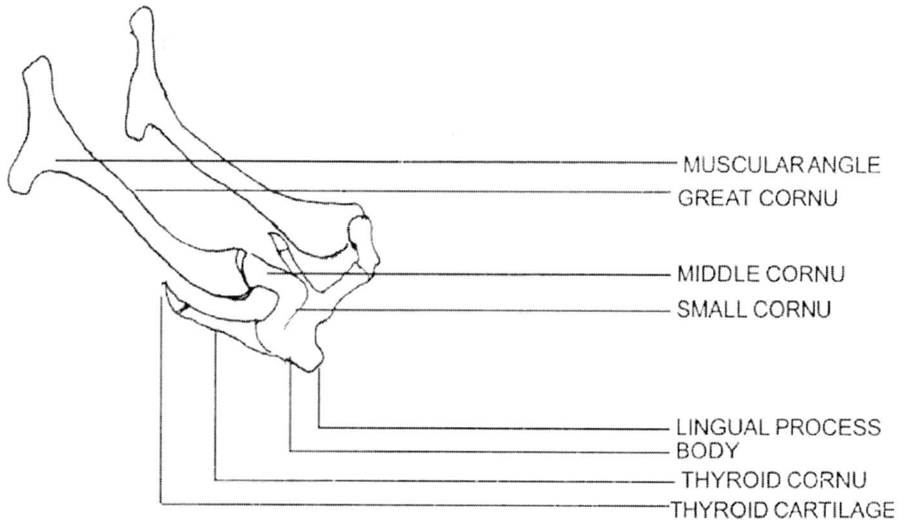

Fig. 2: Hyoid bone

13

Atlas

This vertebra is decidedly atypical in form and structure. The body and spineous process are absent. It has the form of a strong ring, from which two curved plates, the wings, project laterally. The ring incloses a very large vertebral foramen and consistis of two lateral masses connected by dorsal and ventral arches.

The lateral masses (Massae laterales) present two deep oval anterior articular cavities (Foveae articulares craniales) which receive the occipital condyles; they are separated by a wide notch above and a narrow one below. The lateral margin is also notched, and a triangular non-articular depression cuts into the medial part of each cavity. The posterior articular surfaces (Facies articulares caudales) are somewhat saddle-shaped; they are confluent on the ventral arch, but are widely separated dorsally, and do not conform in shape to the corresponding surfaces of the axis.

The dorsal arch (Arcus dorsali,) presents a median dorsal tubercle (Tuberculum dorsale) and is concave ventrally. It is perforated on either side near its anterior margin by the inter vertebral foramen (Foramen invertebrale). The anterior border is deeply notched, and the posterior border is thin and concave.

The ventral arch (Arcus ventralis) is thicker, narrower, and less curved than the dorsal. In its lower surface is the ventral tubercle (Tuberculum ventrale), into which the terminal tendon of the longus colli muscle is inserted. The upper face has posteriorly a transversely- concave articular surface, the fovea dentis, on which the dens or odontoid process of the axis rests.

In front of this is a transverse rough excavation and a ridge for the attachment of the ligamentirm dentis.

The wings (Alae atlantis) are modified transverse processes.They are extensive curved plates which project ventro-laterally and backward from the lateral masses. The dorsal surface is concave. Between the ventral aspect of the wing and the lateral mass is a cavity, the fossa atlantis; in this there is a foramen which opens into the vertebral canal. The border is thick and rough; its position can be recognized in the living animal. Two foramina perforate each wing. The anterior one, the foramen alare, is connected with the intervertebral foramen by a short groove. The posterior one is the foramen transversarium.

Development.-The atlas ossifies from four centers, two for the ventral arch, and one on either side for each lateral mass, wing, and half of the dorsal arch. At birth the bone consists of three pieces-the ventral arch and two lateral parts, which are separated by a layer of cartilage in the dorsal median line and by two ventro-lateral layers. These parts are usually fused at about six months.

Reference: Sisson and Grossman, J.D. (1953). The Anatomy of the Domestic Animals. 4th Edn. W.B. Saunders Co. Philadelphia., P. 127.

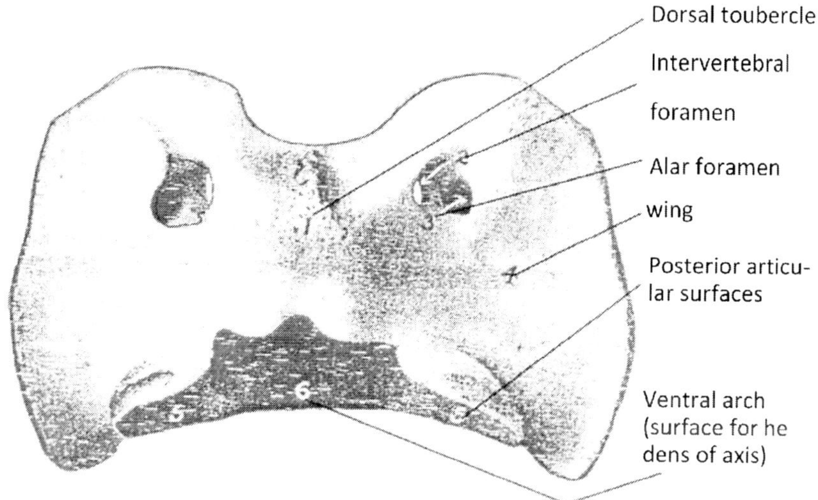

Fig. 1: Atlas of Ox: Dorsal view.

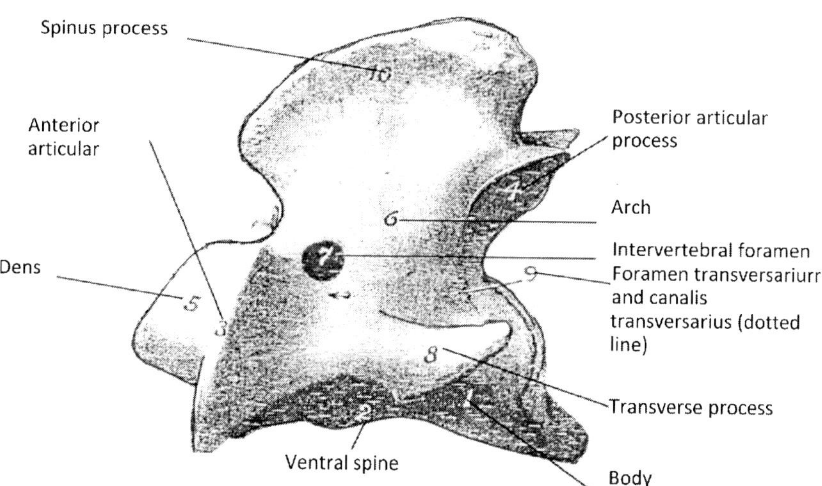

Fig. 2: Atlas of Ox: Dorsal view.

Reference: Sisson and Grossman, J.D. (1953). The Anatomy of the Domestic Animals. 4th Edn. W.B. Saunders Co. Philadelphia., P. 127.

14

The Cervical Vertebre

The cervical vertebrae are 7 in number.

The first and second cervical vertebrae are highly modified in conformity with the special function of support and movements of the head.

The **third, fourth** and **fifth** have the following characters:

The body is long. **Ventral surface** present a median **ventral spine.**

The **dorsal surface** has a flat central area which is narrow in the middle of the vertebrae, and wide at either end. On either side of this area there is a groove which lodges the longitudinal spinal vein.

The **anterior extremity or head** has an oval articular surface which faces forward and downward; it is strongly convex and wider above than below.

The **posterior extremity** is larger and has a nearly circular cotyloid cavity.

The **arch** is large and strong. It is perforated on either side by foramen which communicates with the foramen transverse hum. The vertebral notches are large.

The **articular process** are large. Their articular surface are extensive, oval in outline, and slightly concave.

The **transverse processes** are large and plate like .Each arises by two roots, **one from the arch and one from the body; between these there is foramen transversarium.**

The **spinous process** has the form of a low crest,which widens behind, and is connected by ridges with the posterior articular processes.

The **sixth** cervical vertebra has the following distinctive features

It is shorter and wider than fifth. Arch is large. **Posterior articular processes** are shorter, thicker, and further apart. The **spinous process** is less rudimentary. The **transverse processes** have three branches, third part is thick ,othertwo are short and thicker. The **foramen transversarium** is large; below its posterior end there is a fossa. The **ventral spine** is small and less prominent posteriorly.

The **seventh** cervical vertebra is readily distinguished by the following characters: it is **shorter** and **wider** than others. The **body** is flattened dorso-ventrally and wide. The **arch** and **notches** are large. The anterior articular process are wider and longer than posterior pair. The **spinous process** is an inch or more in height. The **transverse process** is undivided, and has no foramen transversarium. The ventral crest is replaced by a pair of tubercles. In some specimen a large foramen tranversarium is present on one side or both sides.

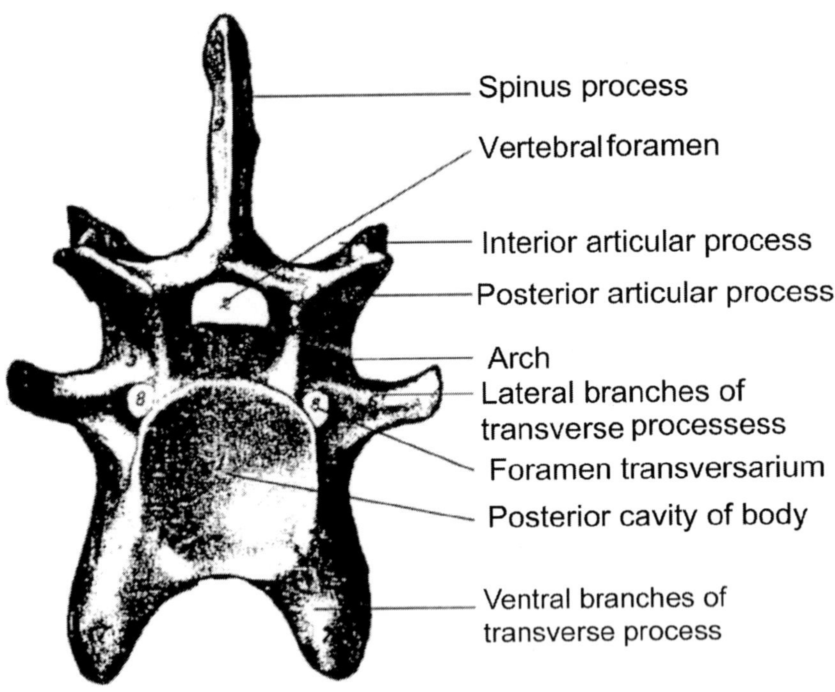

Fig. 1: Sixth cervical vertebra of ox: Posterior view.

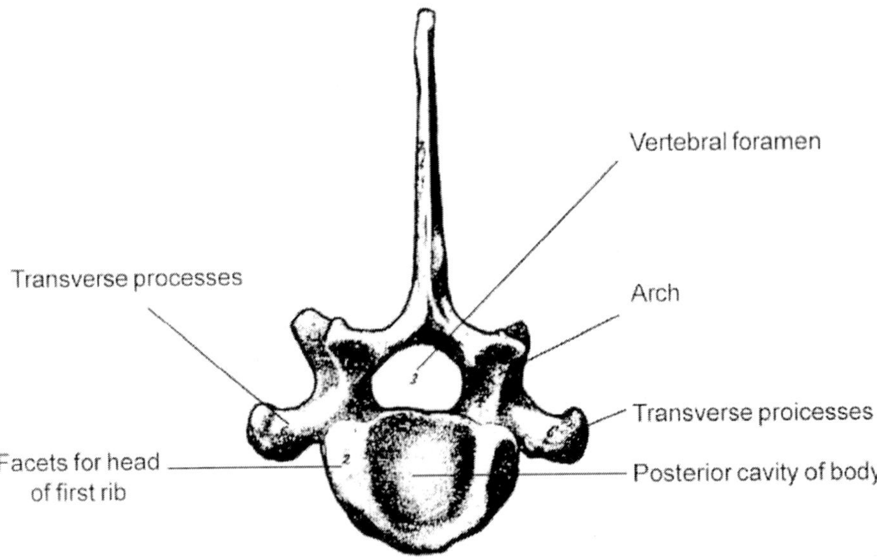

Reference: Sisson and Grossman, J.D. (1953). The Anatomy of the Domestic Animals. 4th Edn. W.B. Saunders Co. Philadelphia., P. 127.

15

Fourth Lumbar Vertebrae and Sacrum of Ox

LUMBAR VERTEBRAE (Fig. 1)

- Lumbar vertebrae, six in number, are much longer than in the horse.
- The body is much constricted in the middle, expanded at either end, and bears a rudimentary ventral crest.
- The articular processes are large, and their facets are more strongly cun/ed than in the horse.
- The transeverse processes ail'curve foPA/ard, borders a.^e thin and irregular and often bear projections of variable size and form..
- The spinous processes are relatively low wide, the last being the smallest; their summits are moderately thickened.

SACRUM (Fig. 2)

- The sacrum is longer than that of the horse. It consists originally of five segments, but fusion is more complete and involves the spinous processes, which are united to form a median sacral crest, with a convex thick and rough margin.
- A lateral sacral crest is formed by the fusion of the articular processes. The pelvic surface is concave in both directions, and is marked by a central, groove (sulcus vasculosus), which indicates the course of the middle sacral artery.
- The ventral sacral foramina are large.
- The wings curved downward and forward.
- The lateral borders are thin, sharp, and irregular.
- The bone does not become narrower posteriorly, so that the apex is usually wider than the part just behind the wings; the posterior end of the median crest forms a pointed projection over the opening of the sacral canal.

Reference: Sisson, S and Grossman, J.D. (1953), The Anatomy of the Domestic Animals. W.B. Saunders co. Philadelphia. Page 128, 129.

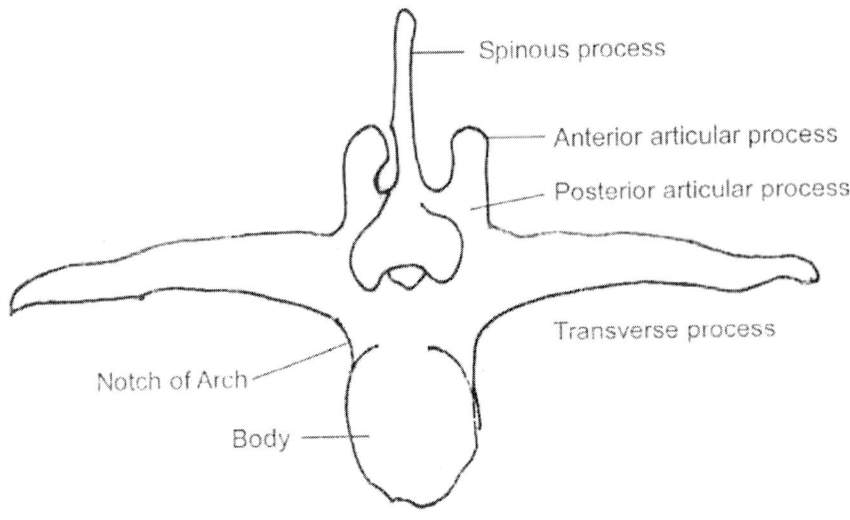

Fig. 1: Fourth Lumber Vertebrae of Ox. Posterior view

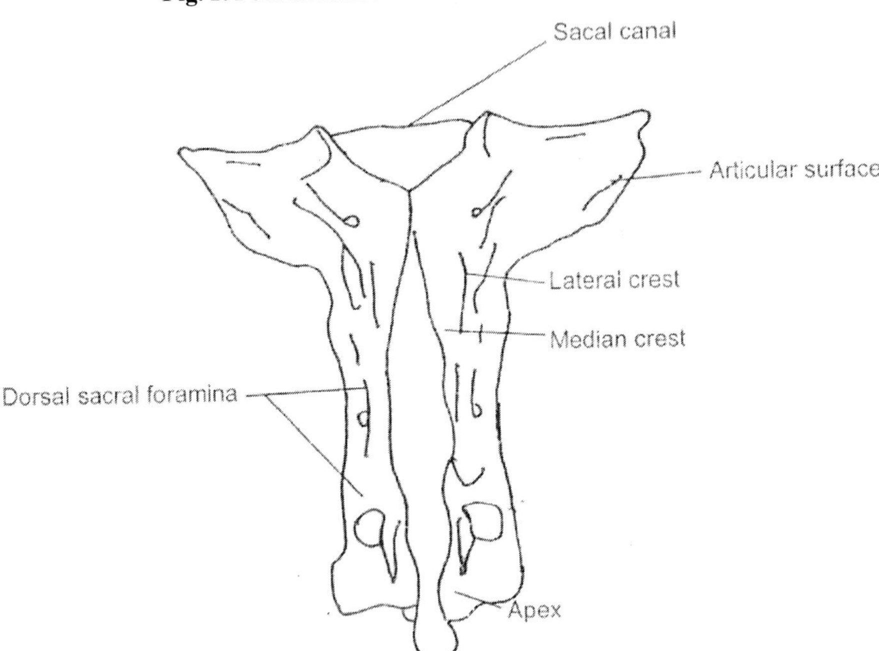

Fig. 2: Sacrum of Ox: Dorsal view

Reference: Sisson, S and Grossman, J.D. (1953), The Anatomy of the Domestic Animals. W.B. Saunders co. Philadelphia. Page 128, 129.

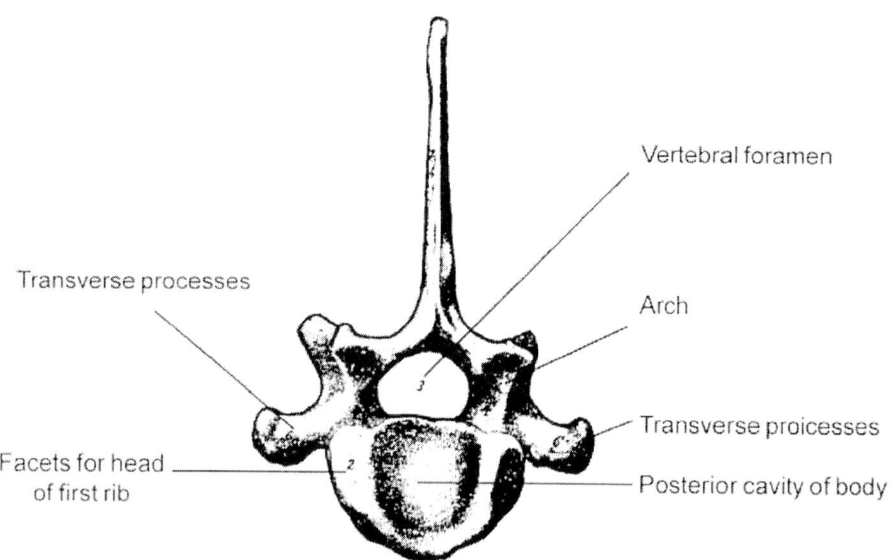

Reference: Sisson and Grossman, J.D. (1953). The Anatomy of the Domestic Animals. 4th Edn. W.B. Saunders Co. Philadelphia., P. 127.

16

Scapula of Ox

The scapula is more regularly triangular than in horse, relatively, wider at the vertebral end and narrower at the distal end. The scapular index is about T.0.6. The spine is more prominent and is placed further forward, so that the supraspinous fossa is narrow and does not extend to the lower part of the bone. The spine is sinuous, bent backward in its middle, forward below. Its free border is somewhat thickened in its middle, but bears no distinct tuber. Instead of little more prominent, and is prolonged by a pointed production, the acromion, from which part of the deltoid muscle arises. The sub scapular fossa is shallow. The areas for the attachment of the stratus muscle are not very distinct. The nutrient foramen is usually in the lower third of the posterior border. The glenoid cavity is almost circular and without any distinct notch. The tuberosity is small and close to the glenoid cavity. The coracoid process is short and rounded. The cartilage resembles that of the horse. The tuberosity unites with the rest.

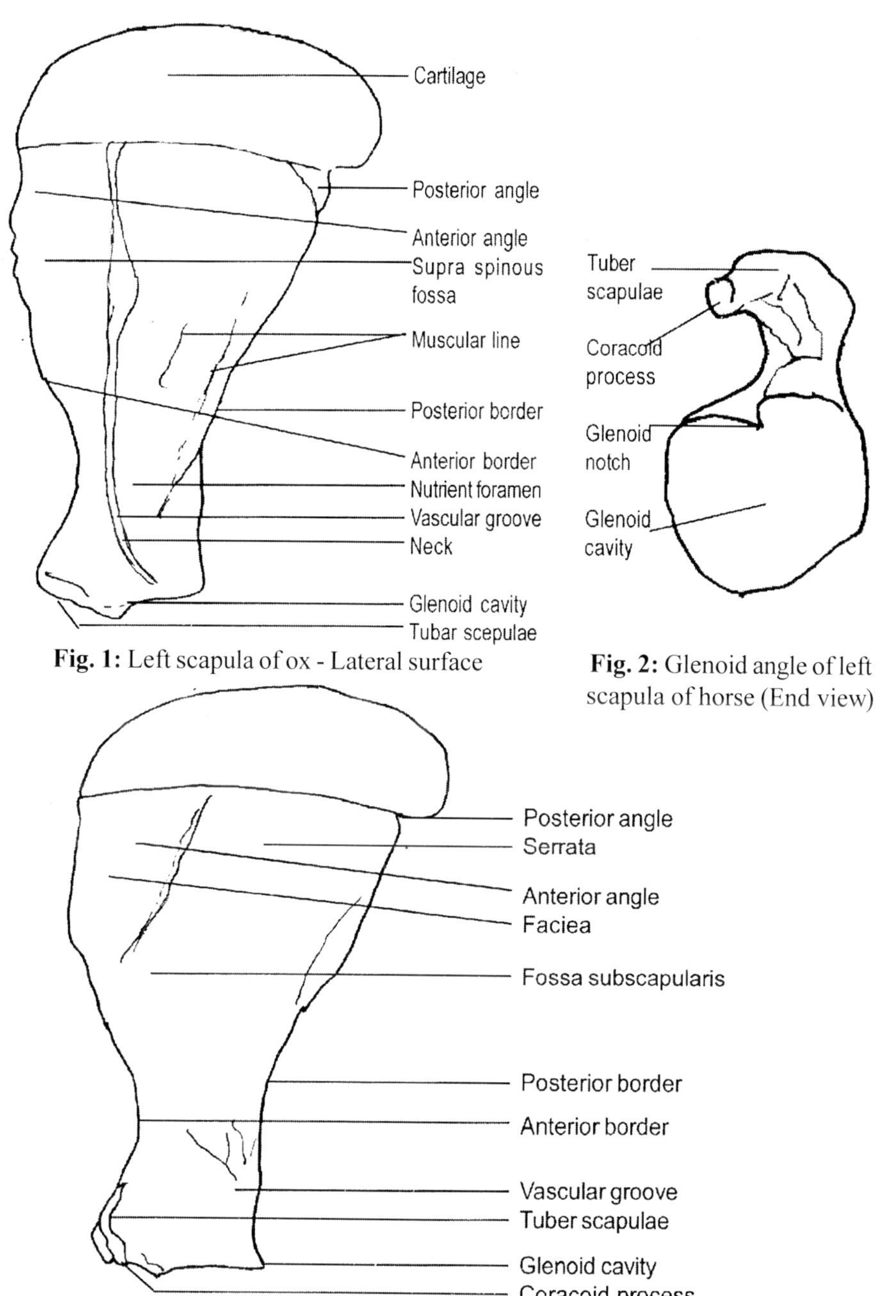

Fig. 1: Left scapula of ox - Lateral surface

Fig. 2: Glenoid angle of left scapula of horse (End view)

Fig. 3: Right scapula of Ox- Costal surface.

Reference: Sisson and Grossman, J.D. (1953). The Anatomy of the Domestic Animals. 4th Edn. W.B. Saunders Co. Philadelphia., P. 146.

17

Carpus and Adjacent Bones of Ox

Fia.1. Left carous and adjacent bones of Ox: Front view:-

1. Ulna
2. Radius
3. Fused second and tliird carpals
4. Ulnar carpal
5. Radial carpal
6. Fourth carpal
7. Fused second and third carpals
8. Metacarpal tuberosity
9. Vascular groove
10. Intermediate carpal bone

Fia. 2. Left carous and adjacent bones of Ox: Lateral view.

1. Distal interosseous space
2. Distal end of radius
3. Styloid process of ulna
4. Accessory carpal
5. Intermeidate carpal
6. Ulnar carpal
7. Fused second and third carpal
8. Fourth carpal
9. Meta carpal tuberosity
10. Fifth (small) metacarpal
11. Fused 3rd and fourth (large) metacarpal

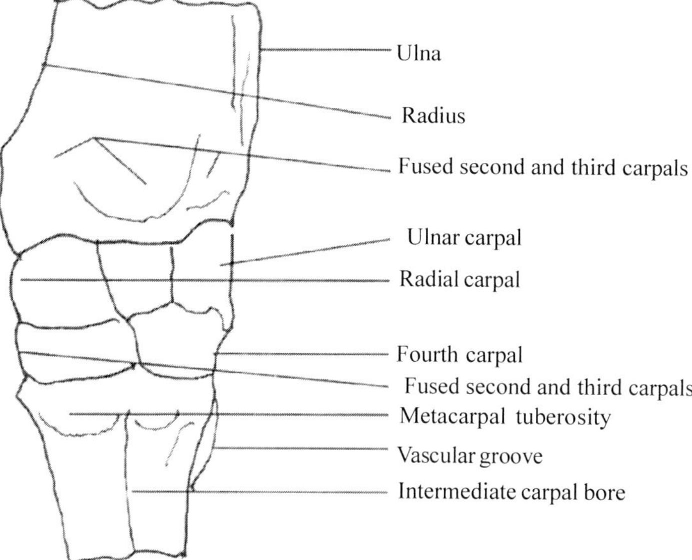

Fig. 1: Left carpus and adjacent bones of Ox; Front view.

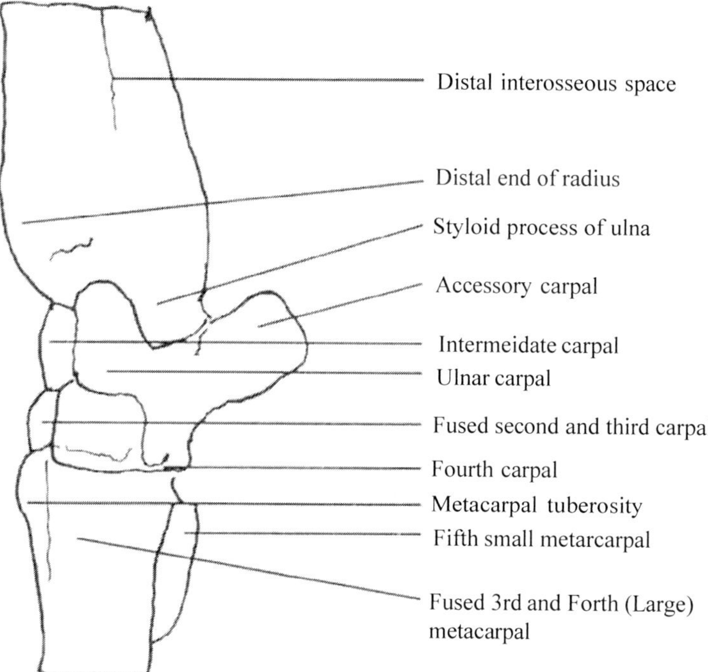

Fig. 2: Left carpus and adjacent bones of Ox; Lateral view.

18

Metacarpal and Metatarsal of Ox

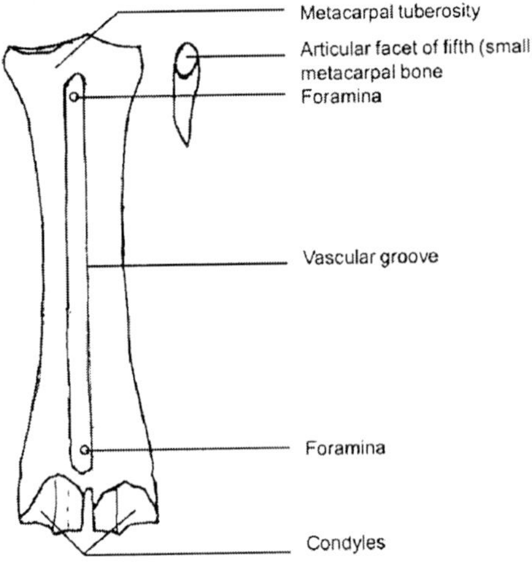

Fig. 1: Left metacarpal bone of ox: front view: the small bone has been moved

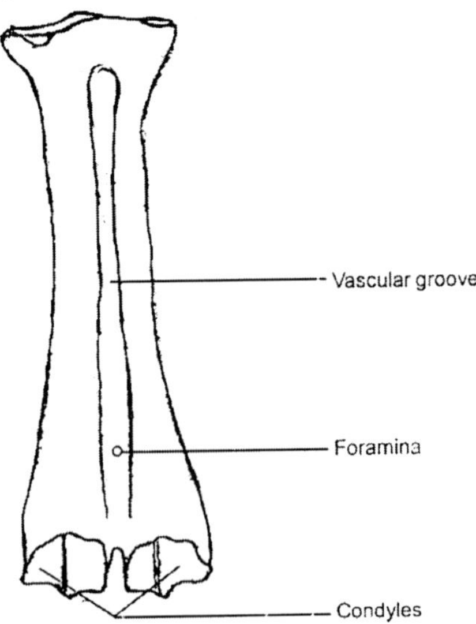

Fig. 2: Large metatarsal bone of ox : dorsal view

19

Bone of Distal Part of Fore Limb of Ox

DIGITS

Four digits are presents in the ox of these two the third and forth -are fully developed and have three phalanges and three sesamoid each.The second and fifth are vestiges.

FRIST PHALANX- (Fig.No.1)

1. The interdigital surface is flattened and its volor parts bears a prominence for the attachment of the interdigital ligaments.
2. The proximal extremity is relatively large and somewhat compressed from side to side.
3. The articular surface is concave from before backword and is divided by sagittal groove in two areas, of which the aboxial one is the larger and higher.
4. Behind tese are two facets for articulation with the sesamoid bones.
5. The distal extremity smaller than the proximal.

SECOND PHALANX (Fig No-2)

1. The proximal articular surface is divided by asagittal ridge into two glenoid cavities.
2. The distal extremity smaller than the proximal.
3. There is a deep depression for ligamentous attachment on the interdigital side.

THIRD PHALANX

1. The dorsal surface is marked in its distal part by a shallow groove, along which there are several foramin of considerable size.
2. It is also ablic transversely rthe Interdigital side being the lower.

3. The volor surface is narrow and slightly concave and present two or three foramina of considerable size.

PROXIMAL SESAMOID

1. Four proximal sesamoid are present two for each digit.
2. The bones of each pair articulate with the corresponding part of the distal end of the large metacarpal bone by their dorsal surface with each other hand with the first phalanx by small facets.

DISTAL SESAMOIDS

The two distal sesamoids are short and their ends are but narrower than the middle.

Reference : Sisson and Grossman, J.D. (1954). The Anatomy of the Domestic Animals. 4th Edn. W.B. Saunders Co. Philadelphia., PP. 149-150.

Bone of Distal Part of Fore Limb of Ox

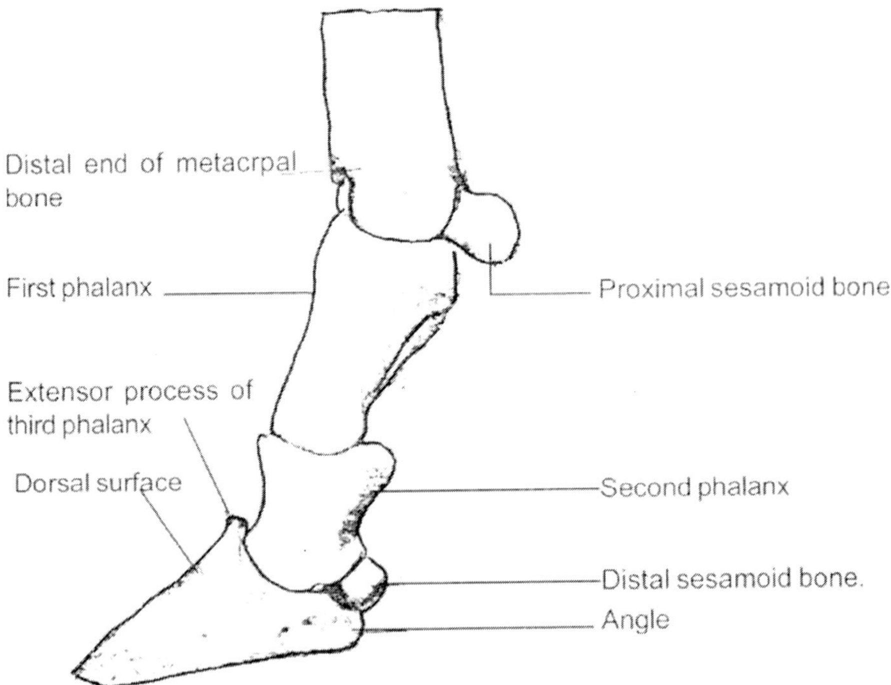

Fig. 1: Bones of distal part of fore limb of Ox: Lateral view.

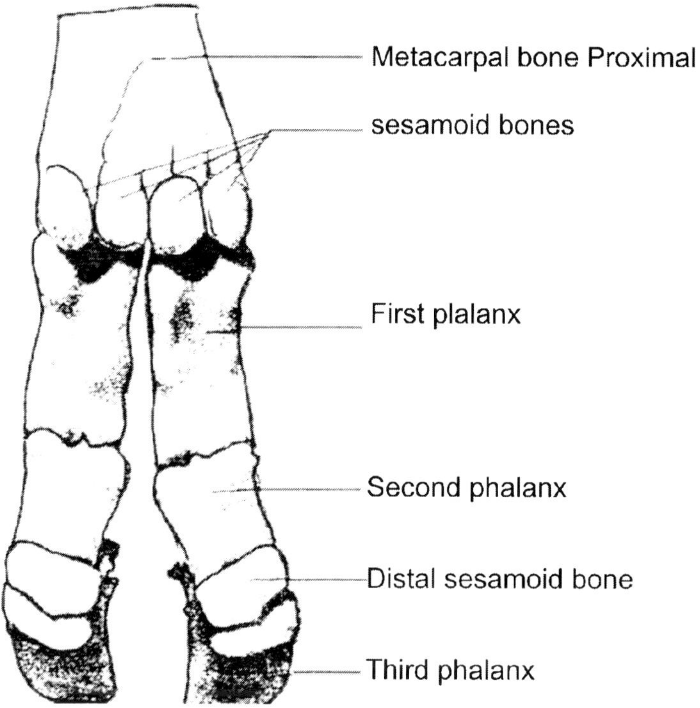

Fig. 2: Bones of distal part of forelimb of Ox: Volar view

Reference : Sisson and Grossman, J.D. (1954). The Anatomy of the Domestic Animals. 4th Edn. W.B. Saunders Co. Philadelphia., PP. 149-150

20

Sacrum of Ox

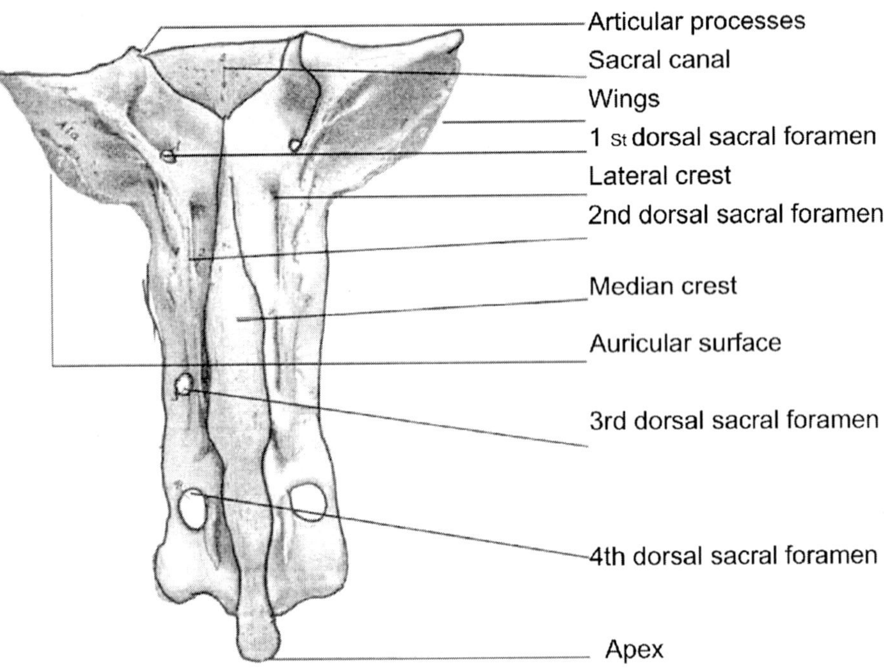

Fig. 1: Sacrum of Ox; Dorsal View

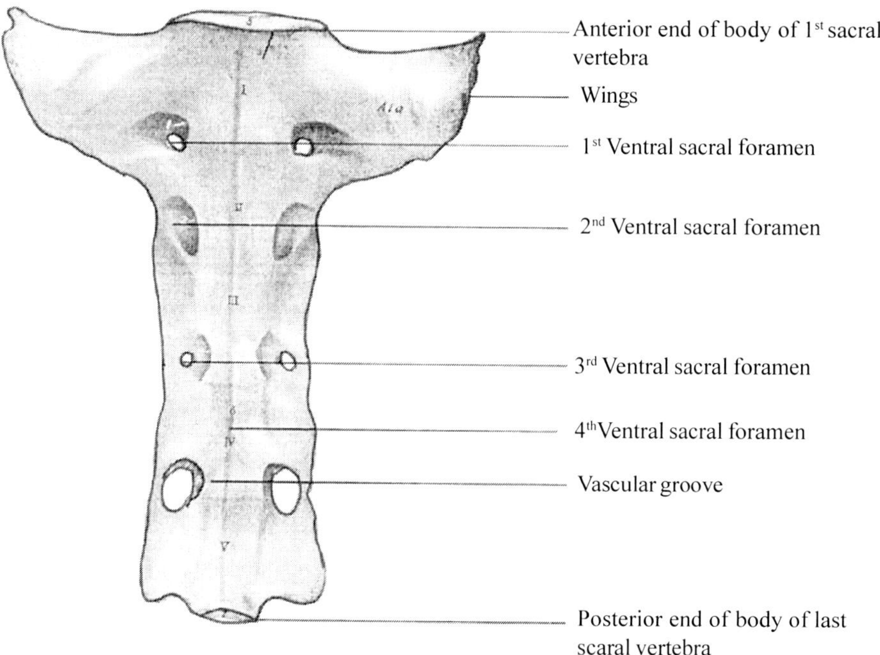

Fig. 2: Sacrum of Ox, Ventral view

21

Bones of the Pelvic Girdle

The ilia are almost parallel to each other and form a much smaller angle with the horizontal plane than in the horses.they are relatively small. The glutei line is prominent and nearly parallel to the lateral border,it joins the ischiatic spine.A rounded ridge separates the two parts of pelvic surface.The surface for articulation with sacrum is triangular. The tuber coxae is relatively prominent and not so oblique as in horses, wide in middle,smaller at either end.Shaft is short and compressed from side to side.

Ischium is large.Its long axis is directed obliquely upward and downward forming an angle of 5o to 60 degree with horizontal plane.The transverse axis is obliquely downward and inward at similar angle so concave from side to side.Ventral surface has rough ridge for muscular attatchment. The ischiatic spine is high and thin and bears a series of vertical rough line. lschiuatic arch is narrow and deep.The tuber ischii is large and three sided bearing dorsal ,ventral, lateral tuberosities.The symphysis bears a ventral ridge which fades out at ischial arch.The acetabular branch of pubis is narrow and is directed laterally,and a little forward.The anterior border is marked by a transverse groove which ends below rough iliopectineal eminence. The symphyseal branch is wide and thin. The acetabulum is smaller than in horses. Rim is rounded and usually marked by two notches. One is directed to deep acetabular fossa and and converted to foramen. The other is anteromedial and small also replaced by foramen or absent.

The obturator foramen is large and elliptical,medial border is thin and sharp.Fusion of three bonesoccur at 7-10 months. Pelvic inlet is elliptical and more oblique than in horses. In a cow conjugate diameter is 9-10 inches and transverse one is 7-8 inches. The dorsal wall is concave in both directions.The ventral wall is deeply concave particularly in transverse direction.the cavity is narrower and axis is inclined upward in posterior part. The outlet has vertical diameter of nine inches measured to 2nd coccygeal vertebra. Aetabulum is little farther to tuber coxae than to tuber ischii.

Reference: Sisson and Grossman, J.D. (1954). The Anatomy of the Domestic Animals.

Bones of the Pelvic Girdle

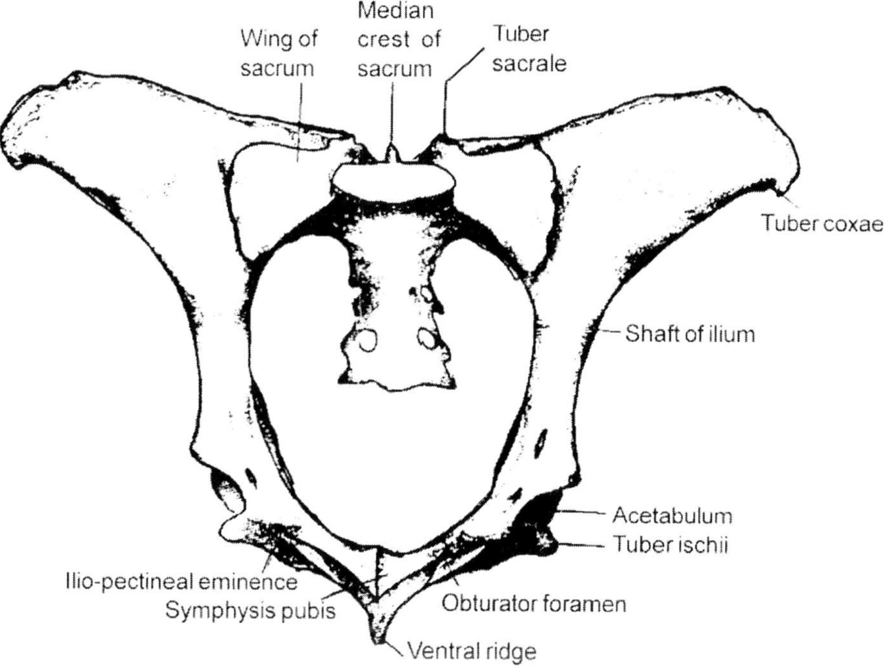

Fig. 1: Pelvic of cow, viewed from in front and somewhat from below.

References: Sisson and Grossman, J.D. (1953). The Anatomy of the Domestic Animals. 4th Edn. W.B. Saunders Co. Philadelphia., P.P. 151-152.

22

Right Os Coxae of Ox; Lateral View

ILIUM

The ilium are almost parallel to each other and form a much smaller angle with the horizontal plane than in the horse. They are relatively small. The gluteal line is prominent and is nearly parallel to the lateral border; it join the ischiatic spine. A rounded ridge separates the two parts of the pelvic surface. The surface for articulation with the sacrum is triangular. The tuber sacrale is truncated, does not extend so high as the vertebral spines, and is separated from the opposite angle by a wider interval than in the horse. The tuber coxae is relatively large and prominent; it is not so oblique as in the horse, and is wide in the middle, smaller at either end. The shaft is short and compressed from side to side.

ISCHIUM

The ishchium is large. Its long axis is directed obliquely upward and backward, forming an angle of about 50 to 60 degrees with the horizontal plane. The transverse axis is oblique downward and inward at a similar angle, so that this part of the pelvic floor is deeply concave from side to side. The middle of the ventral surface bears a rough ridge or imprint for muscular attachment. The ischiatic spine is high and thin, and bears a series of almost vertical rough line laterally. The tuber ischii is large and three-sided, bearing dorsal, ventral, and lateral tuberosities. The ischial arch is narrow and deep. The symphysis bears a ventral ridge, which fades out near the ischial arch.

PUBIS

The acetabular branch of the pubis is narrow, and is directed laterally and a little forward. The anterior border is marked by a transverse groove which ends below the rough ilio-pectineal eminence. The symphyseal branch is wide and thin.

ACETABULUM

The acetabulum is smaller than the horse. The rim is rounded and is usually marked by two notches. One of these is postero-medial and is narrow and deep; it leads to the deep acetabular fossa and is often almost converted into a foramen by a bar of bone. The other notch is antero-medial, small, and sometimes replaced by a foramen or absent.

OBTURATOR FORAMEN

The obturator foramen is large' and elliptical; its medial border is thin and sharp.

Right Os Coxae of Ox; Lateral View

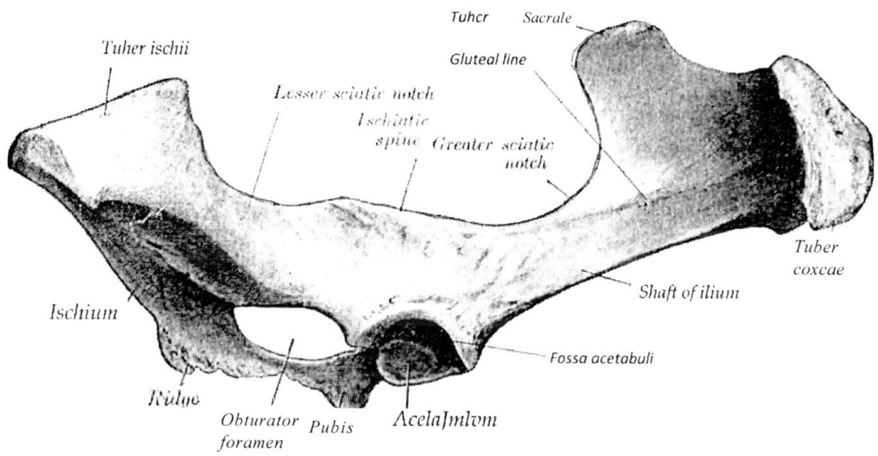

Fig. 1: Right os coxae of ox; Lateral View

Reference : Sissson,S. and Grossman J.D (1954)- Anatomy of the Domestic Animal 4th Edition W.B. Saunders Co. Philadelphia. P. 151

23

Bones of the Hind Limb

FEMUR

1. The femur has a relatively small shaft, which is cylindrical in its middle. The trochanter minor has the form of a rough tuberosity.
2. The trochanteric ridge connects it with the trochanter major. The third trochanter is absent. The supracondyloid fossa is shallow. The proximal extremity is very wide.
3. The fovea capitis is a small depression on the middle of the heacKfor the attachment of the round ligament.
4. The trochanter major is very massive and is undivided; its lateral surface is very rough. The trochanteric fossa is deep. The ridges of the trochlea are less oblique.

TIBIA

1. The tibia resembles that of the horse rather closely, but Is somewhat shorter. The shaft is distinctly curved, so that the medial side is convex.
2. The articular grooves and ridge of the distal end are almost sagittal in direction. The synovial fossa is shallow. The lateral groove Is separated by a sharp ridge which is for articulation with the lateral malleolus
3. The anterior part of the medial malleolus Is prolonged downward and has a pointed end. Laterally there Is a deep narrow groove which separates two prominences.

FIBULA

1. The fibula usually consists of the two extremities only. The head is fused with the lateral condyle of the tibia and is continued by a small, blunt-pointed prolongation below. The distal end remains separate and forms the lateral malleolus.

2. The proximal surface articulates with the distal end of the tibia, and bears a small spine which fits into the groove on that bonfe.
3. The distal surface rests on the fibular tarsal and the medial articulates with the lateral ridge of the tiblal tarsal bone. The lateral surface is rough and irregular.

Reference: Sisson and Grossman, J.D. (1954). The Anatomy of the Domestic Animals. 4th Edn. W.B. Saunders Co. Philadelphia., PP. 149-150.

BONES OF THE HIND LIMB

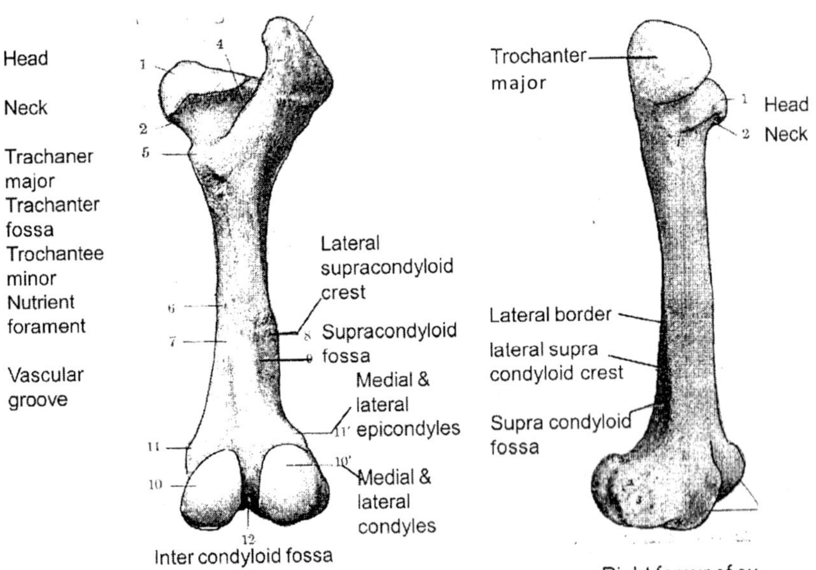

Fig. 1: Right femur of Ox, Posterior view

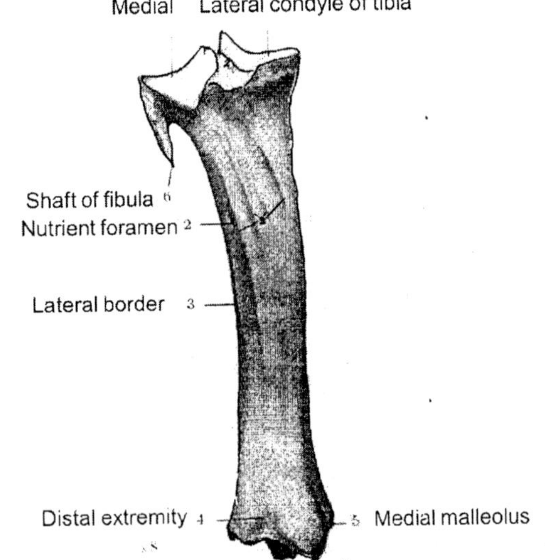

Fig. 2: Left tibia and proximal part of fibula of ox posterior view

References: Sison and Grossman, J.D. (1954).The Anatomy of the Domestic Animals 4th edn. W.B. Saunders Co. Philadelphia., pp. 149-150

24

Tarsus and Adjacent Bones of Ox

- M.mMedial malleolus
- M.I., Lateral malleolus
- T, Tibia
- T. t., Tibial tarsal bone
- T.f., Fibulartarsal bone
- T.c. + 4, Fused central and fourth tarsal bones.
- T.1, First tarsal bone
- T.2+3, Fused second and third tarsal bones
- Mt.2,Small, or second metatarsal bone
- Mt.3+4, Large metatarsal or fused third or fourth metatarsal bone
- 1, Groove for tendon of flexor digitalis longus
- 2, Groove for deep flexor tendon

Tarsus and Adjacent Bones of Ox

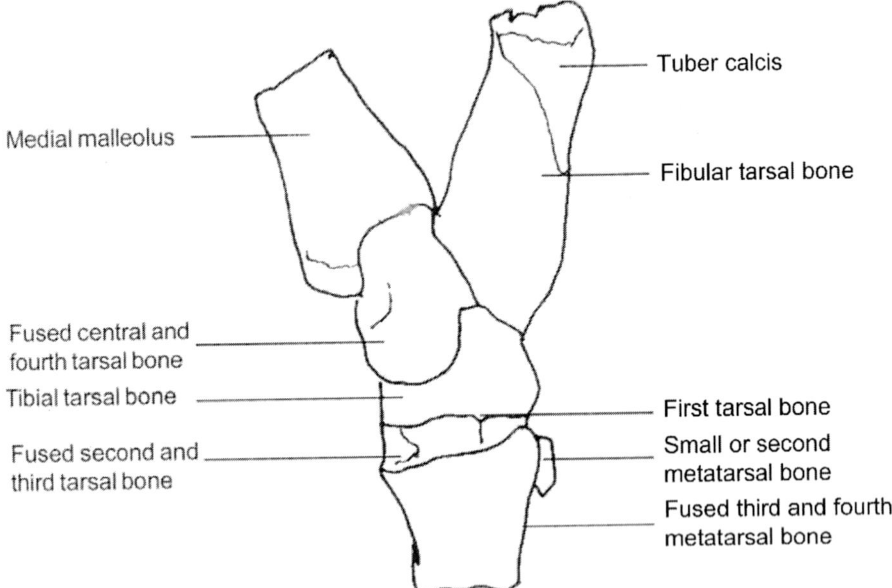

Fig. 1: Right tarsus and adjacent bones of ox- Medial view

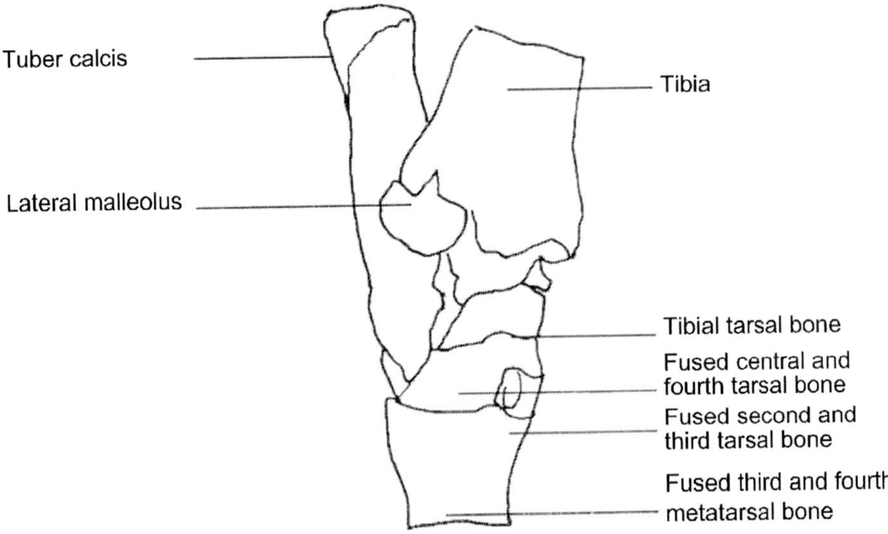

Fig. 2: Right tarsus and adjacent bone of ox - Dorso -Lateral view

Orthopaedics

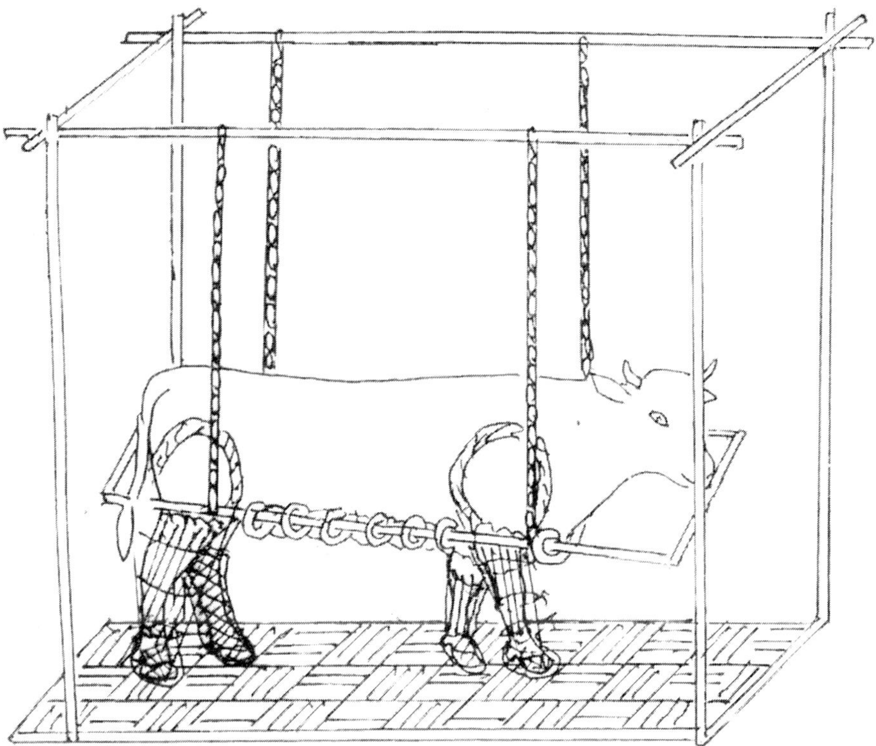

Fig. 3: Orthopaedics

25

Orthopaedic Instruments

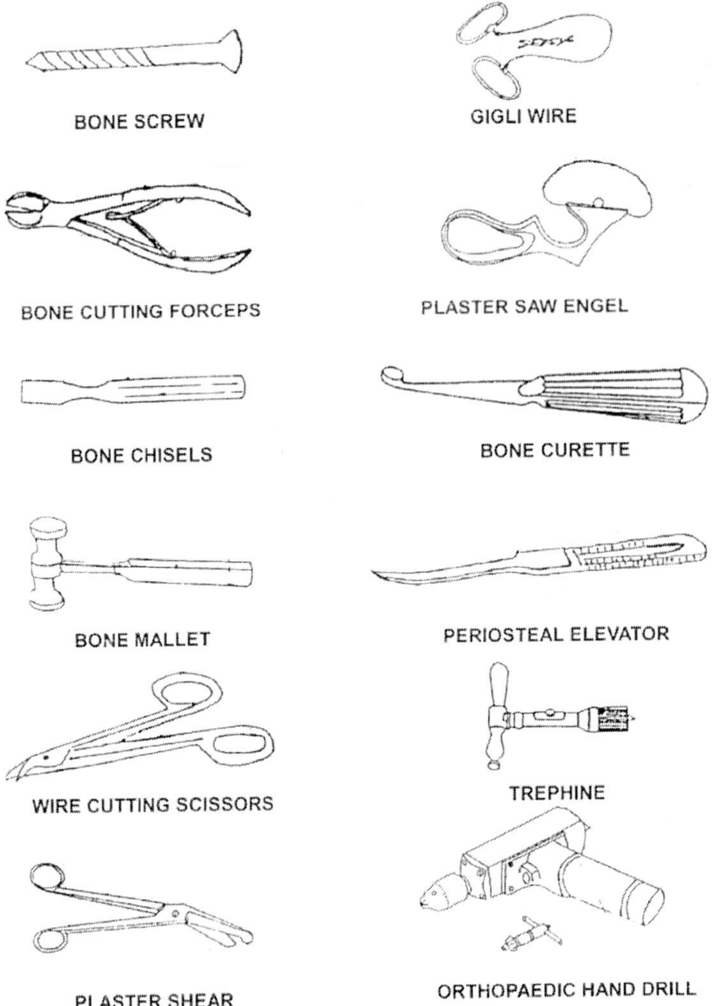

Fig. 1: Orthopaedics Instruments-I

References: Whittick W.G. (1974), Canine Orthopaedics, Lea and Febiger, Philadelphia

Orthopaedics Instruments –II

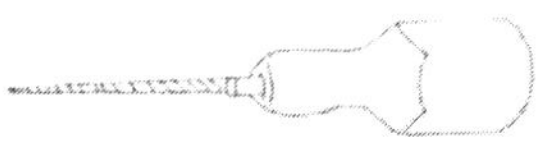

BONE TAP

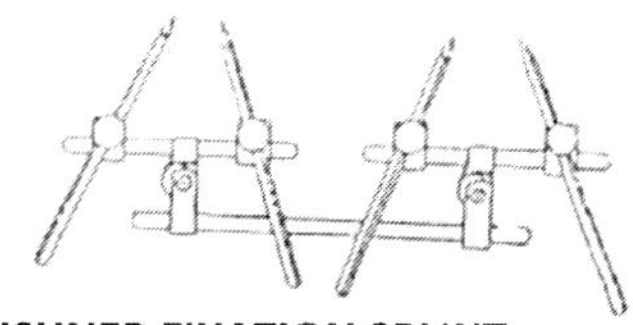

KRISHNER FIXATION SPLINT

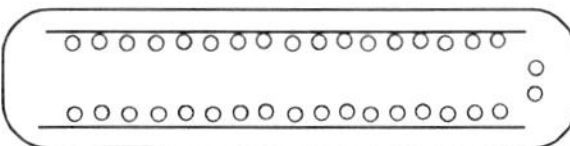

RULERAND PIN GAUGE

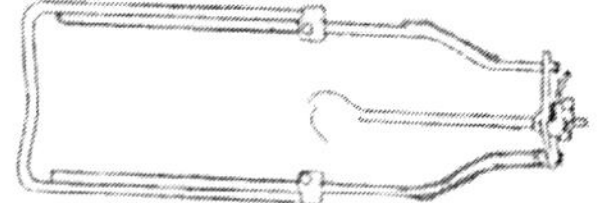

GORDON EXTENDER

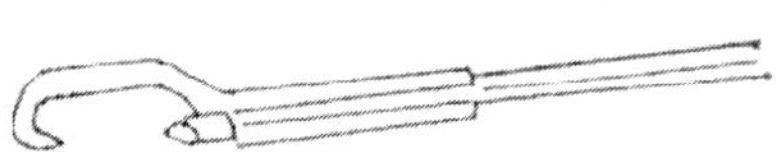

DRILL GUIDE

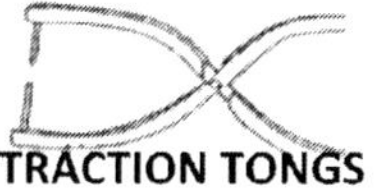

TRACTION TONGS

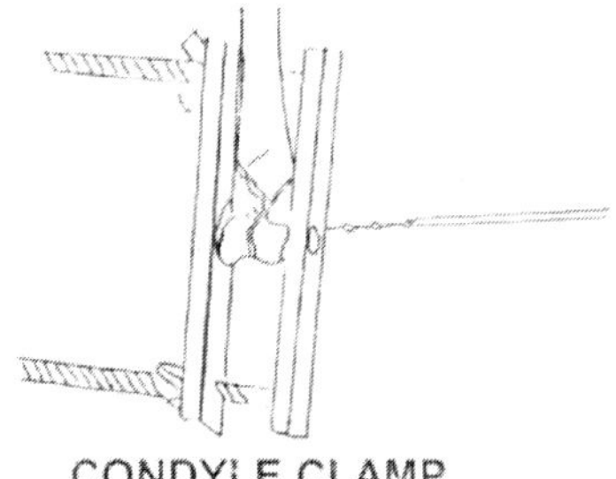

CONDYLE CLAMP

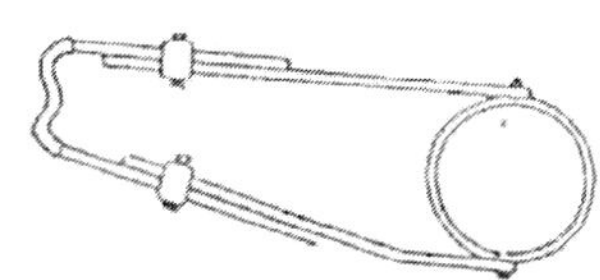

MODIFIED THOMAS SPLINT

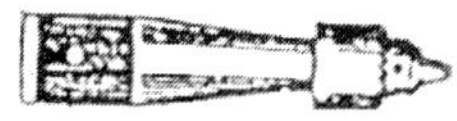

INTRAMEDULLARY PIN DRILL WITH JACOB'S

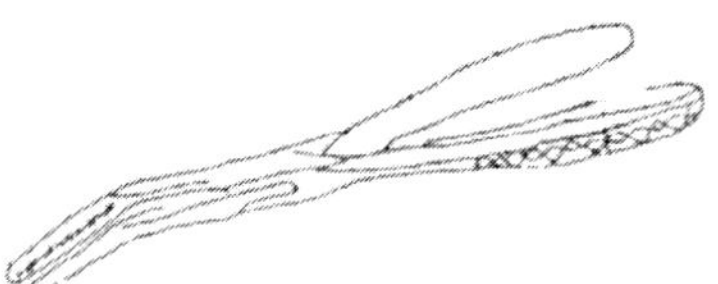

VAN BUREN SEQUESTRUM FORECEPS

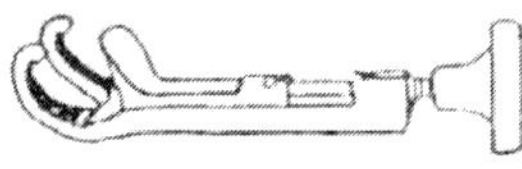

LOMAN BONE HOLDING CLAMP

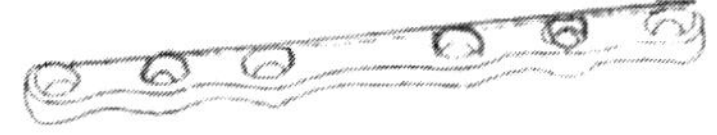

NEUTRALIZATION PLATE

Fig. 2: Orthopaedics Instruments-II

References: Whittick W.G. (1974), Canine Orthopaedics, Lea and Febiger, Philadelphia P.P. -449-462.

26

First Aid in Orthopaedic Patient

First Aid in Orthopaedic Patient

1. Immediately transfer the animal to a safety place.

   The place should be well settled, well ventilated, neat and clean.

   If the fracture site is limb and it is a simple fracture, immediately immobilize the animal with soft cotton padding and plastic scale placed at four sites.

2. If the fracture site is limb and it is a compound fracture, cover the fractured site v/ith th'ck padded clean cotton cloth and few bamboo splint placed on four sides to keep limb straight.

3. Control the bleeding, if bleeding occurs at time of covering of fractured site with thick padded clean cotton cloth.

4. If the fracture site is vertebral column, it is better not to lift the patient vigorously.

5. A patient with vertebral column fracture shouldn't be allowed for standing.

6. The patient shouldn't be attempted to shift to hospital with vehicle. It may cause more trauma to vertebral column.

7. Above all attempt should be made not to disturb the fractured site as well as fractured patient to shift to hospital within vehicle. It may aggravate the condition. It is better to call the physician to patient for treatment.

8. Take help of a doctor for stabilization of first aid procedure.

First Aid in Orthopaedic Patient

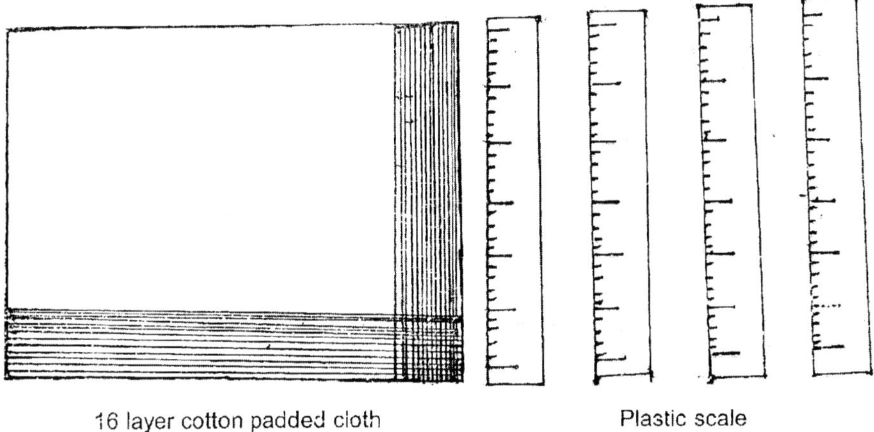

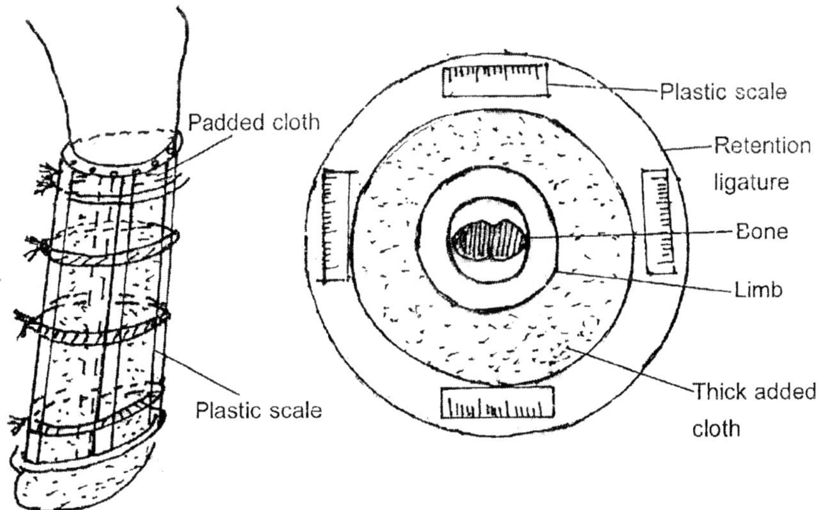

27

Classification of Fracture

- Complete fracture- It is a fracture in which there is complete loss of bone continuity and the bone is divided into two or more fragments (Fig.1).
- Green stick fracture- It is the fracture in which, the cortex opposite to the bending force fractures completely, while the cortex under the force remains in tact, commonly seen in immature animals, (Fig-2)
- Overriding fracture-A fracture in which the fragments lie side by side, causing shortening of limb (Fig-3)
- Transverse fracture-The fracture line here runs transverse to the long axis of bone. Such type of fracture is caused by bending forces (Fig-4).
- Oblique fracture- In this the fracture line runs oblique to the long axis of the bone. Such type of fracture is caused by bending with axial compression (Fig-5).
- Spiral fracture-Here the fracture line spirals along the long axis of bone. Such type of fracture is caused by torsion, twisting or rotational forces e.g. in humorous (Fig-6)
- Comminuted fracture- In this fracture, at least three fracture lines inter connect each other at one point (Fig-7).
- Multiple fracture-In this the bone is broken into 3 or more segments. The fracture lines don't interconnect each other.(Fig-8).
- Avulsion fracture-A fragment of bone at the site of muscle insertion is detached due to its forceful contraction (Fig-9).
- Condylar fracture-Fracture of the condyle either medial or lateral or both (Fig-10)
- Supracondylar fracture- Fracture over both the condyles are fractured off the shaft as a unit (Fig-11).
- Fracture dislocation/Monteggia fracture- When a fracture of bone results into joint instability leading to subluxation or luxation of the joint, it is called as fracture dislocation (Fig-12).

Reference: Gangwar, Naveen Ku. Devi, Kh. S. (2010). General Animal Surgery and Anesthesiology, New India Publishing Agency. New Delhi, PR 77-81.

Classification of Fracture

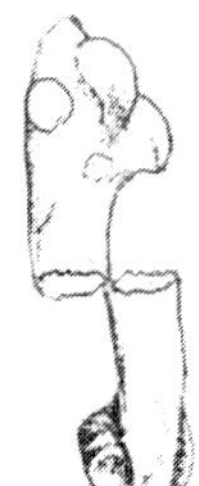

Fig. 1: Complete Fracture

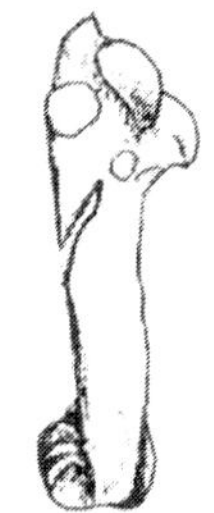

Fig. 2: Green Stick Fracture

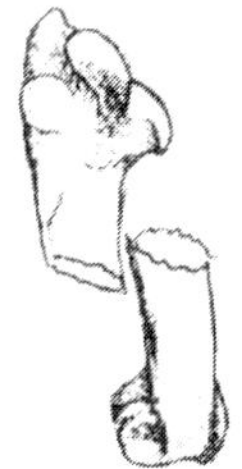

Fig. 3: Over riding Fracture

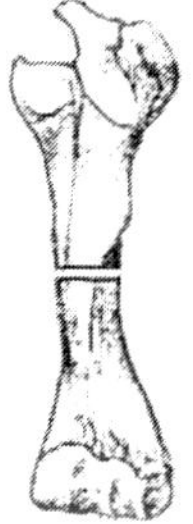

Fig.4 : Transverse Fracture

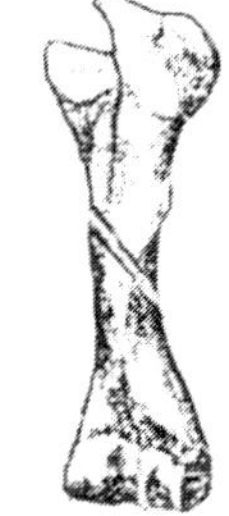

Fig. 5: Oblique Fracture

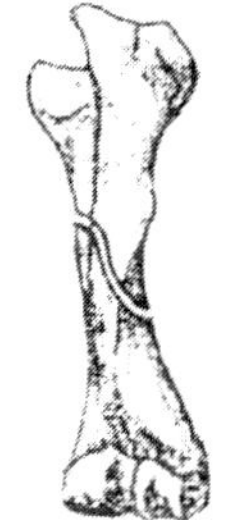

Fig. 6: Spiral Fracture

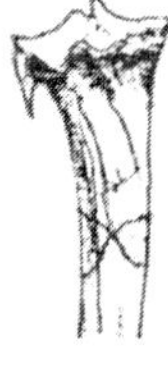

F!g. 7: Comminuted Fracture

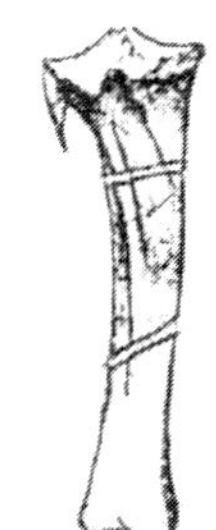

Fig. 8: Multiple Fracture

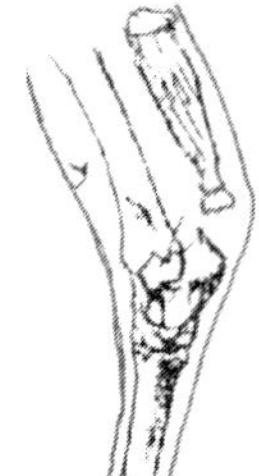

Fig.9: Avulsion Fracture

Fig.10: Condylar Fracture

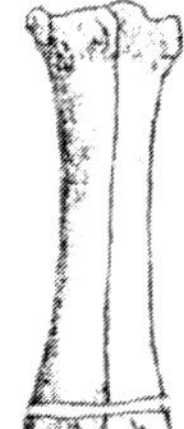

Fig.11: Supra Condylar Fracture

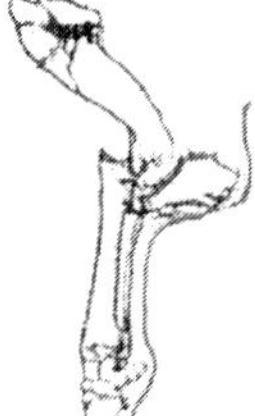

Fig.12: Montegsia Fracture

28

Curve Showing Degree of Inflammation and Time of Application of External Immobilisers

Definition: A fracture is a dissolution of bony continuity with or without displacement of the fragments.

Different stages of fracture: Inflammatory phase, reparative phase, and remodelling phase.

Fundamental steps

1. After fracture, the limb should be kept in temporary immobilisation for 72 days. The temporary immobilisers used may be Thomas splint or bamboo splint or aluminium splint or starch bandage.
2. From 72 hrs. Onwards the limb is immobilised by application of plaster of paris cast.
3. In day of fracture, replastering is done.
4. Too tight pop cast application and not removing plaster at proper time leads to aseptic necrosis.
5. Pop cast removal time:

   New born - 14 days of application

   Young - 21 days of application

   Middle age group - 30 days of application

   Higher age group - 45 days of application

   Tendon repair - 90 days of application
6. Joint above and joint below should be included In plaster cast.
7. Restricted movement within 8 foot x 8 foot to 10 foot x i **o** foot size enclosure.

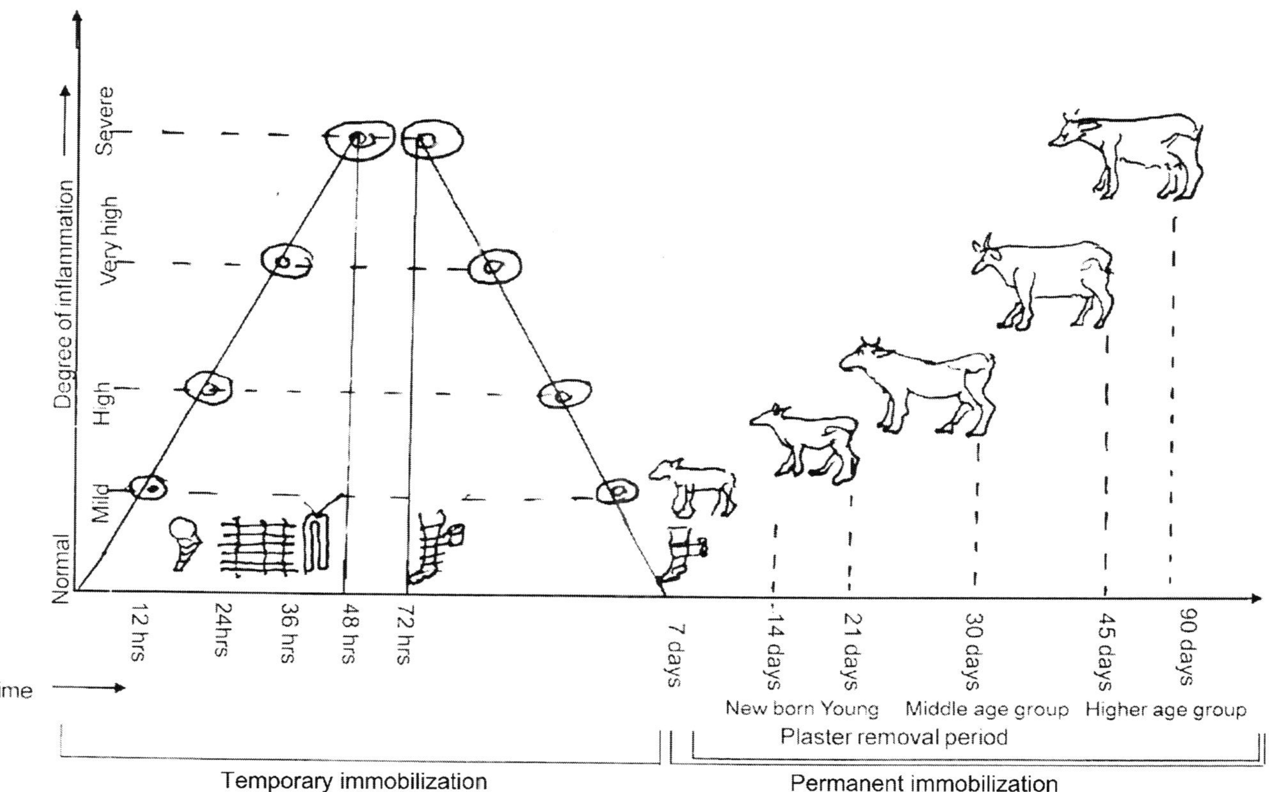

Fig. 1: Showing curve showing degree of inflammation and time of application of external immobilizing devices.

29

Bone Showing Various Level of Fracture and Their External Immobilisation Technique

Aim

To know the various level of fracture & their appropriate method of immobilisation for large animal fracture.

Definition

Fracture is a disolution of bony continuity with or without displacement of the fragments.

Level of fracture

1. Lower level of fracture.
2. Middle level of fracture.
3. Higher level of fracture.
4. Highest level of fracture.

Region

1. Below knee or below hock to foot.
2. Below elbow to knee or below stifle to hock.
3. Below shoulder to elbow or belov/ hip to stifle.
4. Above shoulder to joint and above hip joint.

Method of immobilization

1. Pop cast immobilization, conjoined 'U' plate
2. Pop cast immobiolization + Thomas splint.

3. Intramedullary pinning + Thomas splint.
4. No satisfactory treatment only velpeau - spling.

Sl.No.	Level of fracture	Region	Method of immobilization + conjoind 'U' plate
1.	Lower level	Below knee or belov/ hock to foot.	Pop cast immobilization.
2.	Middle level	Below elbow to knee or below stifle to hock.	Pop cast immobiolization + Thomas splint.
3.	Higher level	Below shoulder to elbow or below hip to stifle.	Intramedullary pinning + Thomas splint.
4.	Highest level	Above shoulder to joint and above hip joint.	No satisfactory treatment only velpeau - spling.

Table showing various level of fracture & appropriate method of external immobilisation

Various Level of Fracture With Their Appropriate Treatment

Definition : Fracture is a dissolution of bony continuity with or without displacement of the fragments.

Classification:- 1) Highest level fracture 3) Middle level fracture
2) Higher level fracture 4) Lower level fracture

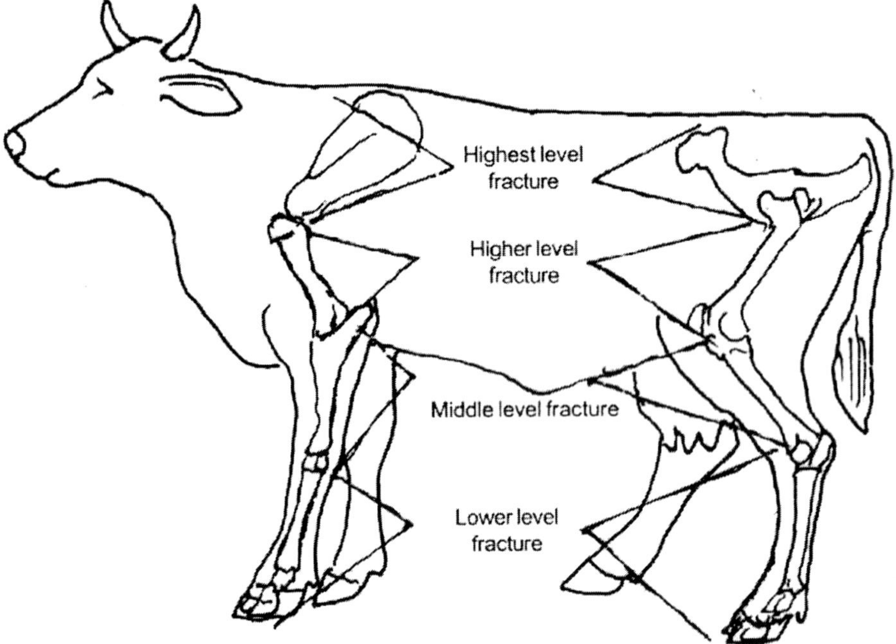

Fig. 1: Showing level of fractures in large animal.

Level of fracture	Region	Method of immobilization
1. Lower level fracture	Below knee or hock to feet	POP cast immobilization-conjoined 'U' plate
2. Middle level fracture	Below elbow to knee or Below stifle to hock	POP cast immobilization +Thomas splint
3. Higher level fracture	Below shoulder to elbow or below hip to stifle	Intramedullary pinning + Thomas splint
4. Highest level fracture	Above shoulder joint and and above hip joint	No satisfactory treatment, only modified velpeau sling

30

Fracture Immobilizing Bandages

Fig. 1: Cotton Bandage

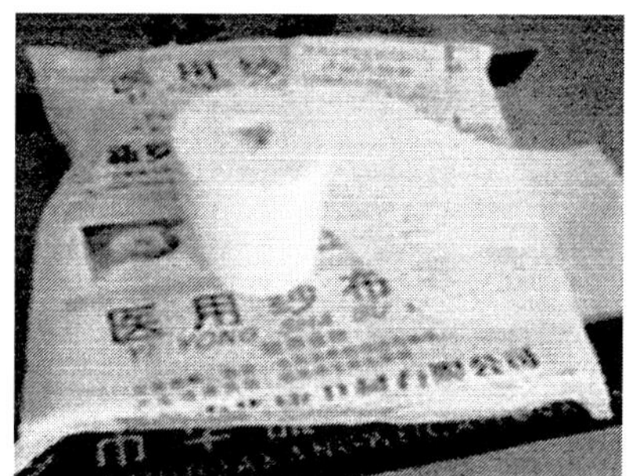

a. Plane Cotton Bandage

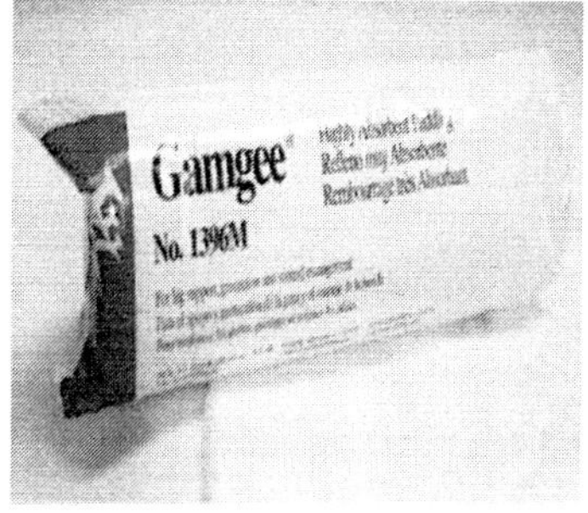

b. Gamgee Bandage

Fig. 2: Adhesive Tape Bandages

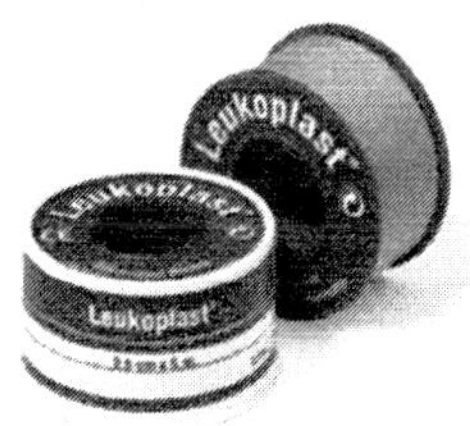

a. Leukoplast

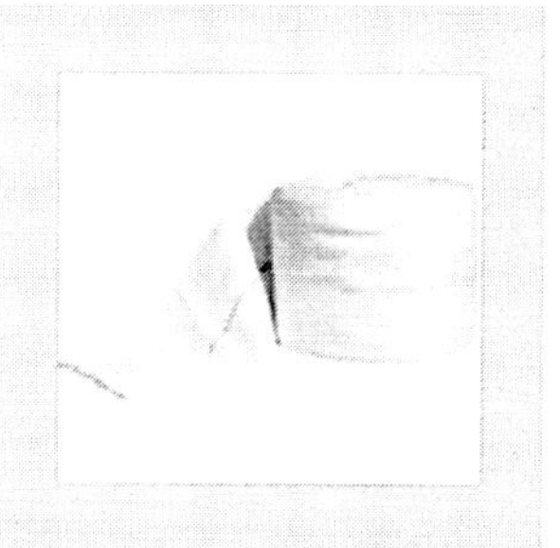

b. Micropore Tape

Fig. 3: Plaster Bandages

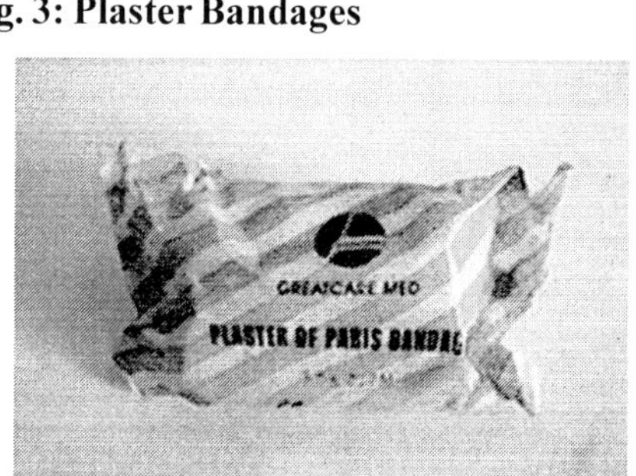

a. POP Bandages

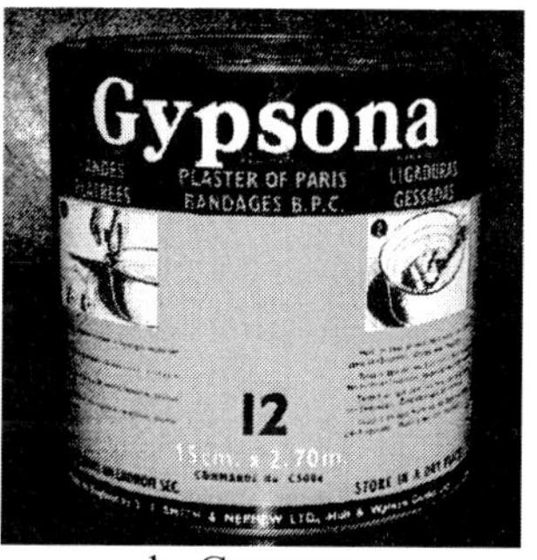

b. Gypsona

Fracture Immobilizing Bandages - II

Fig. 4: Cast Bandages

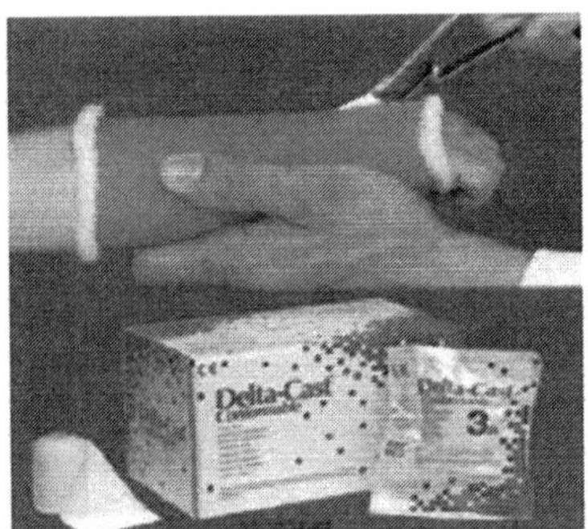

a. Fibre glass cast

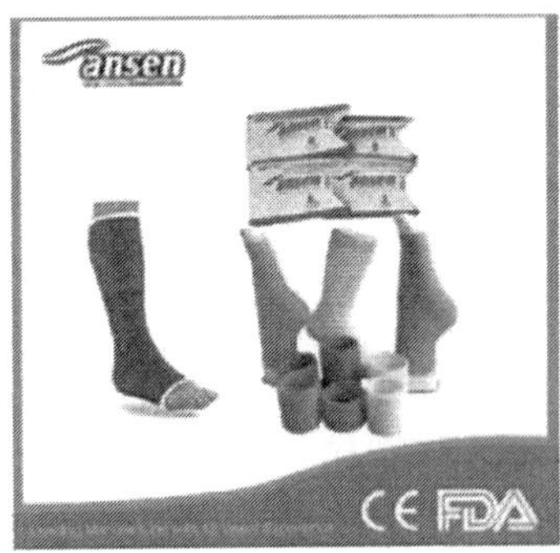

b. Polyester cast

Fig. 5: Fibre glass cast

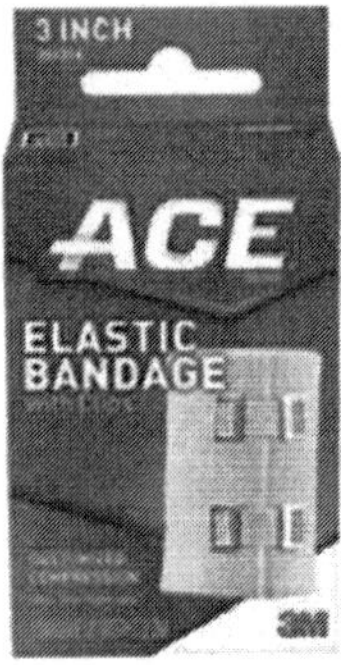

a. Elastic bandages

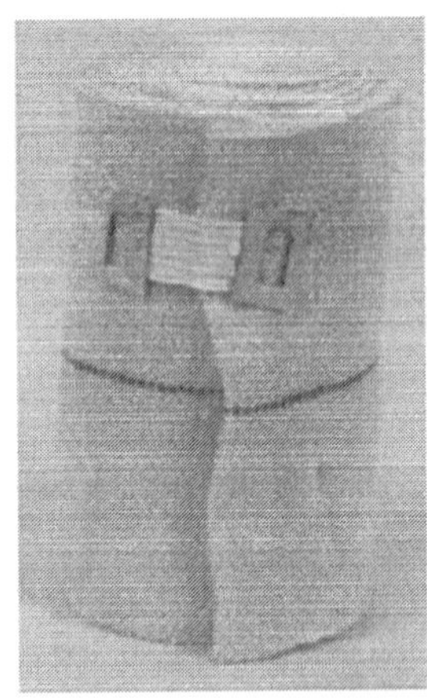

b. Crepe Bandage

Fig. 6: Robert-Jones Bandages

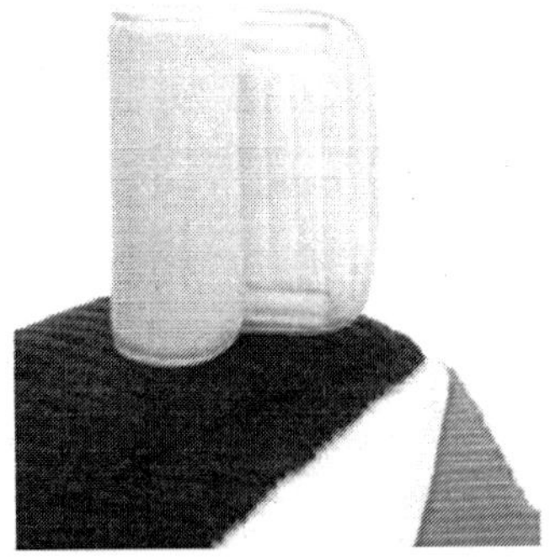

a. For Horse

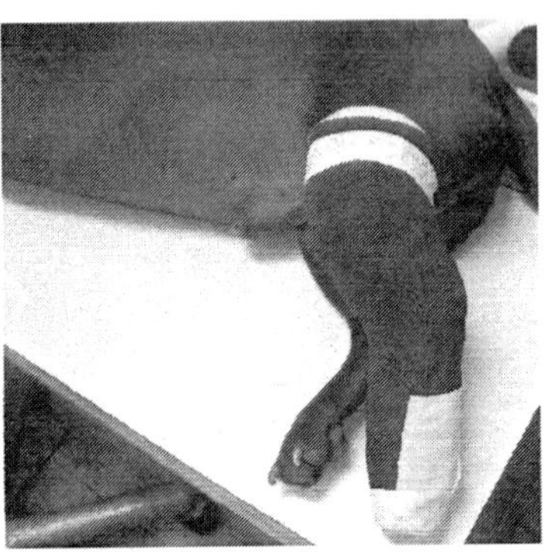

b. For Dog

31

Various External Immobilizer for Large Animal Fracture Repair

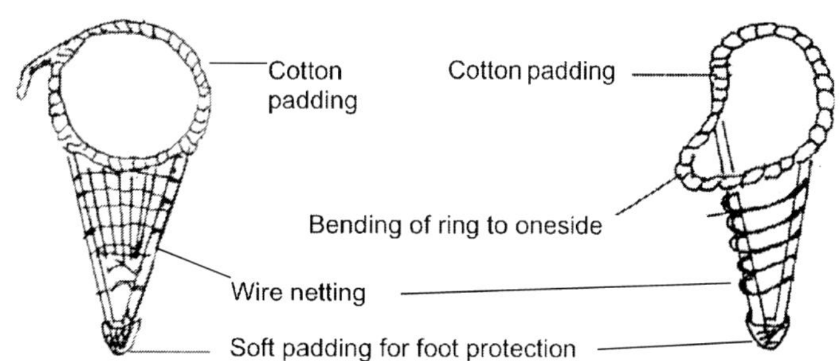

Fig. 1: (a) and (b) Modified Thomas splint.

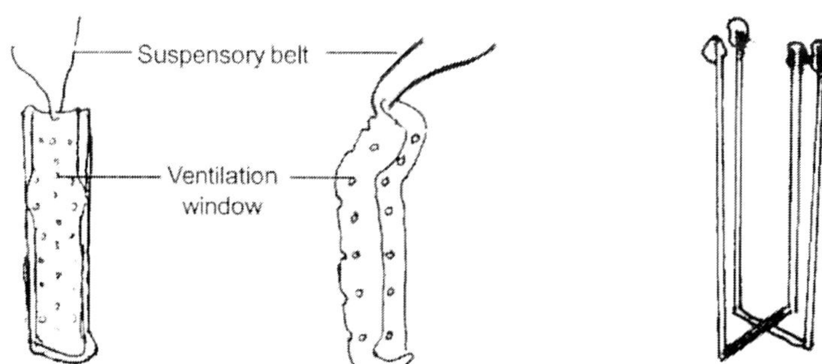

Fig. 2: (a) Caudal halfcast for forelimb

Fig. 2: (b) Caudal halfcast for hindlimb

Fig. 3: Metal conjoined U plate

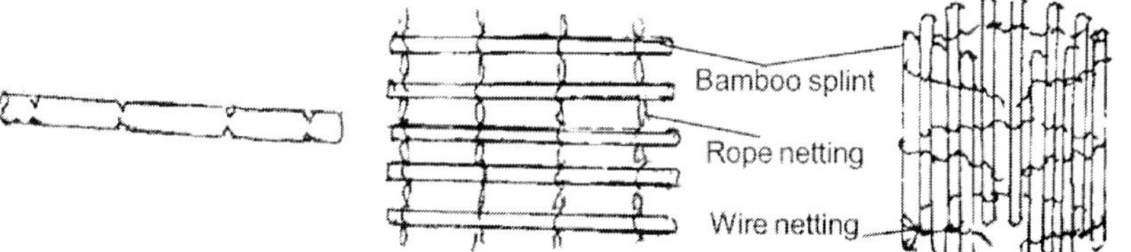

Fig. 4: (a) Bamboo

Fig. 5: (b) Rope netted

Fig. 6: (c) Wire netted

32

Immobilization of Fracture by Temporary Immobilizer

Indication: To know different types of immobilizer for large animal fracture management.

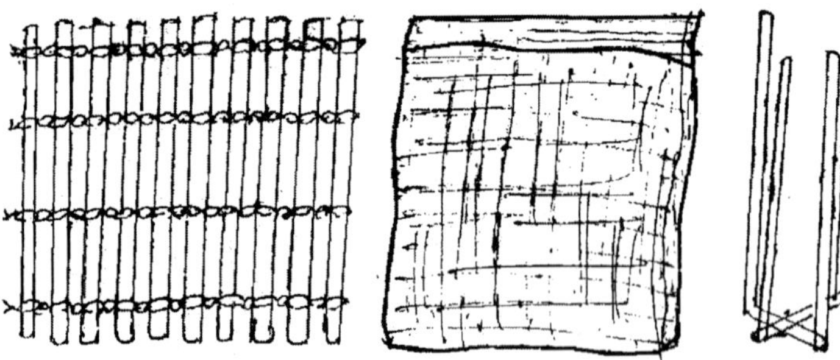

Fig. 1: Netted Bamboo splint

Fig. 2: 16-20 layer cloth padding

Fig. 3: Conjointed U-Plate

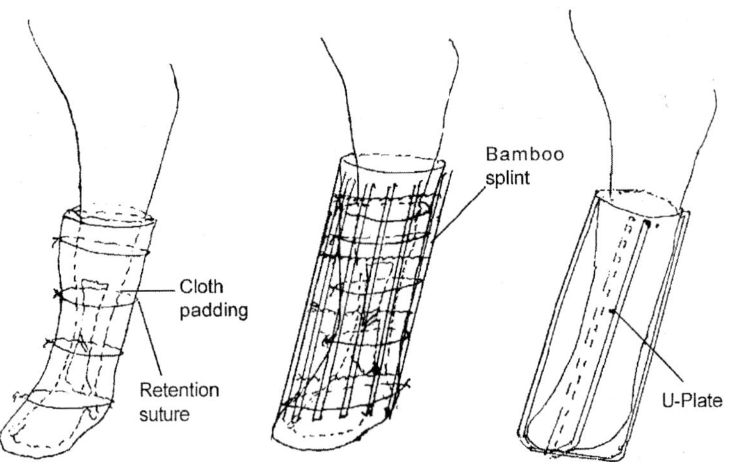

Fig. 4: Application of cloth padding over fracture site

Fig. 5: Application of bamboo splint over fracture site

Fig. 6: Application of conjoined U-Plate over fracture site

33

Pop Bandaging Technique

Indication -To know the method of POP bandaging technique.

Method of preparation of POP bandage rolls-

A gauze bandage of 6" or 4" width is spread on a clean floor. Plaster of paris powder is spread uniformly over the entire length of bandage & is folded into roll bandage. In this way 4-6 bandage rolls are prepared.fig-1(a)&(b)

Method of preparation of pop bandage splints

The length of the prepared pop splint is determined by measuring the entire length of fractured bone along with the joint below and above the fractured site) are measured. This much of length of gauze is spread for splint preparation.

POP powder is impregnated upon gauze. The gauze is again spread over this much of length in this manner sprinkling of POP powder & overlapping gauze bandage upto 4-6 layer are continued [fig-1 (b)]

Procedure of POP cast application

The fragments of bone at fractured site are organized systematically by traction and counter traction by external manipulation before application of POP cast.

The POP splints are placed by overlapping each other.2 POP splints for metacarpal/ metatarsal region & 4 POP splints for radius-ulna and tibio-fibula region are placed on anterior and posterior side along with medial and lateral side by overlapping each other. Fig-3(a) & 3(b).

POP splint rolls are dipped inside luke warm water before application of POP bandage wrapped in diagonal manner from fractured site going up and down several times till the thickness of POP cast reaches at 1 cm thick.Fig-2(b)

The cross-section of part along with the placement of POP splint over a small area and large area has been shown.Fig-3(a) & 3(b).

The wet POP cast is pressed and managed over the depression and prominence before it gets hardened tight.This is kept in position undisturbed half an hour till it becomes hard.

To strengthen the weak POP cast, green bamboo splints are generally placed at 4 side. Fig-4(b).

The cross-section of limb with POP cast bandage has been depicted.

Date of plaster and expected date of removal is noted over POP cast with a pen.

Foot should be covered to avoid hypostatic congestion.

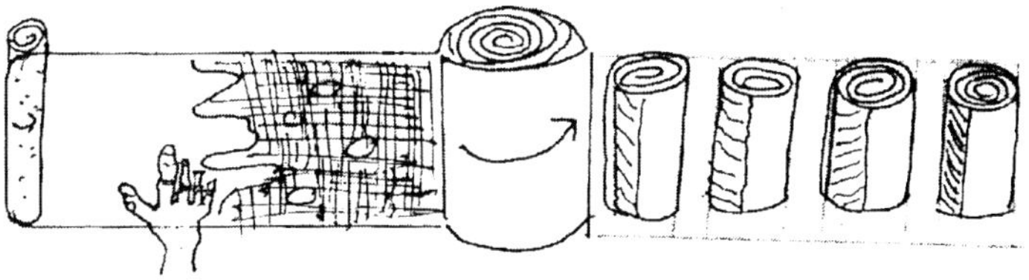

Fig. 1: (a) Pop bandage roll preparation

Four bandage roll

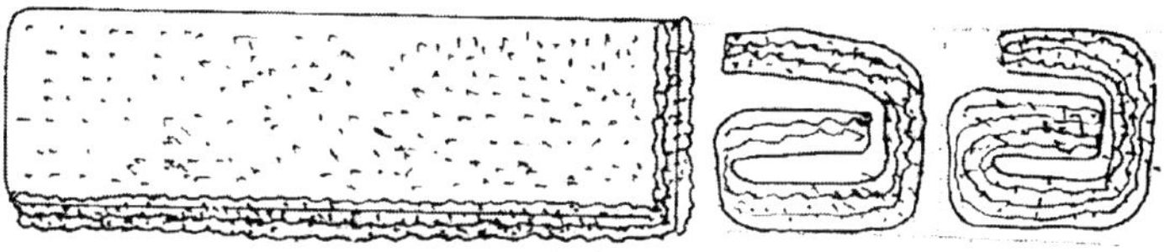

4 to 6 Layer bandage impregnated with POP powder.

Arrangement of POP splint (2-4 nos.)

Fig. 1: (b) Pop slint preparation

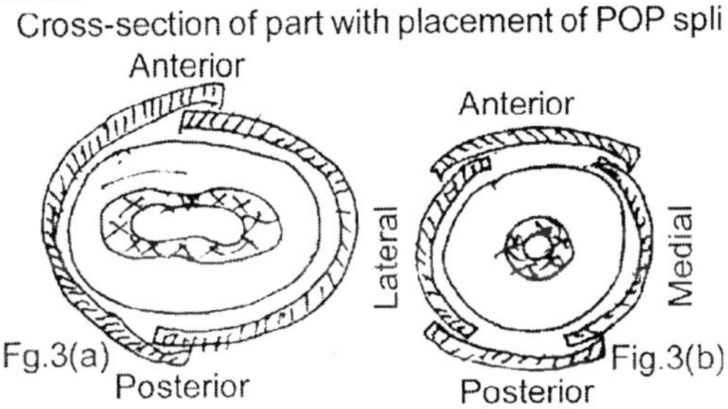

Cross-section of part with placement of POP spli

Anterior

Anterior

Lateral

Medial

Fg.3(a)

Posterior

Posterior

Fig.3(b)

Fig. 3: (a) Metacarpal/Metatarsal - 2splints

Fig. 3: (b) Radius ulna / tibia fibula-4 splints

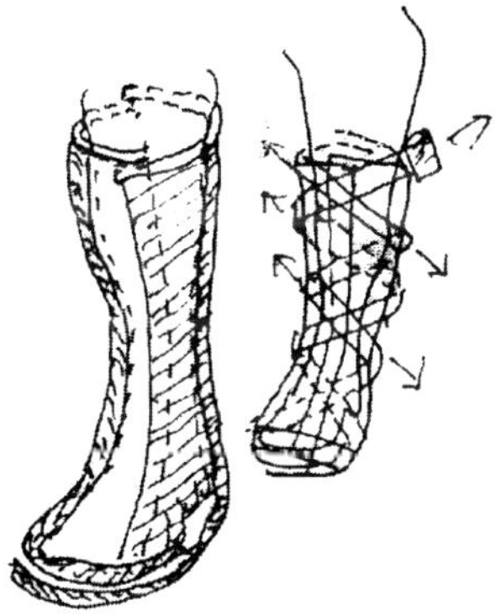

Fig. 2: Placement of POP splint over the fractured region at anterior & posterior surface

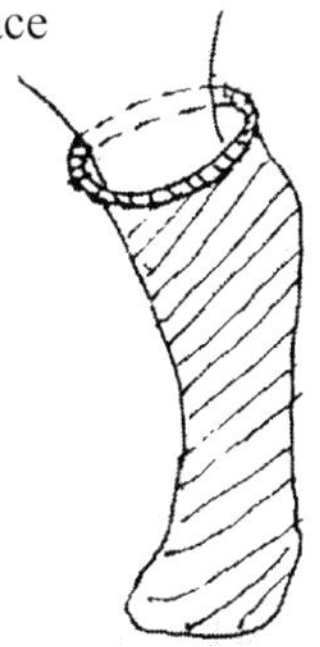

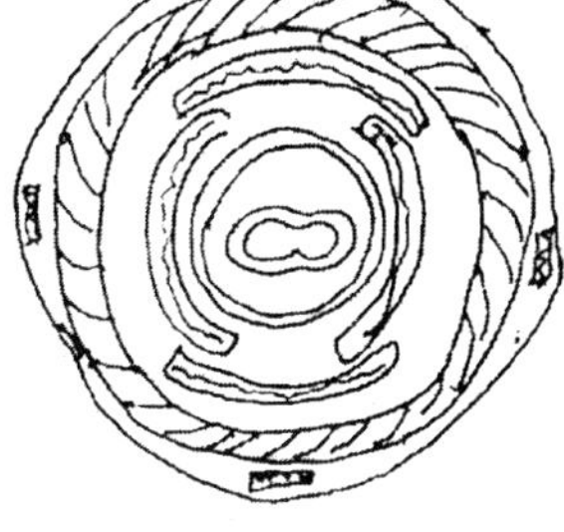

Fig. 4: (a) Complete POP bandage application upon limb

Fig. 4: (b) Cross section of POP application

34

Length to be Covered by P.O.P Cast for Immobilization of Fracture of Different Sites

Aim

To know the portion of limb to be covered by P.O.P cast bandage for immobilization of fore limb (Fig 1a) & hind limb (Fig 2a) bone fracture.

As per general rule, joint below and joint above should be covered.

Recommendation

Lower level fracture (Below knee / hock region fracture)

i. **Fore limb** : - Length to be covered by PoP cast → above knee & covering foot below (Fig 1b)

ii. **Hind limb** : - Length to be covered by POP cast → above hock & covering foot below (Fig 2b)

Middle level fracture (Radius ulna / tibia fibula fracture)

i. **Fore limb** : - Length to be covered by POP cast sufficiently above elbow joint to below knee joint (Fig 1c).

ii. **Hind limb** : - Length to be covered by POP cast → above stifle joint to below hock joint (Fig. 2c).

Length to be Covered by P.O.P Cast for Immobilization of Fracture of Different Sites

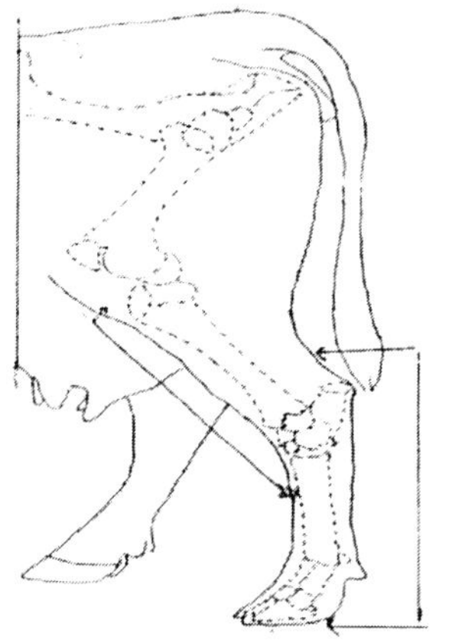

Fig. 1a: Length to be covered by POP Cast for immobilisation of Metatarsal and Tibio fibular fracture

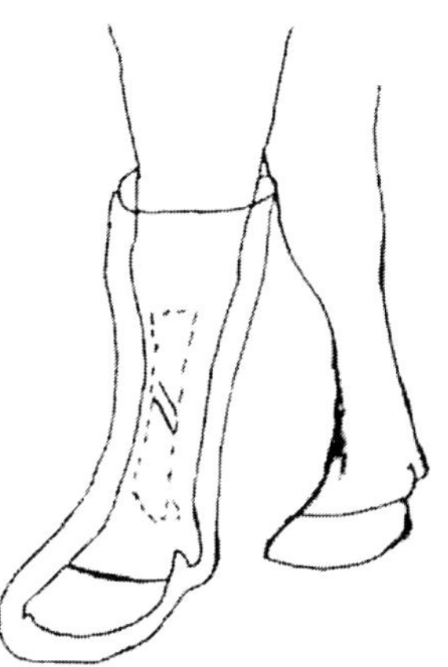

FIg. lb: Above Carpus to below foot

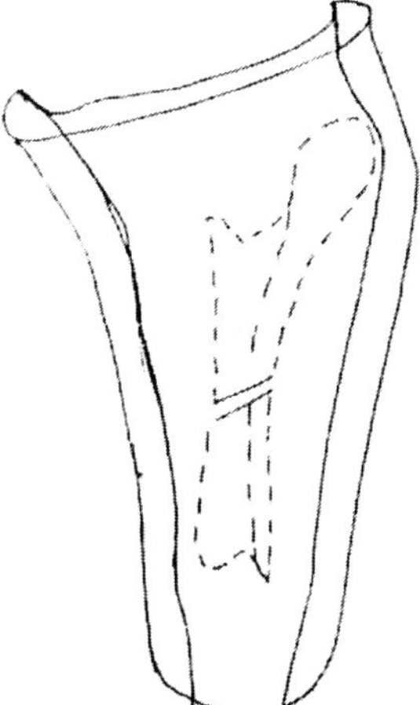

Fig.lc: Above elbow to below foot

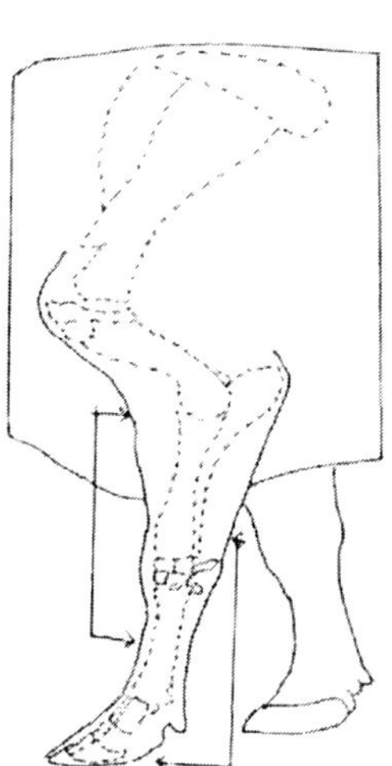

Fig.2a : Length to be covered for POP Cast for immobilisation of Metacarpal and Radius ulna fracture

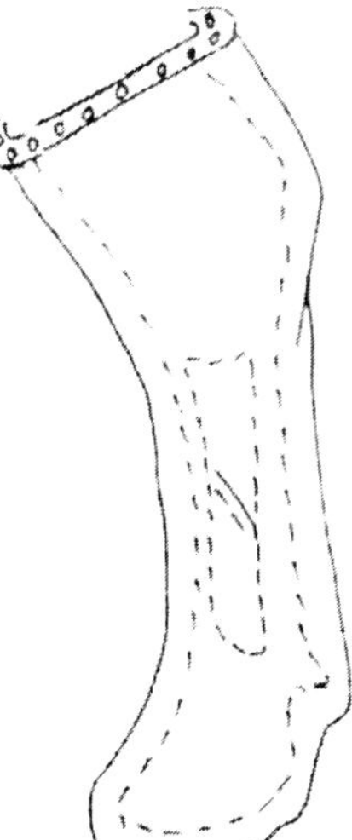

Fig. 2b: Above hock to below foot

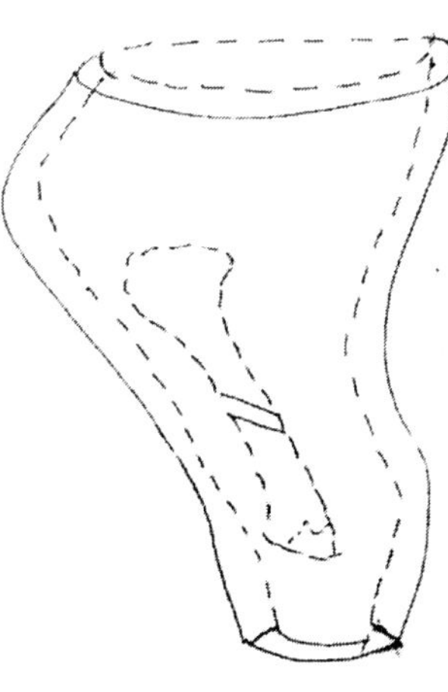

Fig. 2c: Above stifle to below hock

35

Reinforced Pop Cast with Padded Bamboo Splints

Objective

The poor quality of Plaster Of Paris makes the cast weak. For its strengthening, 4pieces of padded green bamboo splints are placed within POP cast along its four sides.

Requirements

4 green bamboo splints which are padded soft at both the ends

Procedure

1. POP cast is applied as per the usual procedure and kept in position for half an hour for hardening.
2. A poor quality POP powder makes a weak, easily fragile and wet bandage
3. In presence of weak POP cast, 4 green bamboo splints are taken which can cover the entire length of POP cast. (Fig. 1)
4. To avoid injury to skin, the green bamboo splints are softened with cotton padding placed at both endings and as well as at middle part. (Fig.2)
5. These 4 green bamboo splints are placed on 4sides of POP cast and again a bandage roll is wrapped over it. (Fig.3)

Post-operative Care

Soiling of the area is kept in check and POP cast is removed after 3-4 weeks.

Reinforced Pop Cast with Padded Bamboo Splints

AIM : Technique of strengthening POP bandage by application of four bamboo splints on anterior, posterior, lateral and medial sides.

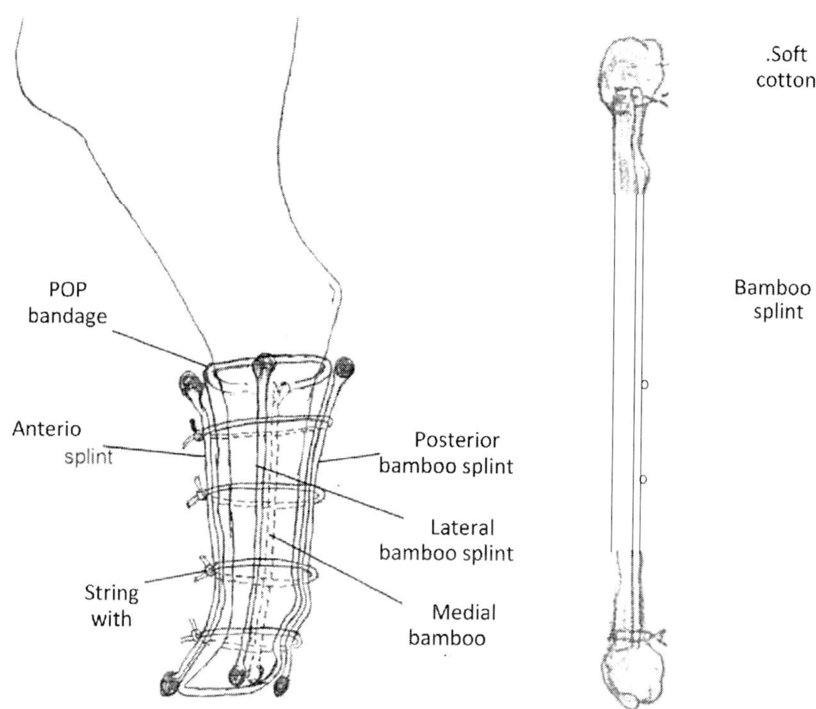

Fig. 1: Application of bamboo splint over POP bandage

Fig. 2: Bamboo splint with soft cotton

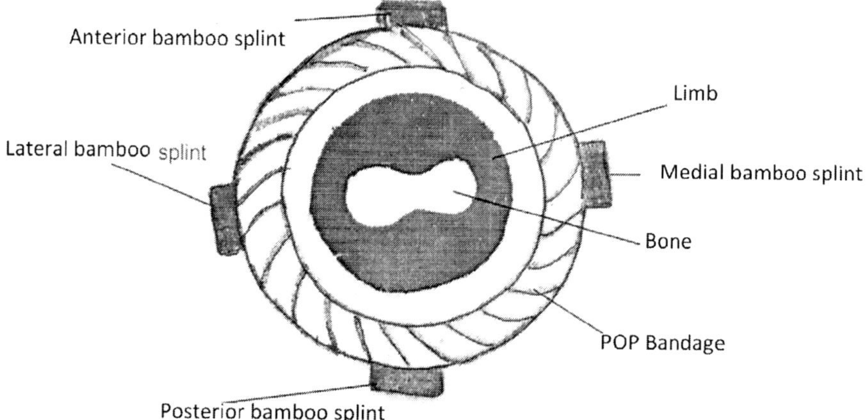

Fig. 3: Cross section of limb with POP bandage and bamboo splints

36

Pop Cast With Window for Compound Fracture

Definition

Compound fracture is a type of fracture in which a broken piece of bone protrudes to outside rupturing the skin with a risk of further infection.

Procedure of management

1. Clean and flush thoroughly the exposed bone using sterile NS followed by sterile medicated NS (NS with antibiotic or antiseptic). Figure (1)
2. Mop dry the wound thoroughly.
3. Apply topical antiseptic or antibiotic.
4. Put the bone inside the part.
5. With a sterile artery forcep fix a flushing catheter within the wound at its higher level. Figure (2)
6. Cover the wound over fracture site with sterile soft padded absorbent cotton padding. Figure (2)
7. The joint below and above of the fracture site covered with thick layered padded cloth before application of POP cast. Figure (3)
8. POP cast is wrapped as per the conventional procedure over the fracture site covering the joint below and above. Figure (4).

Post operative care

1. Infusion of local and topical antibiotic or antiseptic through flushing catheter for 5-7 days post operation.
2. After 7 days catheter should be pulled out.
3. Animal Is kept within restricted movement within limited space.
4. POP cast is removed after 3-4 weeks of immobilisation.

Pop Cast With Window for Compound Fracture

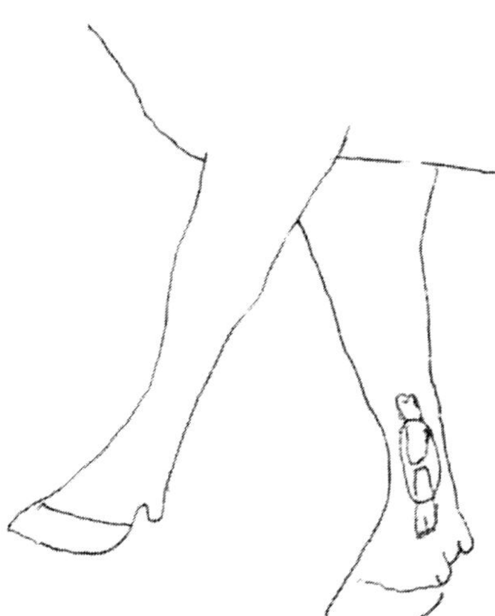

Fig. 1: Compund fracture

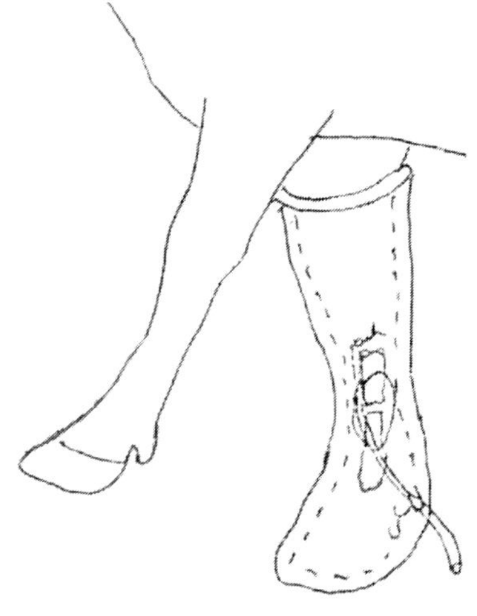

Fig. 2: Fixation of flushing catheter and higher level of wound and application of soft padded absorbent cotton padding

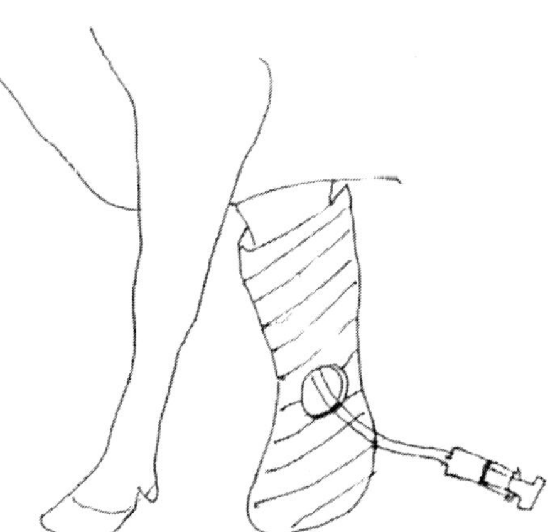

Fig. 3: Wrapping of thick padded cloth

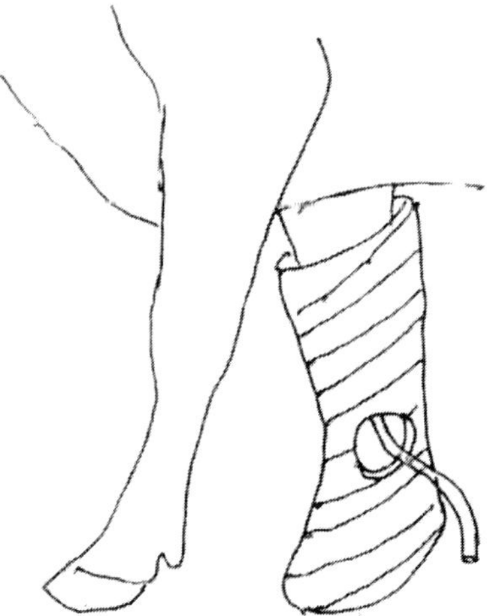

Fig. 4: POP cast with window for compound fracture

37*

Materials used for Immobilization of Fractured Limb with Gum Bandage

*Table starts from next page.

Aim: To prepare a list of materials used for ammobilisation for fractured limb with gum bandage.

Materials required

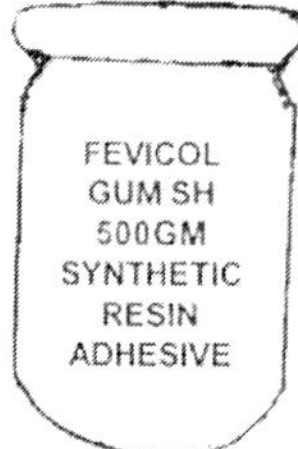

Fig. 1: Fevicol gum-500gm.

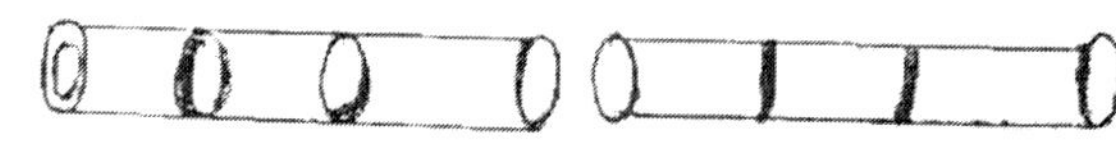

Fig. 2: Green Bamboo 4-1. **Fig. 3:** Dry bamboo 4-1

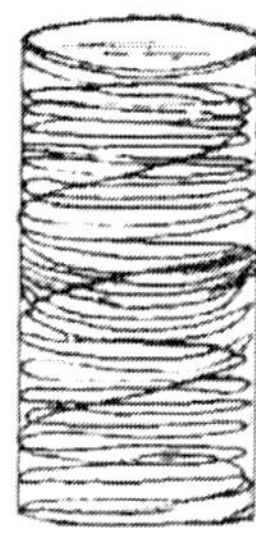

Fig. 4: Jute string 300-400 gm

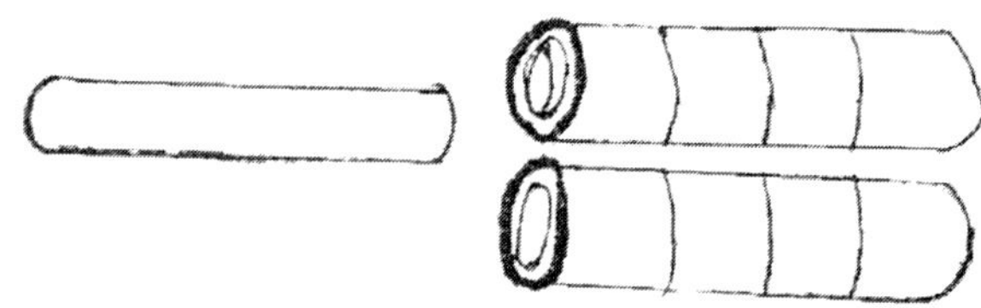

Fig. 5: Bucycle tube 2'-1 **Fig. 6:** Bandage 3-4 roll

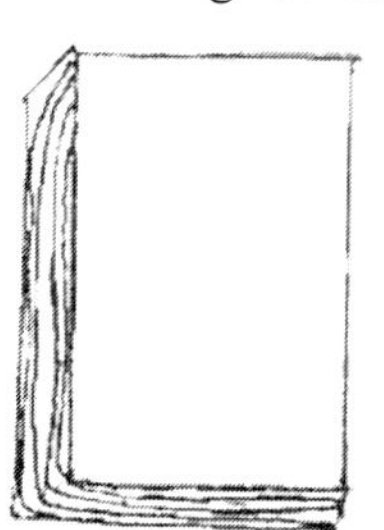

Fig. 7: 8-16 layer thick cloth

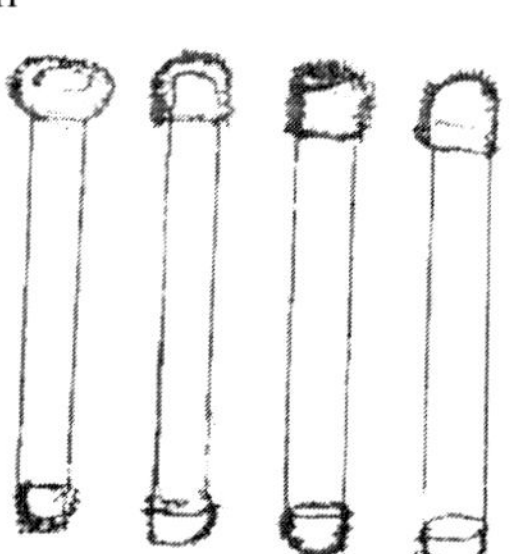

Fig. 8: Green bamboo splints -4

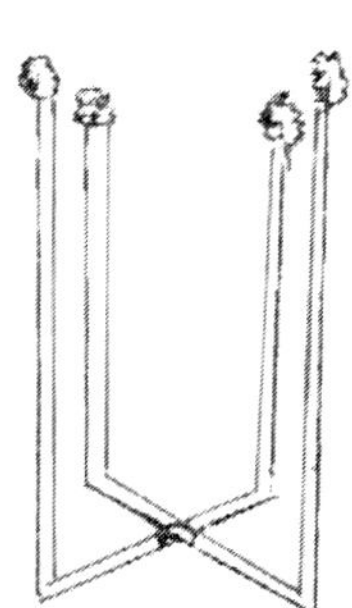

Fig. 9: Conjoined - U plate

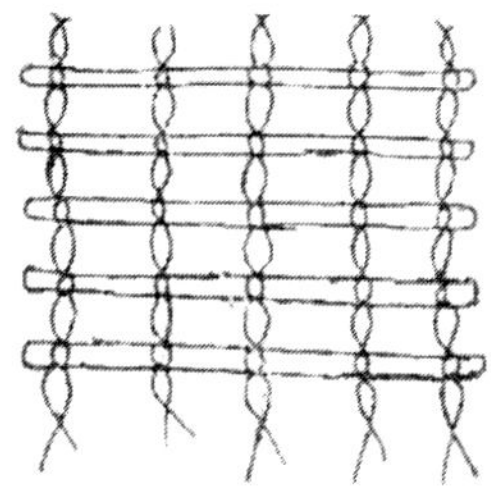

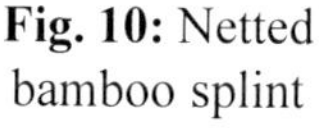

Fig. 10: Netted bamboo splint

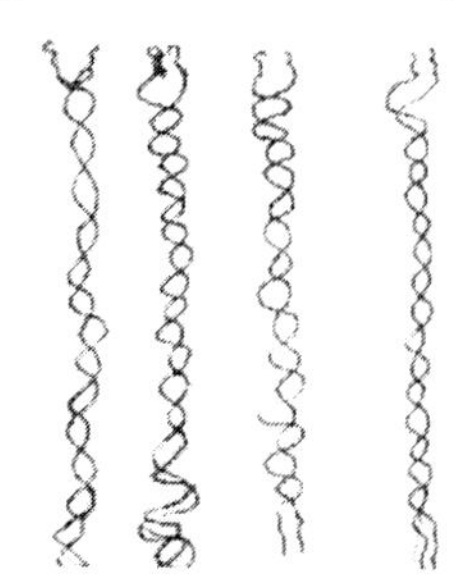

Fig. 12: Double braided jute thread-10

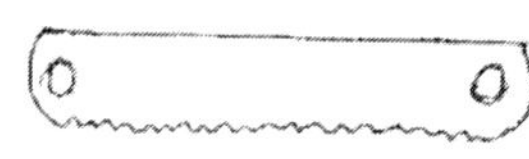

Fig. 11: Saw blade-2

38

Arrangement of 16 Layer Padded Cloth

Indication

Fracture in case of large animals, act as soft padding

Procedure

1. A single piece of long cotton cloth is taken which is separated into two equal halves on the middle line (Fig. 1).
2. One of the 2 parts is taken and folded to form a bilayer padded cloth (Fig 2)
3. The bilayer padded cloth to further folded to form 4 layer padded cloth and subsequently to S and 16 layer padded cloth (Fig. 3).
4. The 16 layer padded cloth is thus used around the fractured limb from the joint above to joint below.
5. The other half of the doth from Fig 1 is then separated into further 2 parts horizontally (Fig. 4)
6. The pieces thus formed are folded to form 2 layer, 4 layers and 8 layers Cloth paddings in order to cover the ends of netted bamboo splints longitudinally and retention Is done with ropes.

Use

Fevicol gum (adhesive) is applied over the fractured site and the 16 layer cloth is wrapped over it around one and half round on the limb including the joint.

Arrangement of 16 Layer Padded Cloth

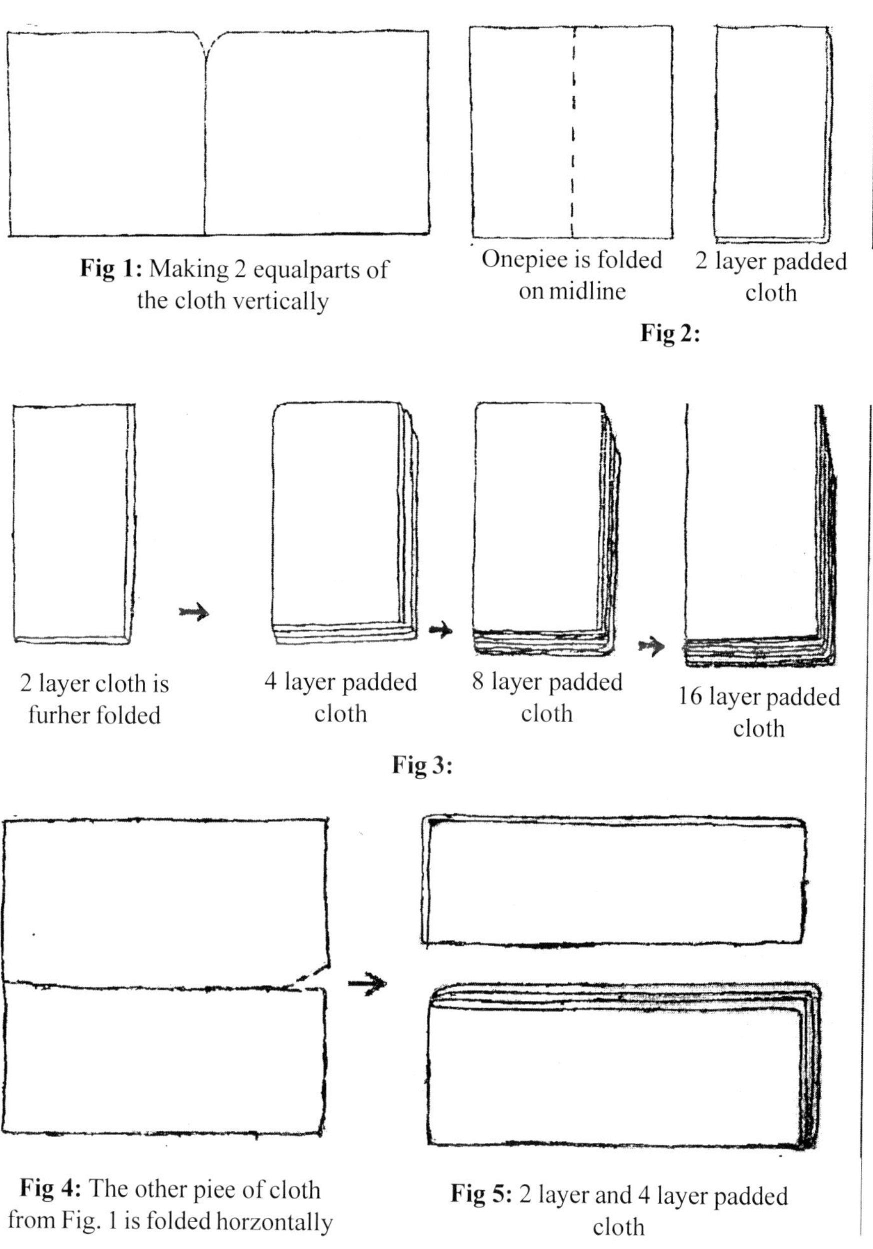

Fig 1: Making 2 equalparts of the cloth vertically

Fig 2:

Fig 3:

Fig 4: The other piee of cloth from Fig. 1 is folded horzontally

Fig 5: 2 layer and 4 layer padded cloth

39

Fabrication of Netted Padded Bamboo Splint

Procedure for Netted Padded Bamboo Splint

1) Marking of the bamboo splints is done maintaining equal distance (Fig.1).
2) At both the edges of the marking, grooving of the bamboo splints is done for perfect tieing of the plastic rope (Fig.2).
3) The bamboo splints are tied with the help of plastic rope maintaining 1 finger space between each bamboo splint (Fig.3).
4) Soft 8 layer padding of cotton is provided at both the ends of the netted bamboo splint in order to avoid injury (Fig.5).
5) The width of the netted padded bamboo splint should be upto one and half times of the limb's circumference (Fig.6).

Fabrication of Netted Padded Bamboo Splint

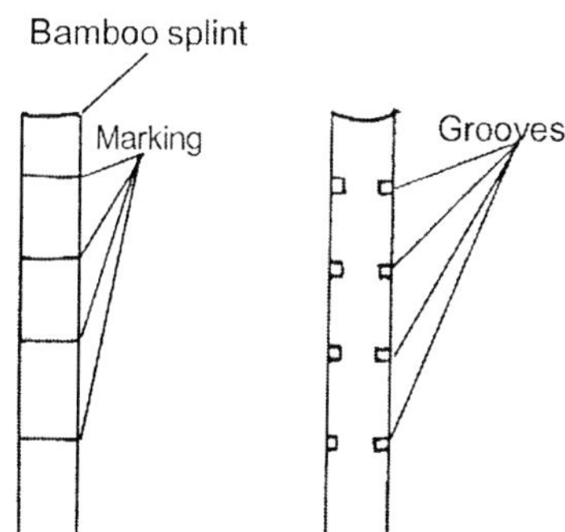

Fig 1: Marking of the bamboo splint

Fig 2: Grooving of the bamboo splint

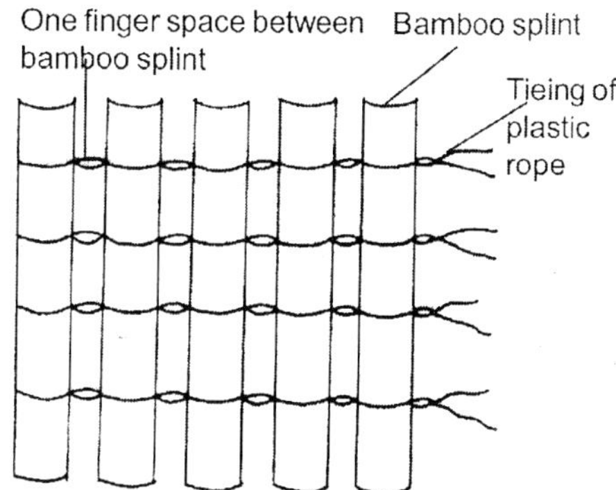

Fig 3: Procedure for netting the bamboo splint

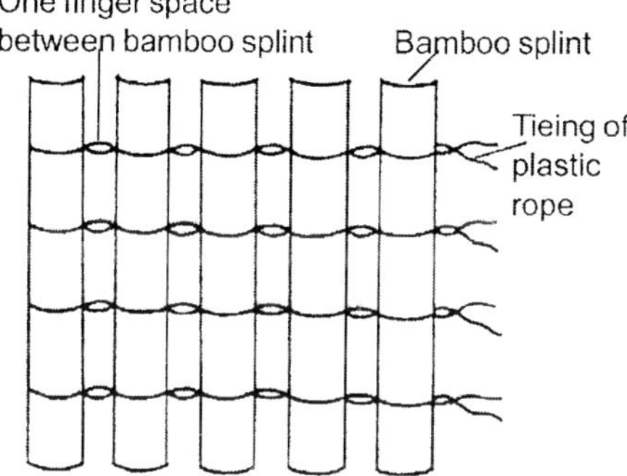

Fig 4: Netted bamboo splint (Complete)

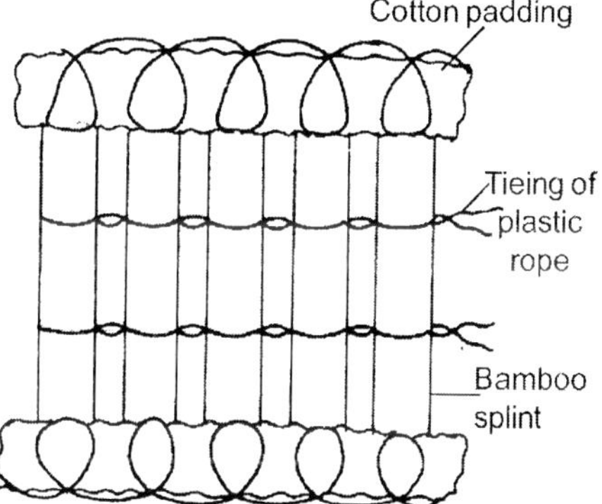

Fig. 5: Padding over the bamboo splint (to avoid injury)

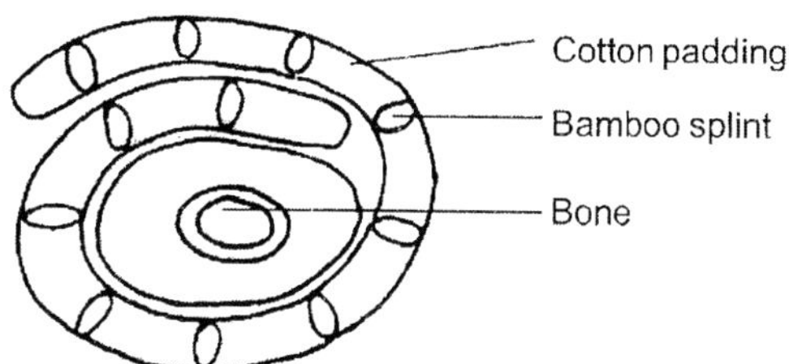

Fig 6: Width of netted padded bamboo splint ($1^1/_2$ rounding of bamboo splint over bone).

40

Fabrication of Single U-Plate and Conjoindu-Plate Using Green Bamboo, Cane, Bread Twiser and Iron Rod

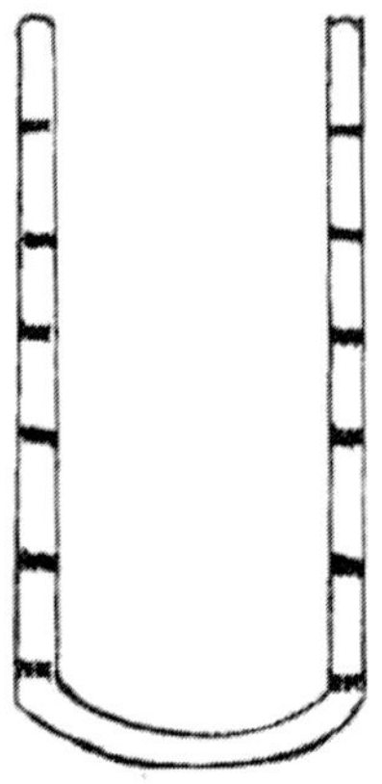

Fig. 1: U-Plate with green bamboo structure

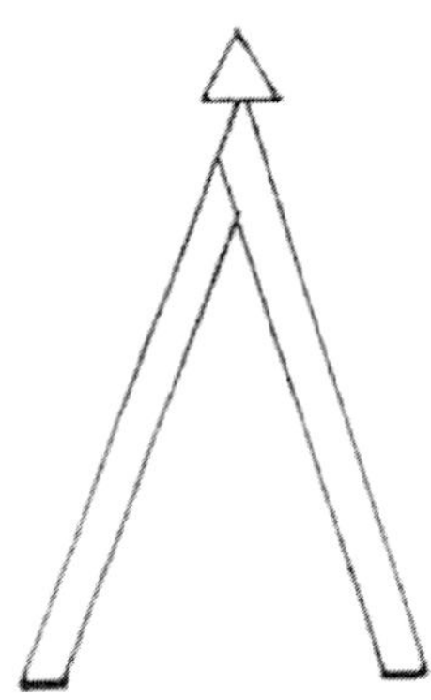

Fig. 2: Bread Twiser

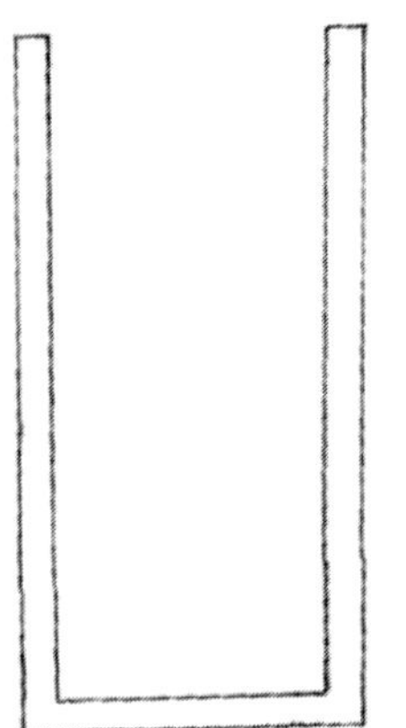

Fig. 3: U-Plate with bread twiser for fore-limb

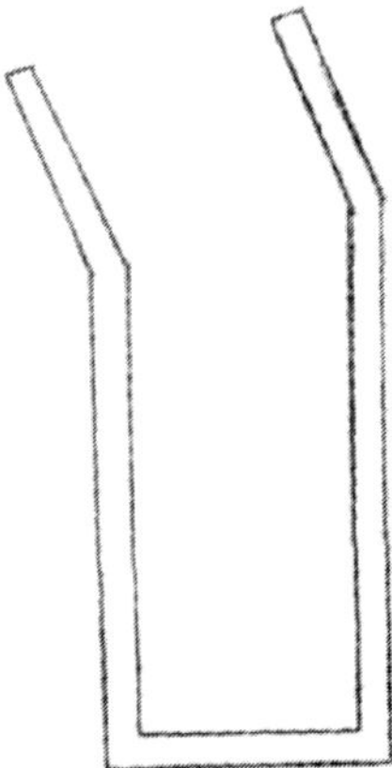

Fig. 4: U-Plate with bread twiser for hindlimb

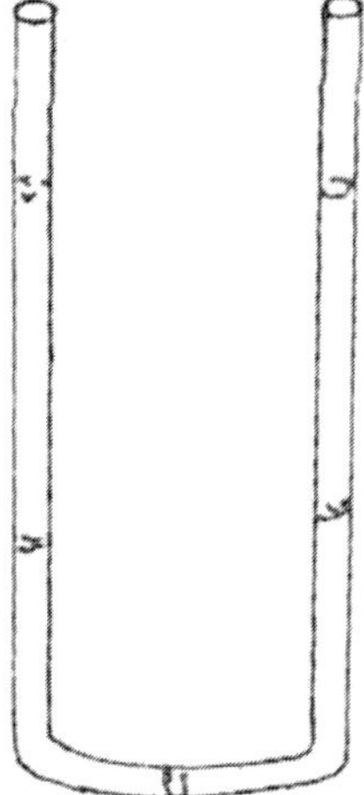

Fig. 5: U-Plate with cane

Fig. 6: Conjoint U-plate with metal of 6mm/ 8mm iron rod.

41*

Liberal Application of GUM over the Fracture Area for Immobilisation

*Table starts from next page.

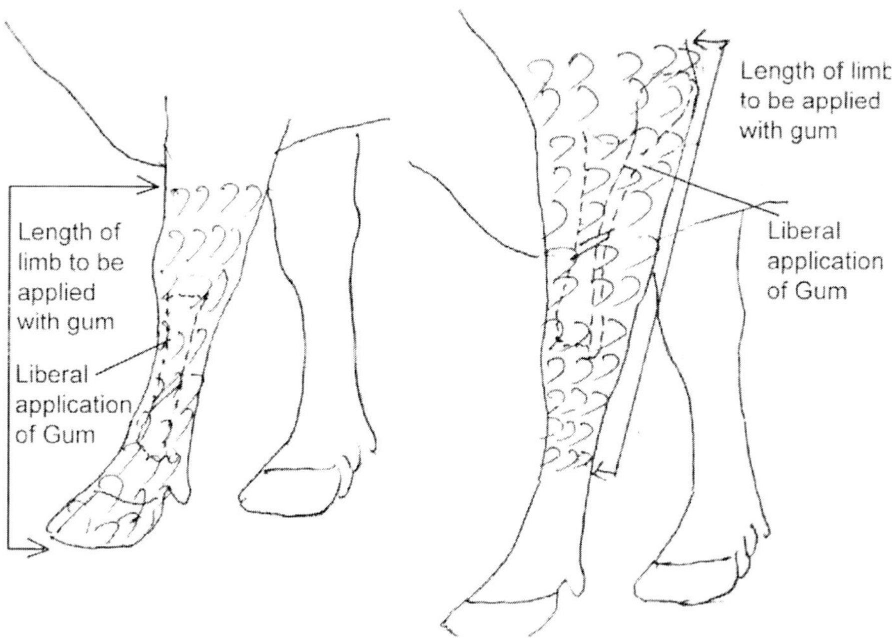

Fig. 1: Fracture of Metacarpus

Fig. 2: Fracture of Radius Ulna

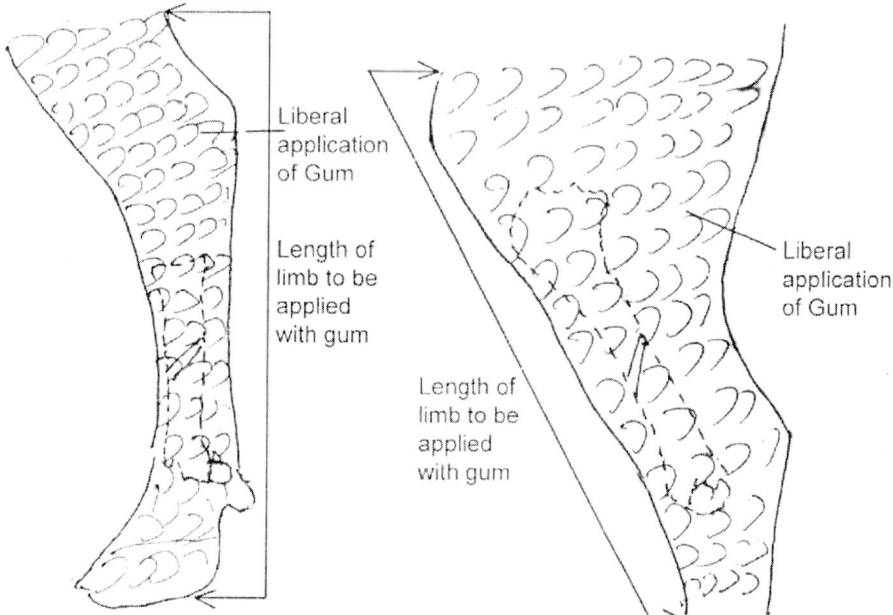

Fig. 3: Fracture of Metacarpus

Fig. 4: Fracture of Tibio Fibula

42

Application of Cotton Padded Cloth and its Retention for Immobilization of Fracture Site

Purpose-To now the technique of application of thick layer sterile absorbent protective cotton padding over fractured site and its retention with thread ligature in order to protect the bone from further damage

Site-Generally area joint above and joint below of fractured site of bone needs to be covered with a thick layer for perfect immobilization of fractured bone.

Procedure

1. The length of the limb to be covered with padded cloth is measured. Fig 1

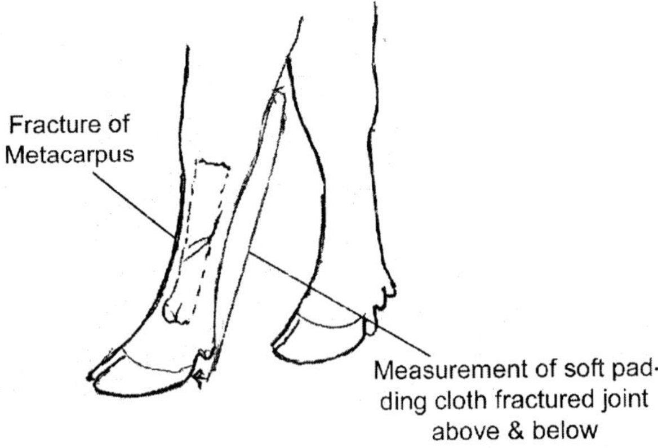

Fig. 1: Length of fractured limb to be covered with padding

2. A thick 16 layer of cloth is prepared by folding of a long cloth up to the measured length. Fig 2

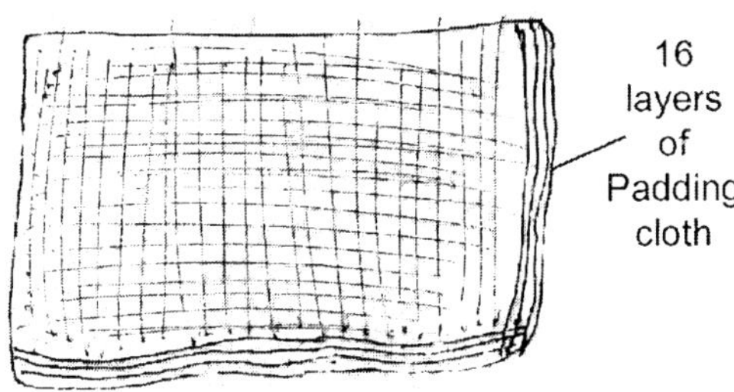

Fig 2: 16 Layer of thick sterile absorbent protective cotton padding

3. Addhessive gum is applied over the limb as well as upon the padded cloth.
4. The bone at the fractured site are brought to exact apposition and alignment by traction and counter traction.Fig 3
5. Fracture site is covered with thick padded cloth up to 2 layer thick. Padded cloth is placed at apposition by thread ligature at sites. Fig 4

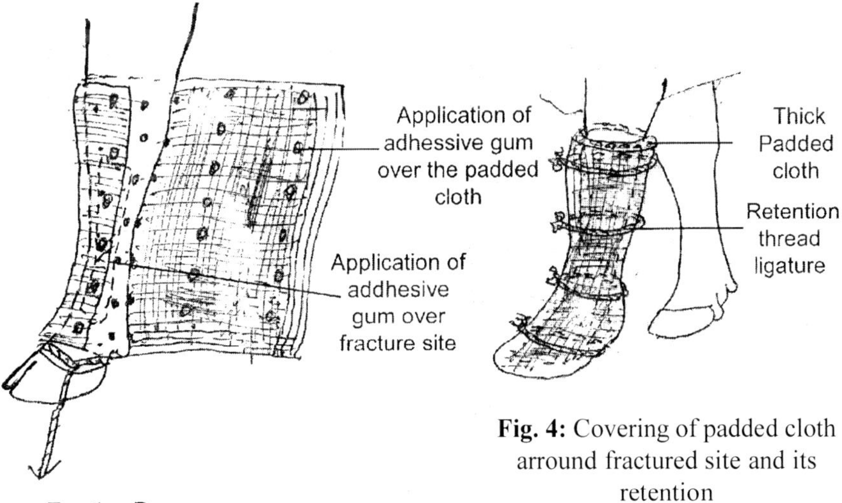

Fig. 3: Application of padded cloth over fractured site after application of traction

Fig. 4: Covering of padded cloth arround fractured site and its retention

43

Application of First Layer Padded Cloth & Its Retention with Thread

Aim: To know the technique of application of first layer padded cloth and its thread

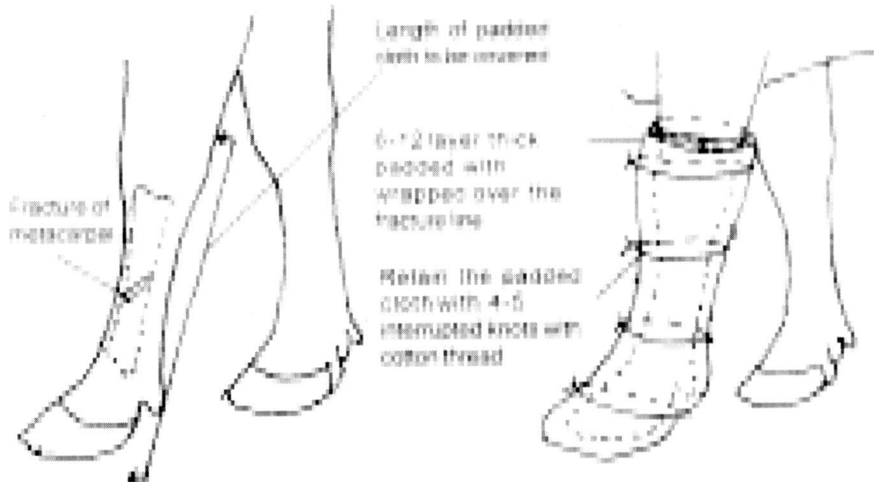

Fig. 1: (A) Simple fracture of metacarpal and length of padded cloth to apply

Fig. 1: (B) Wrapping with padded cloth and its retention

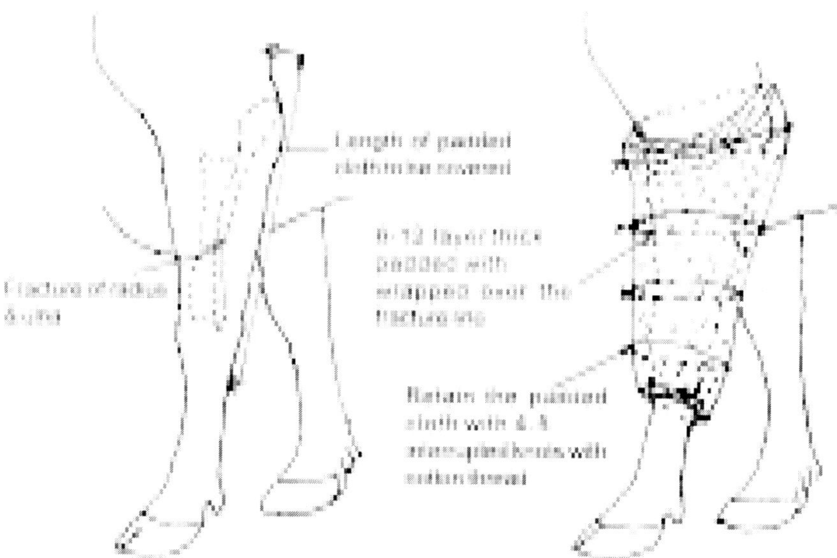

Fig. 2: (A) Simple fracture of radius and ulna & length of padded cloth to be applied

Fig. 2: (B) Wrapping with padded cloth and its retention

44

Liberal Application of Gum Over the 1st Layer Padded Cloth

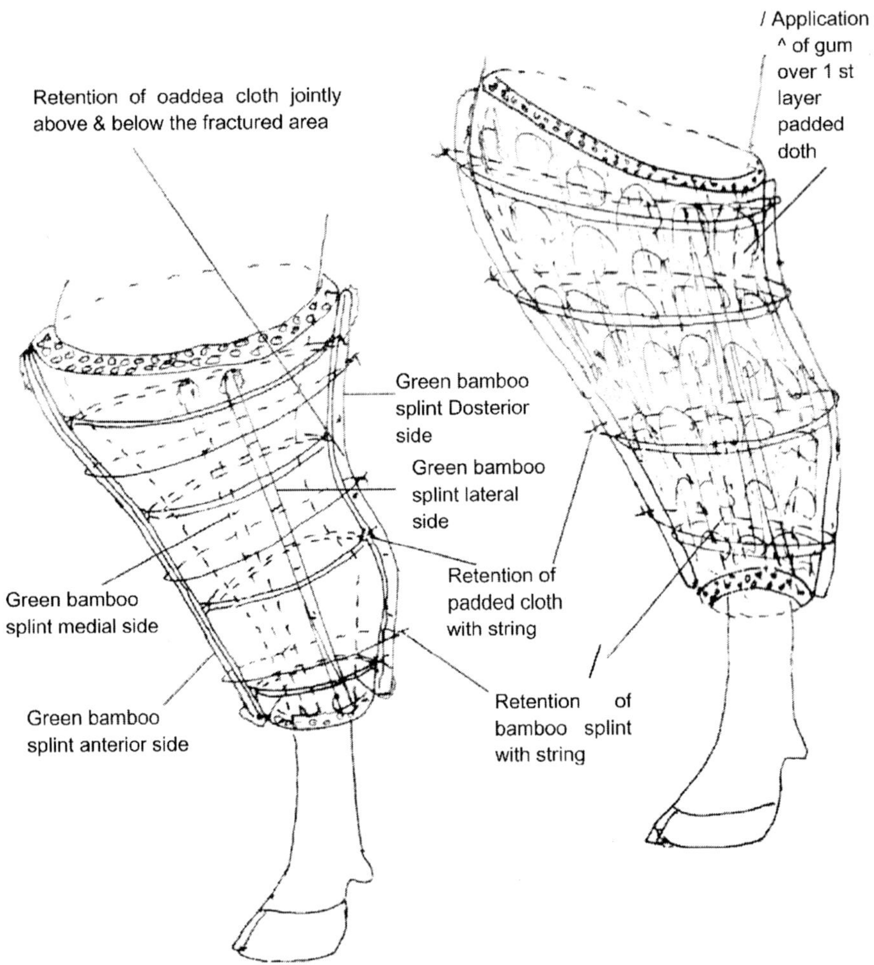

Fig. 1: 1st layer padded cloth over the tract ured area.

Fig. 2: Liberal application of gum over the 1st layer padded cloth

45

Reinforcement of Gum Bandage with Padded Netted Bamboo Splint

Purpose

To strengthen gum bandage in order to keep the fracture perfectly immobilized.

Materials required

Soft cotton padding, Adhesive gum, netted bamboo with soft padding, retention ligature.

Technique

1. The fracture limb is covered with padded cloth.
2. The padded cloth is kept in position using adhesive gum and retention ligatures (Fig. 2)
3. Netted bamboo splint is prepared and both the end of netted bamboo splint are soften using cotton padding (Fig.1).
4. Adhesive gum is applied over the netted padded bamboo splint at several places in order to fix the bamboo splint with bandage cloth perfectly. (Fig. 3)
5. The netted padded bamboo splint is covered over the previous gum bandage upto more than one and half-circle around the fracture site. (Fig. 3 & 3a)
6. The netted bamboo splint is tied with moderate pressure over the padded gum bandage with several double strand jute rope. (Fig. 4).

Post operative care

1. A course of parental antibiotic.
2. Pain relieving medicine for 3-5 days.

3. Animal kept in restricted movement.
4. Coaptation bandage is removed after 1 month.

Reinforcement of Gum Bandage with Padded Netted Bamboo Splint

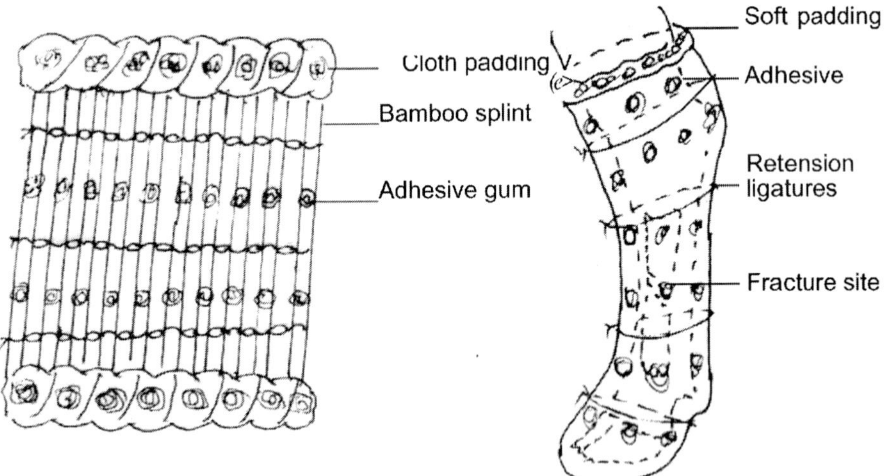

Fig. 1: Netted padded bamboo splint applied with adhesive gum at several places for coaptation.

Fig. 2: Protection of fracture site with soft bandage cotton padding with application of adhesive gum for strengthening with netted padded bamboo splint

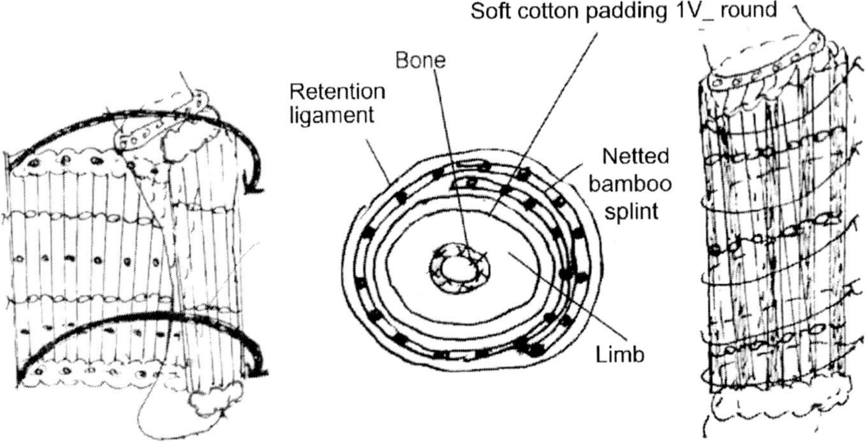

Fig. 3: Strengthening of fracture site with netted padded bamboo splint wrapping with soft padding.

Fig. 3: (a) Wrapping of netted padded bamboo splint over the fracture site one & half round.

Fig. 4: Final coaptation bandage,

46

Fixation of Protective Rubber Slipper Over Foot

CORPUS

1. Fixation of rubber slipper over the foot, after application of fracture, immobilising devices the foot is protected with rubber slipper to avoiding soiling and affection of foot (Fig. No-1).
2. The foot protection the protective rubber slipper is applied given to both their foot (Fig No.2).
3. Gum bandage, immobilised limb (Fig No.3).
4. As well as POP cost application (Fig No. 4).
5. The rubber could be given anterior to posterior derection to avoid entering of soiling towards the foot.
6. The slipper retain in position with due to splint.

Fixation of Protective Rubber Slipper Over Foot

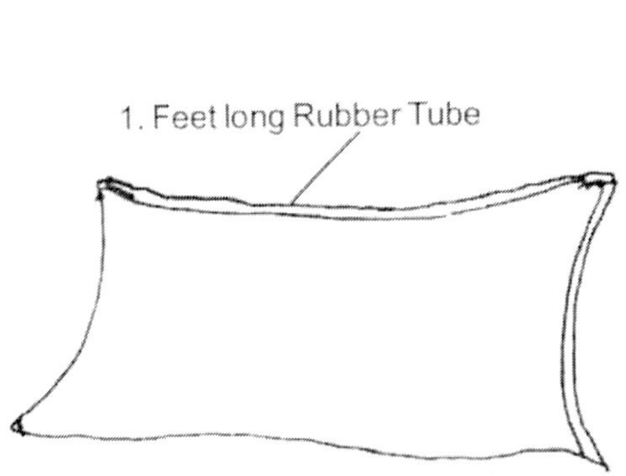

Fig. 1: Protective Rubber tube (1 Feet long cycle tube)

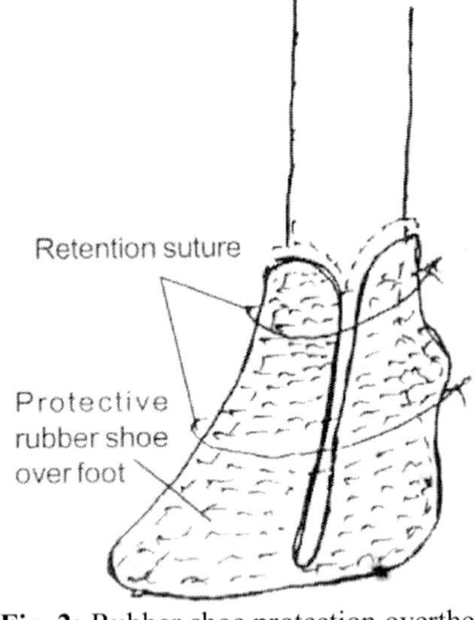

Fig. 2: Rubber shoe protection overthe foot before thomas splint fixation

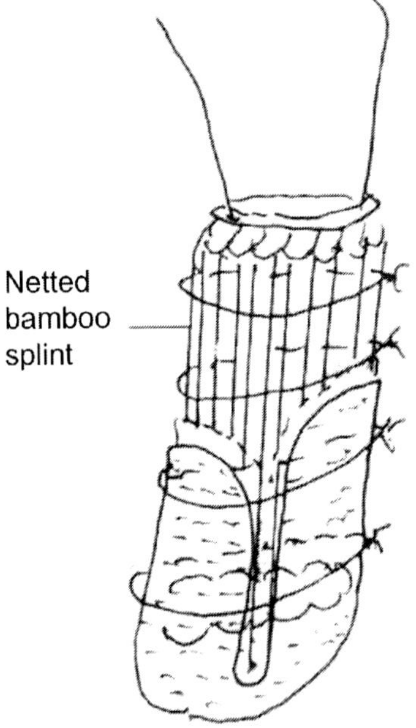

Fig. 3: Protective rubber shoe over netted bamboo splint

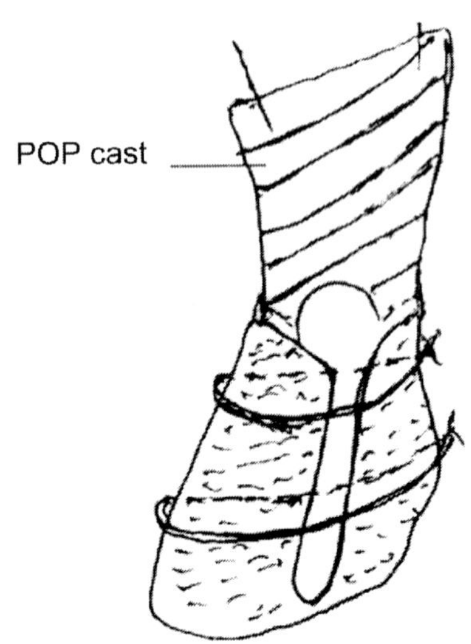

Fig. 4: Rubber shoe protection over POP cast immobilisation.

47

Classification of Fracture & Its Repair in Large Animal

Classification of fracture and its repair in large animal practice by external completion method.

Aim

To know the different level of fracture limbs. In order to access their method of repair (Fig.1).

Level 1 & fracture

The various levels of limb fracture of large animal has been classified in 4 different

levels.

1. Lower level fracture is generally fracture of the metacarpal and metatarsal bone and its lower level bones come under this level fracture. Cast immobilization from upper level of carpas of tarsal covering foot along with conjoint U-plate application are satisifactory method.
2. Middle level fracture suture of radius ulna, carpas and carpo-metacarpa joint is forelimb and fracture is tibio-fubula, tarses and dislocations of tarso metatarsal joint. Then comes under this type of fracture. Cast application sufficiently have and below these joints of these bone along with Thomas splint application are the most reliable method.
3. Higher level fracture and fracture of humerus and femur bone have been classified this group for which intramedullary pinning or Thomas splint has been advocated are the satisfactory treatment.

Highest level fracture

Fracture of scapula shoulder dislocation, fracture of pebic girdle and dislocation has been classified under this. A modification of response sling application with gum bandage along with rest has been satisfactory method of treatment.

Classification of Fracture & its Repair in Large Animal

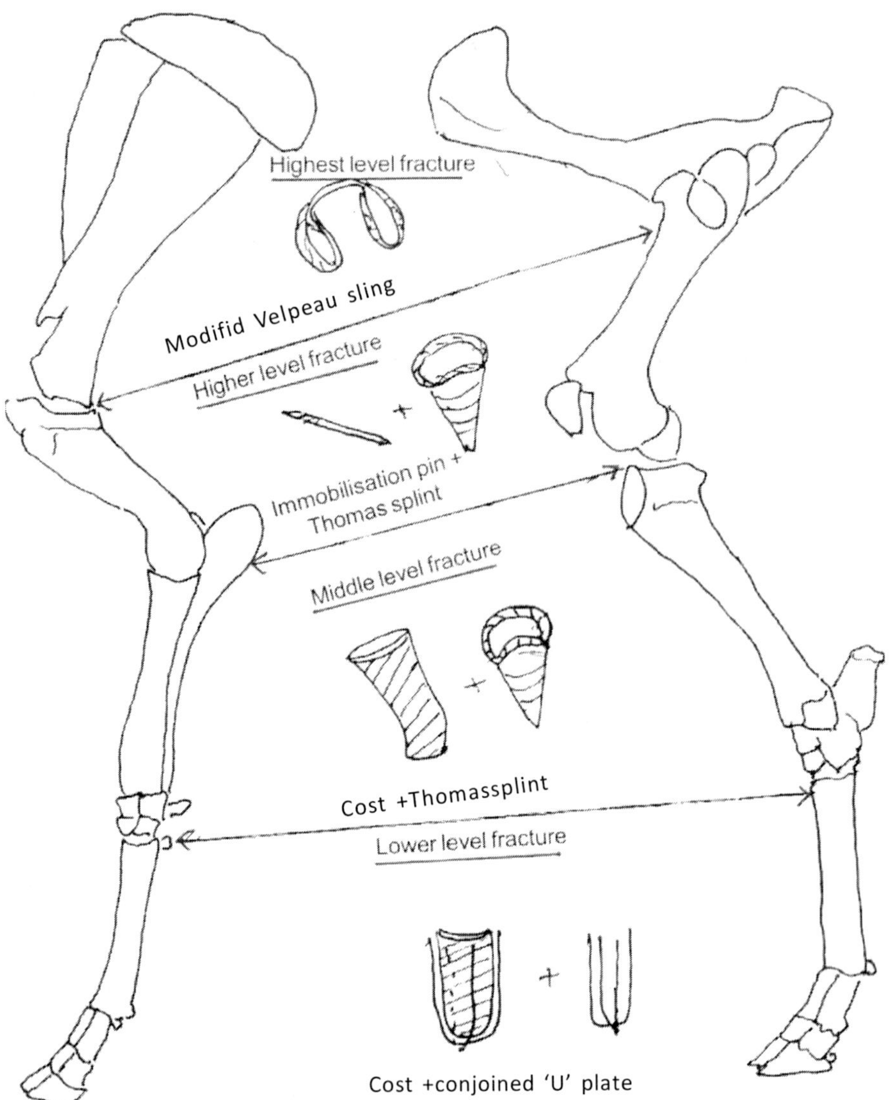

Fig. 1: Showing different levels of fracture and their appropriate method of treatment.

48

Lower Level Fracture and Its Repair

DEFINITION

Lower level fracture in animals include any fracture of the region from knee joint to foot in forelimb and from hock joint to foot in hind iimbs.

CFERA'nVE PROCEOURE-H ere the principle of treatmient is application of cast and conjoint metal 'U' plate over the fractured site. Permanent immobilization of the limb should be done only after 7 days to subside.

a) Length to be covered-Forelimb-above knee joint and below foot.

   Hind limb-above hock joint and below foot, (as shown in fig.1)

b) Padding-6-12 layer thick padded cloth should be vmapped applying gum.s throughout the doth area, over the fracture, it should not be too tight but it should be strong. Sloughing off the hoof may result due to hypostatic congestion; hence the hooves should not be left open. (Cotton pad as shown in fig.2)

c) Retention-The padded cloth should be retained with 4-5 interrupted knots with cotton thread.

d) Netted bamboo splint -After measuring the length to be covered, a netted bamboo splint should be made with the help of bamboo and rope which should cover the complete diameter of the fracture site along with overlapping(as given in fig 3).The netted bamboo splint is to be applied over the padded cloth at the fracture site .

e) Conjoint metal U plate-TA^o 6mm iron rods should be taken measuring the length of the limb respectively. The metal rods should be bent to form 2 separate U plates (accordingly given in fig.4).A rubber tube should be kept at the distal end below hoof before application of the metal U plate.

POST OPERATIVE CARE

1) Advice to the owner to give an incision on the bandage if the animal shows any signs of discomfort.

2) Anti-inflammatory injection to be administered to the patient for minimum 3 days.

3) Complete rest and provision of soft bedding to the patient.

4) Removal of the plaster after 15 days in calves ;21 days in young animals,30 days in middle age groups and 45 days for higher age groups.

Lower Level Fracture and its Repair

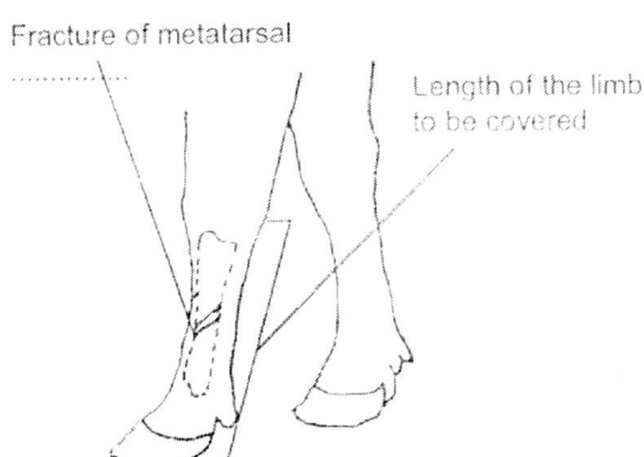

Fig. 1: Length of limb to be coverd

Fig. 2: Thick cotton pad (16 layer)

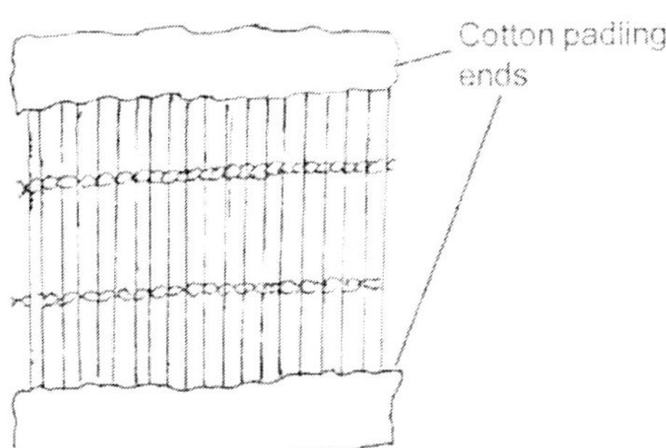

Fig. 3 Netted bamboo splint

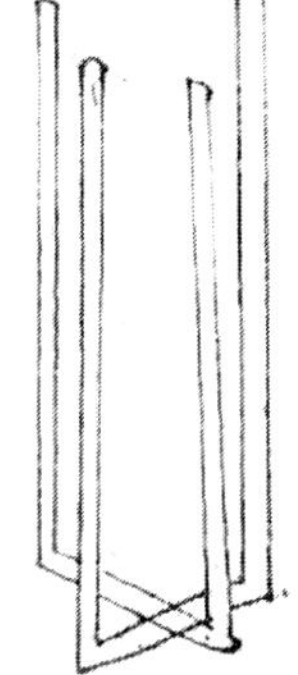

Fig. 4: Conjoint metal U plate

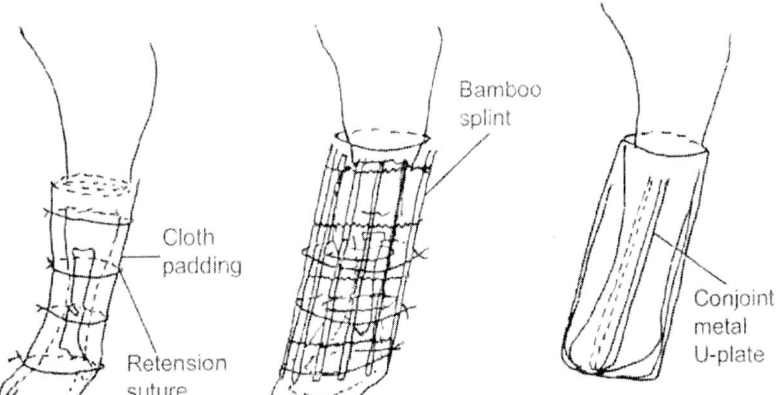

Fig. 5: Retention of cotton pad

Fig. 6: Bamboo splint application

Fig. 7: Conjoint metal U plae application

Immobilization of Metacarpus Compound Fracture Using Netted Bamboo Spilint and Conjoint Angular Metalic Splint (CAMS)

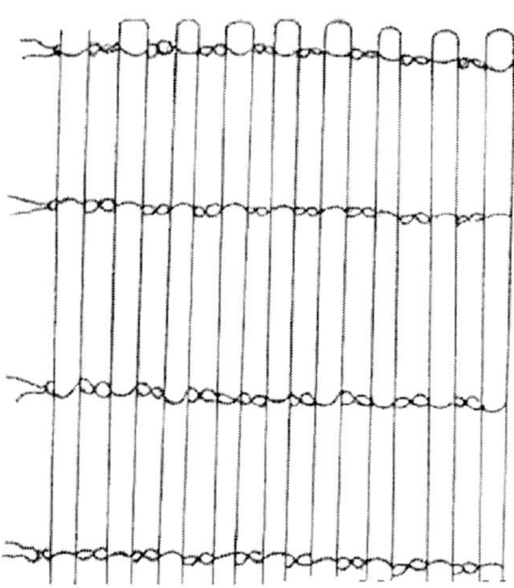

Fig. 1: Netted bamboo splint

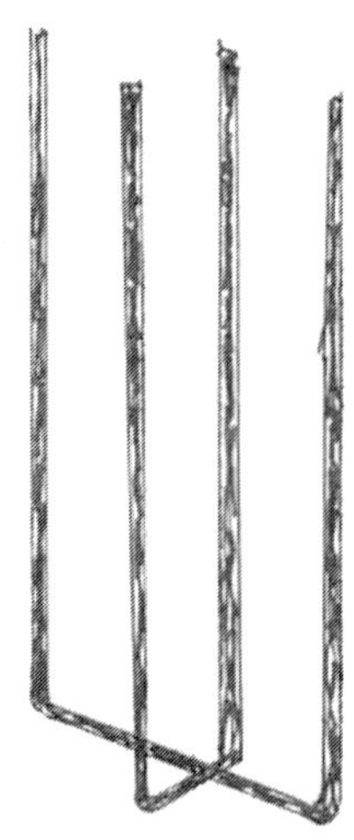

Fig. 2: Conjoint angular metalic splint

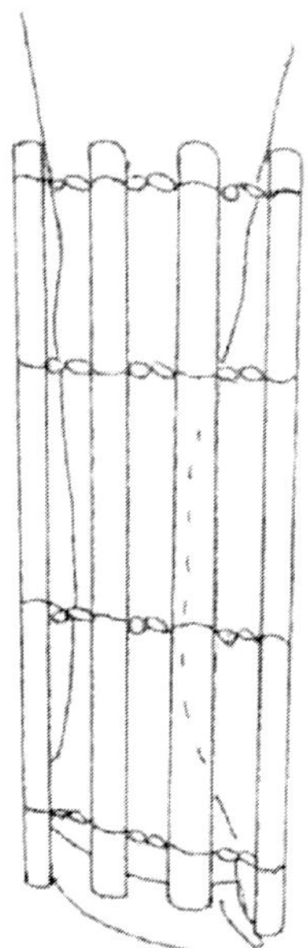

Fig. 3: Netted bamboo splint application upon metacarpus compound fracture

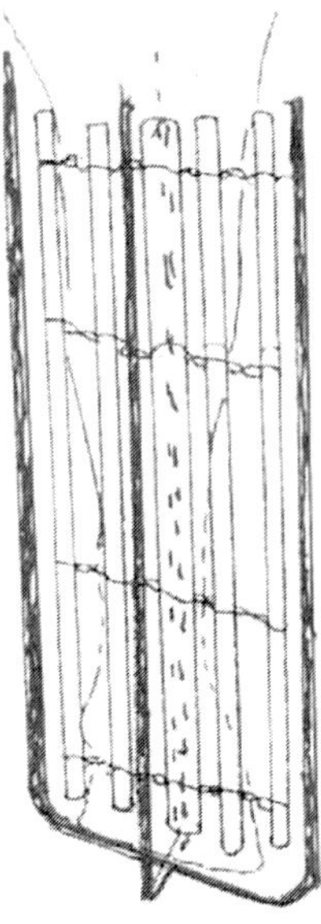

Fig. 4: Complete immobilization of metacarpus compound fracture

Reference: Behera, S.S. (2013). Thesis submitted to Odisha University of Agriculture and Technology.

"Don't ampute my limb for compound fracture"- Animal

49

Treatment of Lower Level Fracture (HINDLIMB)

Aim

To know the immobilization technique for fractured metatarsus.

The fractured metatarsus comes under lower level fracture whose immobilisation is cast as well as conjoined U-Plate application. (Fig. 1).

Requirements

1) Thick padded cloth (Fig. 2(a)
2) Padded netted bamboo splint (Fig. 2(b)
3) Conjoined U plate (Fig. 2(c)

Procedure

1) The bone of fracture site is corrected by traction and counter traction.
2) Thick padded cloth of joint below and joint above length is covered around the fractured site and retained in position with string (Fig. 3).
3) Padded netted bamboo splint applied with gum adhesive is covered over the thick cotton padding cover and retain in position with thread (Fig. 4).
4) After that rubber slipper covered over the foot.
5) Finally the conjoined U plate is fixed over the entire coamputation bandage (Fig. 5).

Reference: Amaresh Kumar, (2004). Veterinary Surgical Techniques. Vikash Publishing House, New Delhi. PR 368-371.

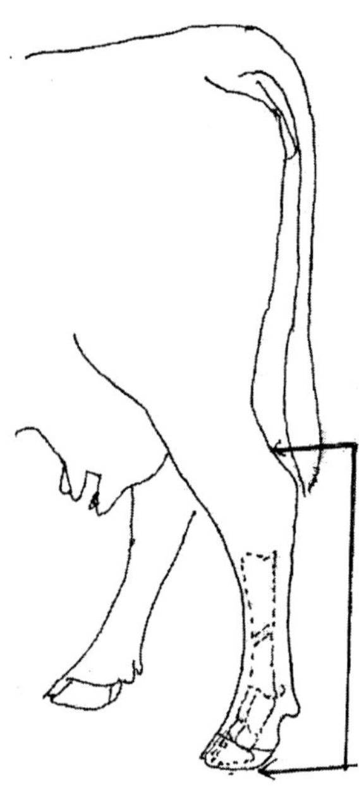

Fig. 1: Length of hte limb at the fracture site to be covered with coamputational bandage

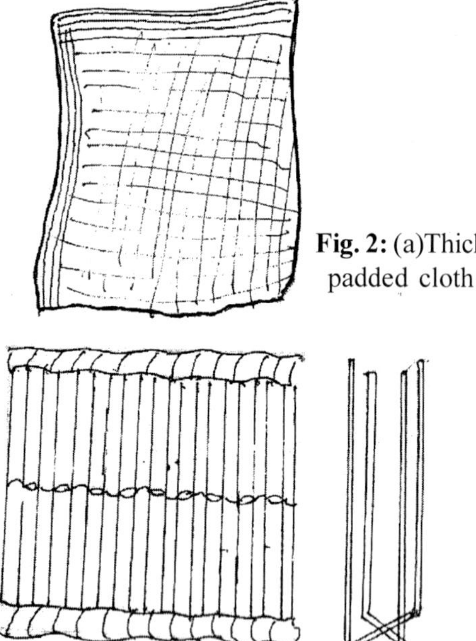

Fig. 2: (a)Thick padded cloth

Fig. 2: (b)Padded netted bamboo splint

Fig. 2: (c)Conjoined U plate

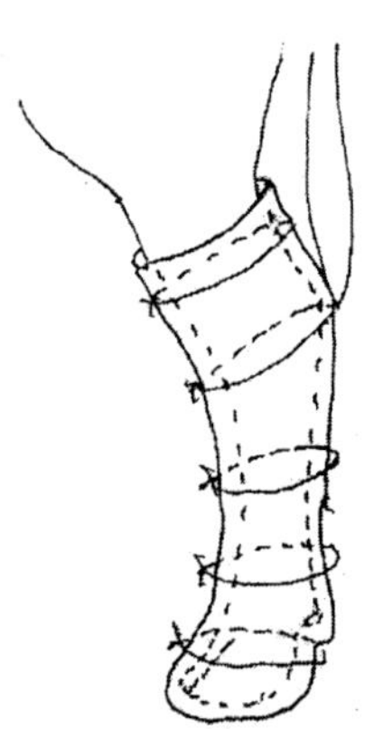

Fig. 3: Protection of fracture site with thick padded cotton cloth

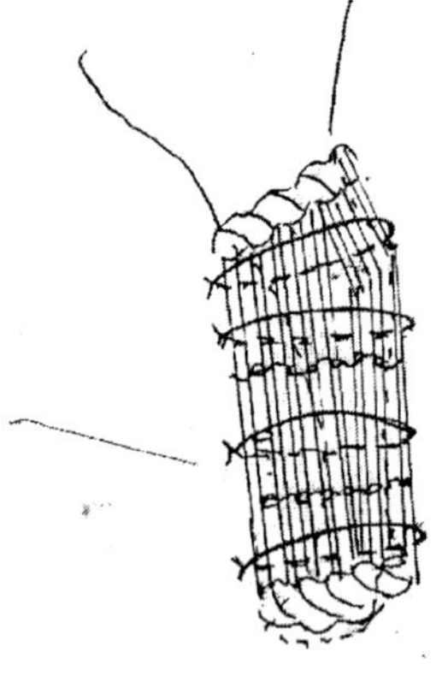

Fig. 4: Strengthening of protective cloth with padded netted bamboo splint

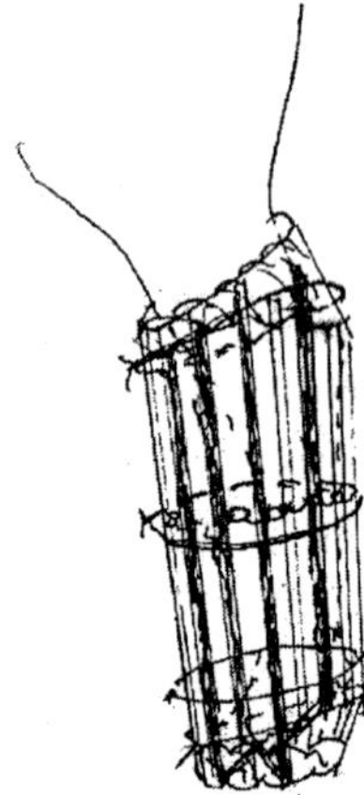

Fig. 5: Fitting of conjoined U plate at the fracture site

References: Amaresh Kumar, (2004). Veterinary Surgical Techniques. Vikas Publishing House, New Delhi. pp 368-371.

50

Lower Level Fracture

Fracture of meta-carpals and meta-tarsals comes under lower level fracture. Padded cloth and netted bamboo splint along with conjoint U plate has been considered as standard method of repair.

(1) The fractufe is a lower level fracture involving the meta-carpal and meta-tarsal bones. (Fig.1 & Fig.2)

(2) The fracture site is immobilized extending joint below and joint above level initially with cloth or cotton padding.(Fig.3)

(3) Netted bamboo splint Is applied over it for support involving joint above and joint below which should not be too tight or too loose.(Flg.4)

(4) Splints are retained in position by thread with knots. The ends of bamboo splint kept padded to avoid skin damage.(Fig.4)

(5) More strength is given to immobilisation by application of conjoint U-plate.Conjoint U-plate is a U shaped metallic plate used for lower level fracture immobilisation. (Fig.5 & Fig.6)

(6) At the end the entire bandage is covered with cloth or a bandage roll.The hoof should also be bandaged to avoid damage due to improper blood circulation.(Flg.6)

Application of Bamboo Splint and Conjoint U-Plate in Lower Level Fracture

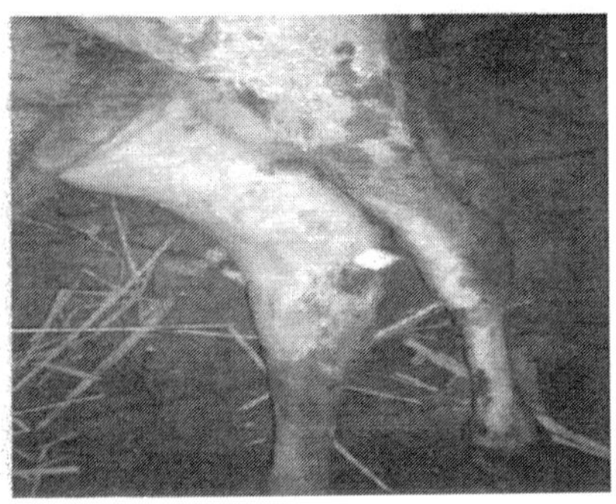
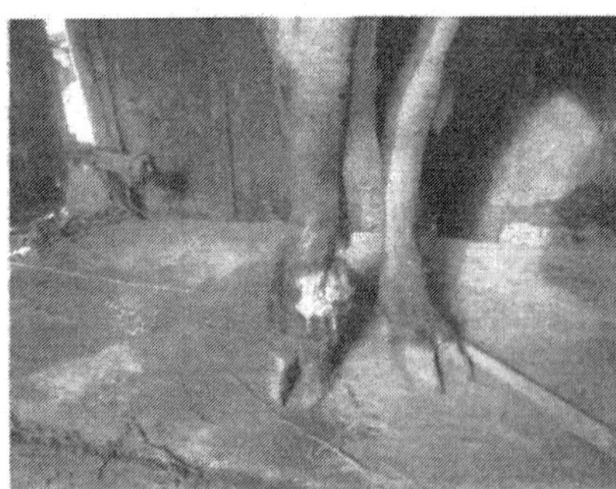
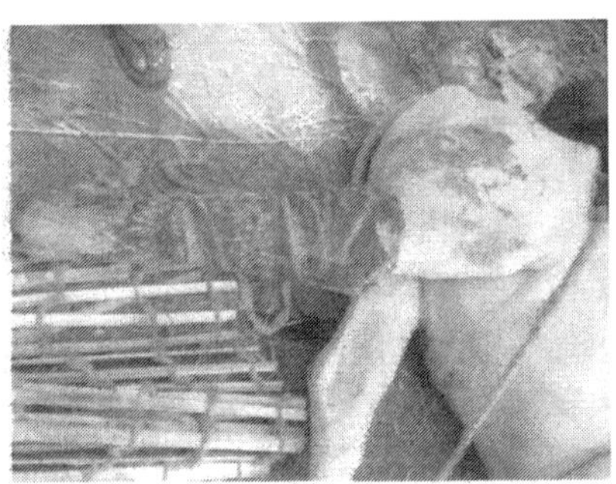
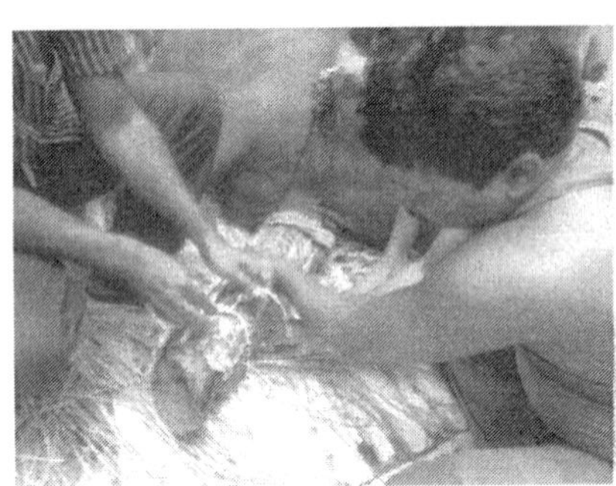
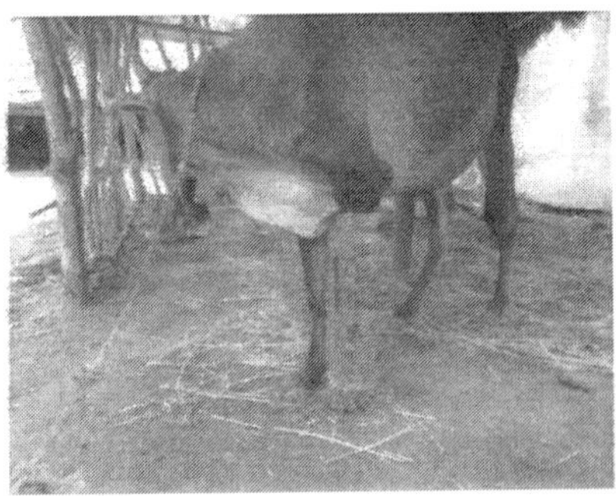
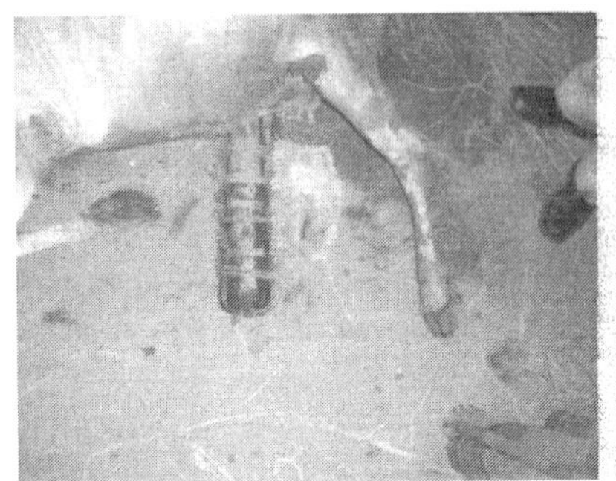

Management of Metacarpal Fracture by Bamboo Splint and Pop Cast

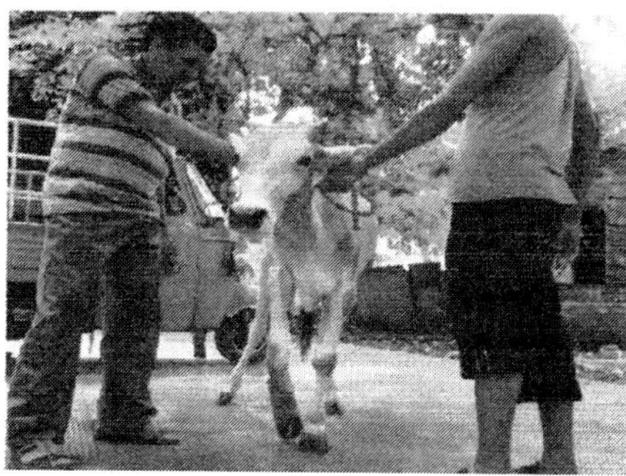

Fig. 1: Unable to bear weight on the fractured limb b.

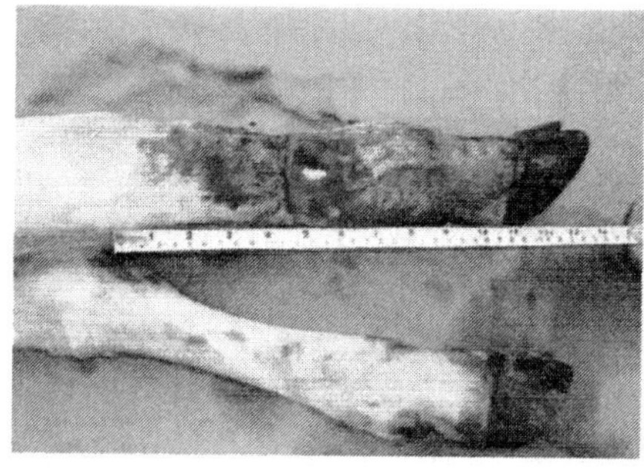

Fig. 2: Measurement of affected limb b (length).

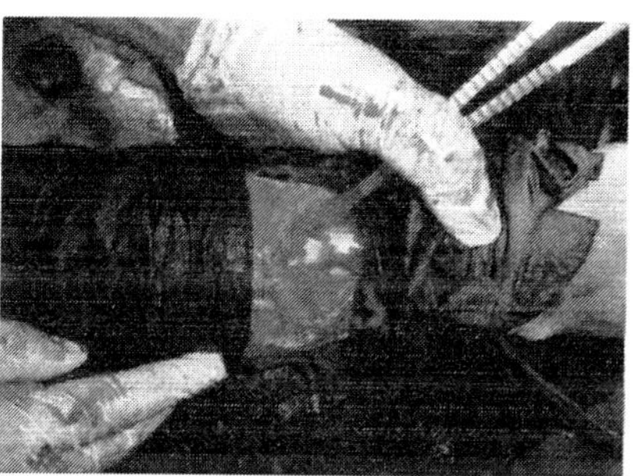

Fig. 3: Alighment of the fractured bone fragment

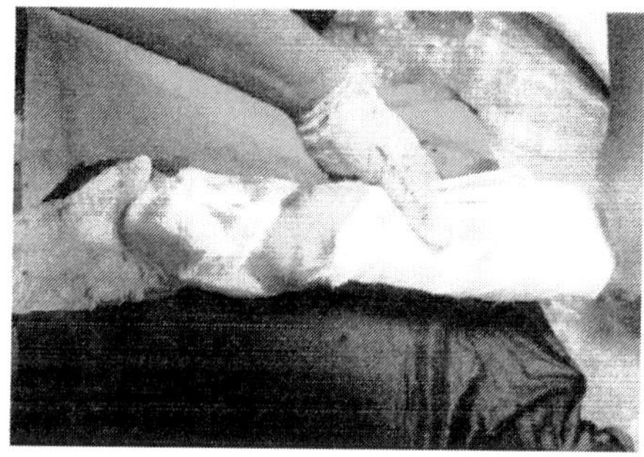

Fig. 4: Bandaging

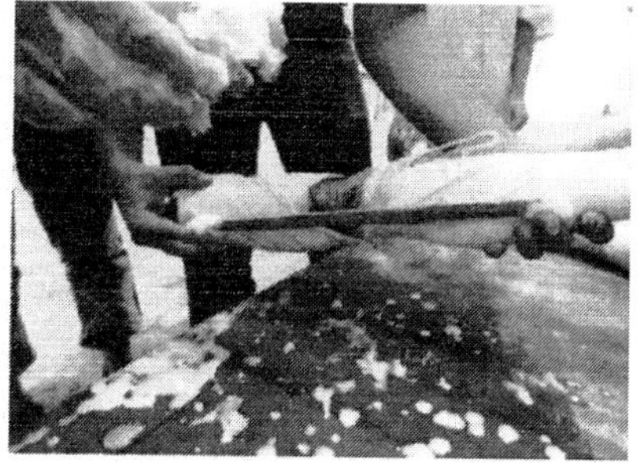

Fig. 5: Application of POP cast reinforced with bamboo splint.

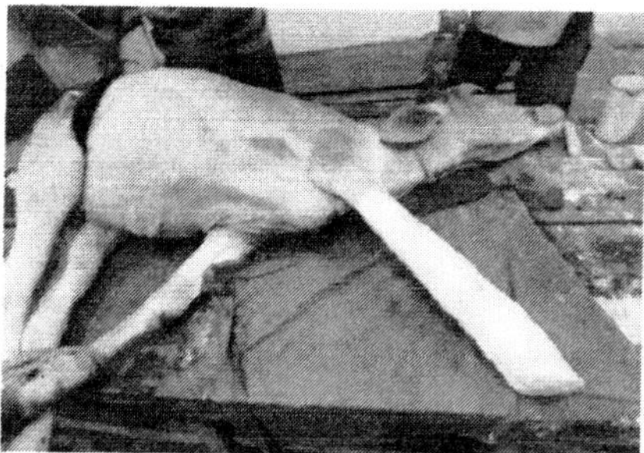

Fig. 6: After completion of surgical procedure

Management of Metacarpal Fracture by Bamboo Splint

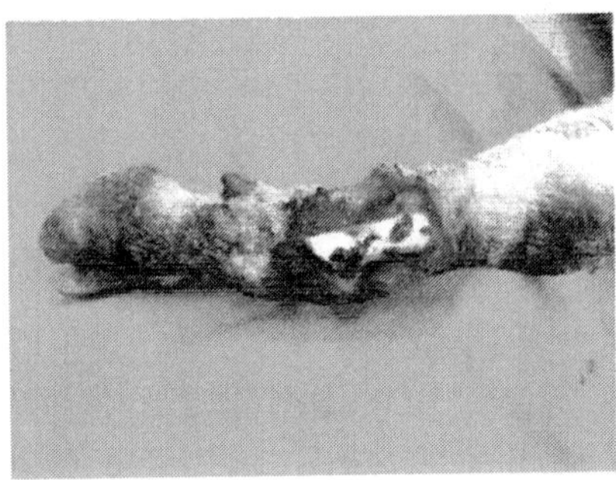

Fig. 1: Compound MC fracture

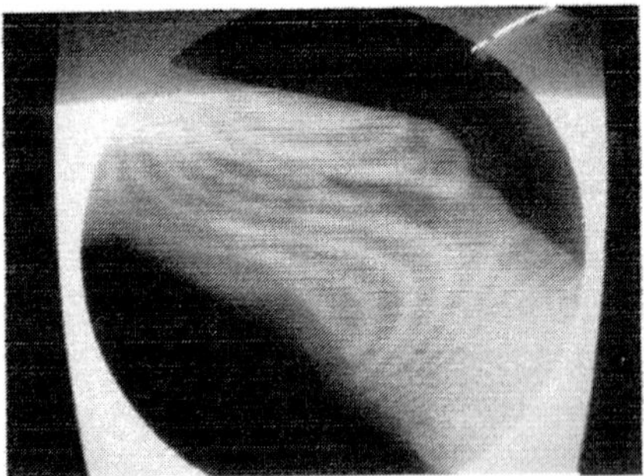

Fig. 2: Over riding of fracture fragment on radiograph.

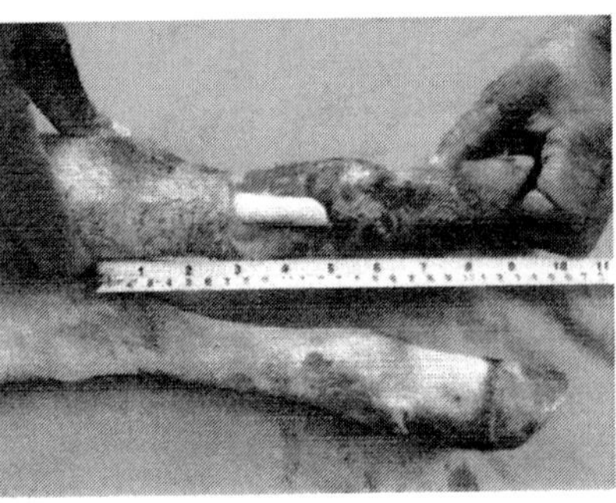

Fig. 3" Measurement of affected limb (length).

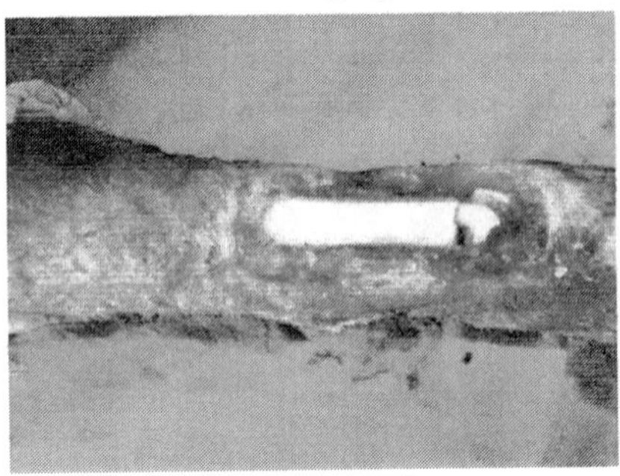

Fig. 4: Alinment of the fractured bone fragment

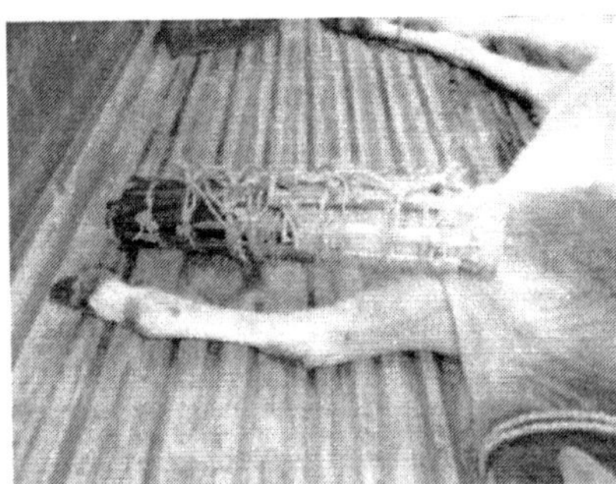

Fig. 5: Temporary immobilizer application

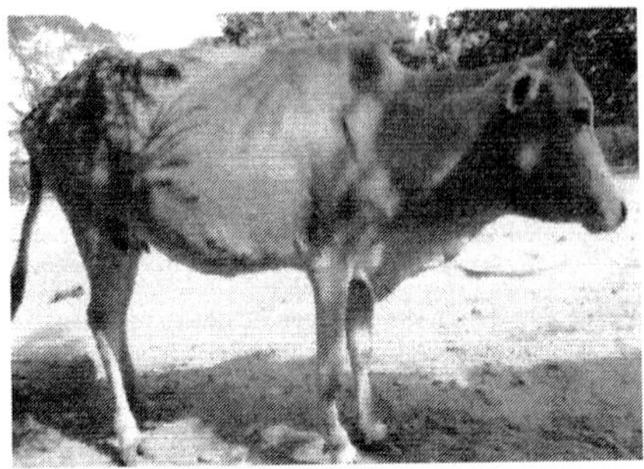

Fig. 6: Weight bearing on the affected limb after healing

Management of Metatarsal Fracture by Camd and Pop Cast

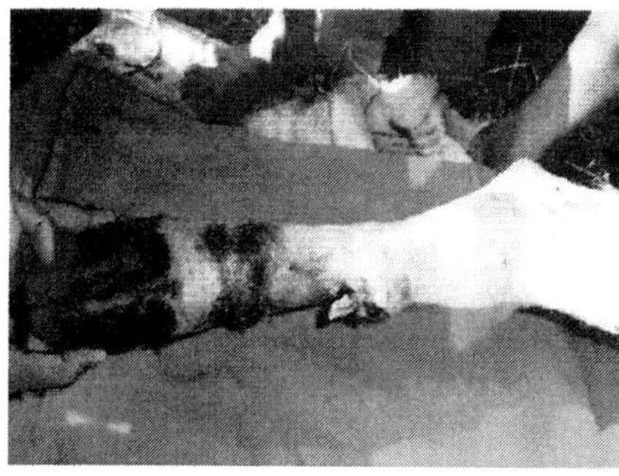

Fig. 1: MT fracture in a deshi cow

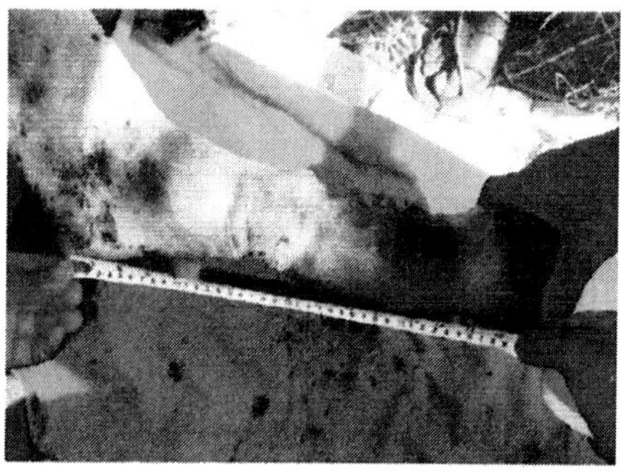

Fig. 2: Measurement of affected limb of right MT fracture in a bull.

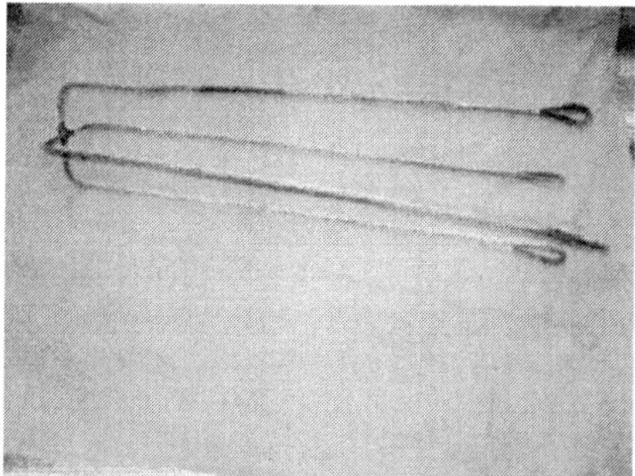

Fig. 3: Fabrication of conjoint angular metallic device (CAMD)

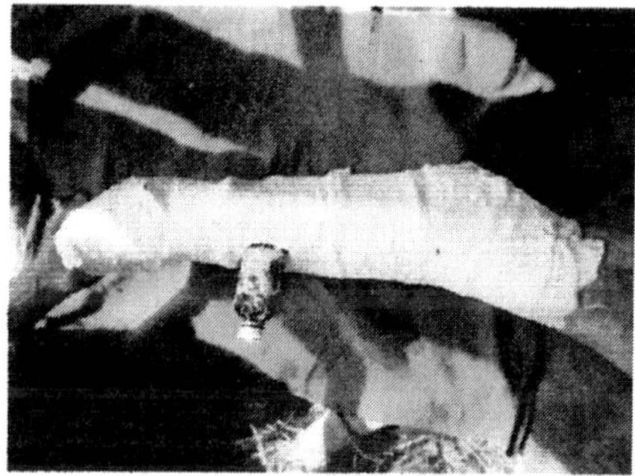

Fig. 4: Permanent immobilization with POP cast reinforced with CAMD

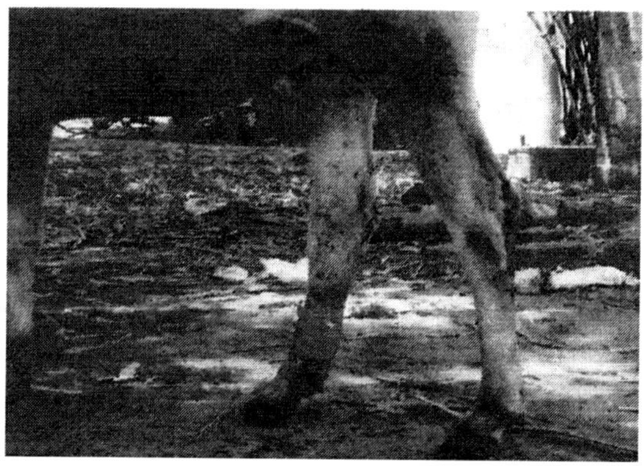

Fig. 5: After complete healing

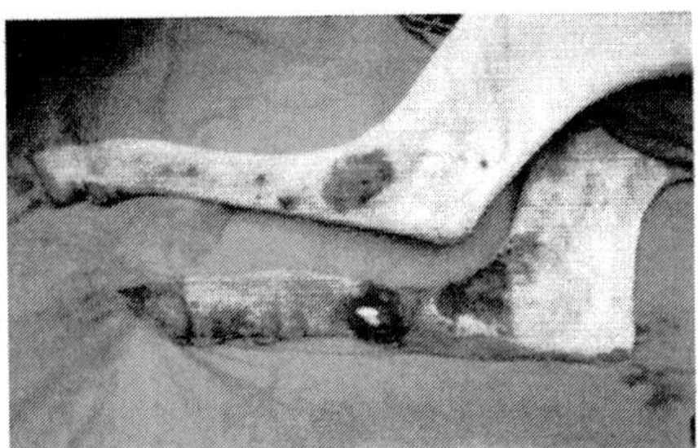

Fig. 6: Left MT fracture of cow.

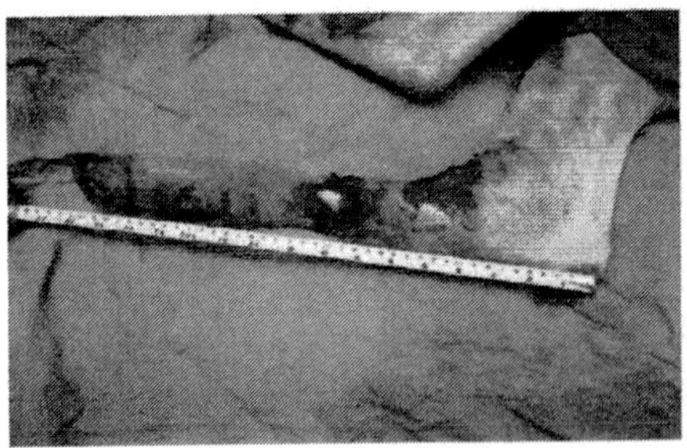

Fig. 7: Measurement of affected limb (length)

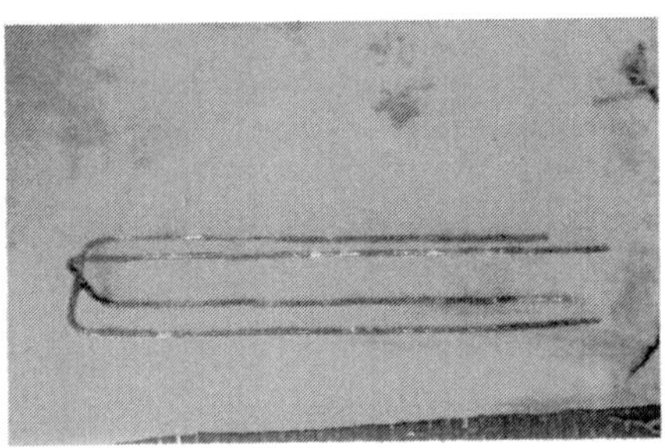

Fig. 8: Fabrication of conjoint angular metallic device (CAMD).

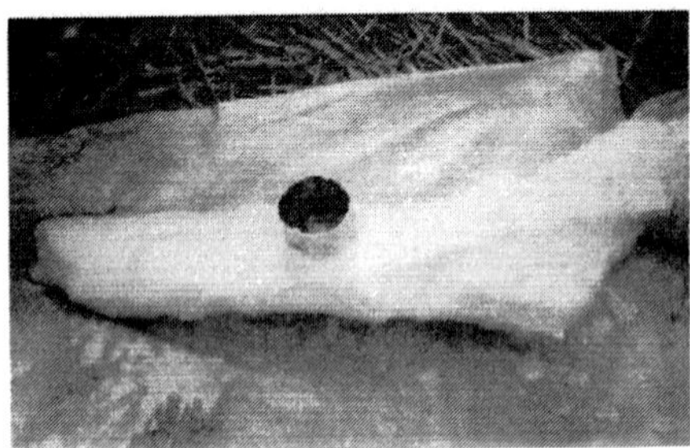

Fig. 9: Permanent immobilization with POP cast rein forced with CAMD.

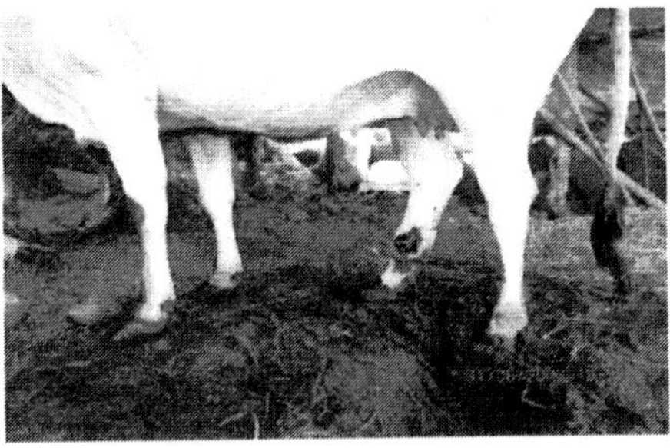

Fig. 10: After complete healing

51

Middle Level Fracture Repair

Definition

Fracture of radius-ulna & tibia-fibula comes under middle level fracture.

Methods of Fracture Repair

External coagtation bandage along with thomas splint application.

Technique for Fracture Repair

Animal controlled with lateral recumbency with fractured limb upward.

Procedure

1. For immobilisation of these fracture the area 3-4" below the knee or hock. 3-4" above the elbow or stifle needs to be immobilised by coaptation bandage, Fig -1
2. The fractured bone are brought into apposition by traction and counter traction by passing a rope around the axilla & groin & arround hoof.
3. Gum is applied upon the fractured site covering 3-4" below the knee & 3-4" above the hock for radius- ulna and 3-4" below the hock & 3-4" above the stifle joint for tibia fibula, Fig -2.
4. A 16 layered thick cloth of this length is wrapped around the fractured position of the limb. The cloth is retained with thread knot at several places, Fig -3
5. 4 green bamboo splints are kept on the 4 sides of the limb over the cloth padding and retained with thread knots.Fig -4
6. Gum is applied over the above application. Again the entire application is covered with a gauze bandage.
7. A netted bamboo splint of this measured length is wrapped arround the cloth bandage & tied in position with string.Fig-5

8. Now the above coaptated fractured limb is further immobilised within a thomas splint & retained in position.fig-6

Management of Middle Level Fracture

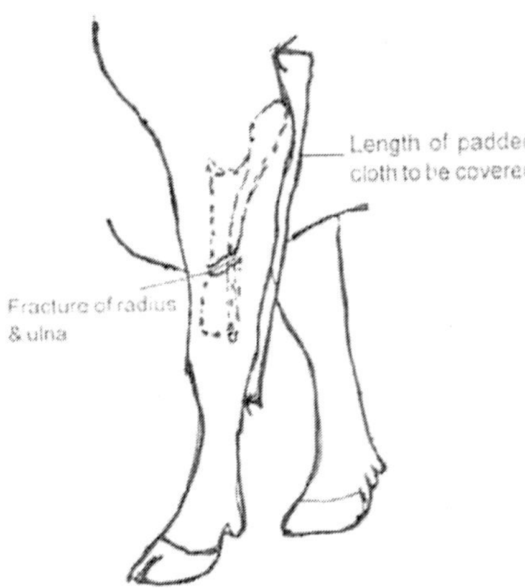

Fig. 1: Simple fracture of radius and ulna & length of padded cloth

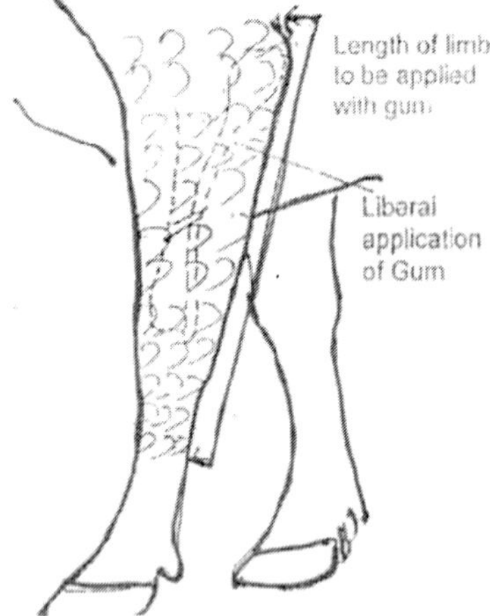

Fig. 2: Application of gum over the fracture site

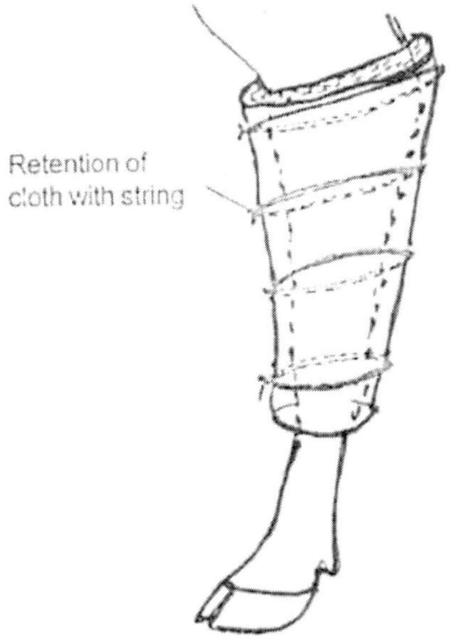

Fig. 3: Padded cloth around the fracture

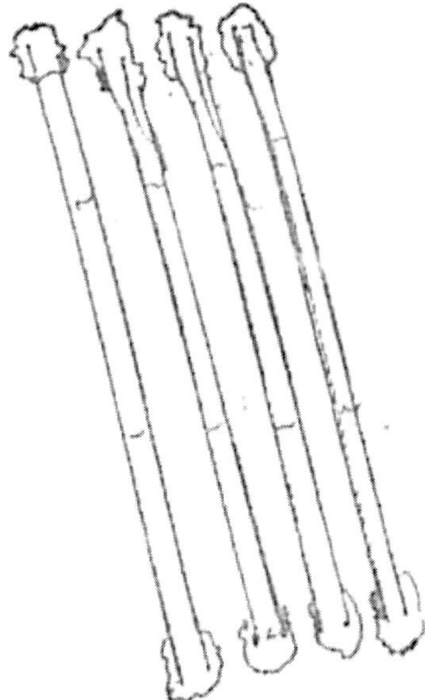

Fig. 4: Four padded bamboo splint

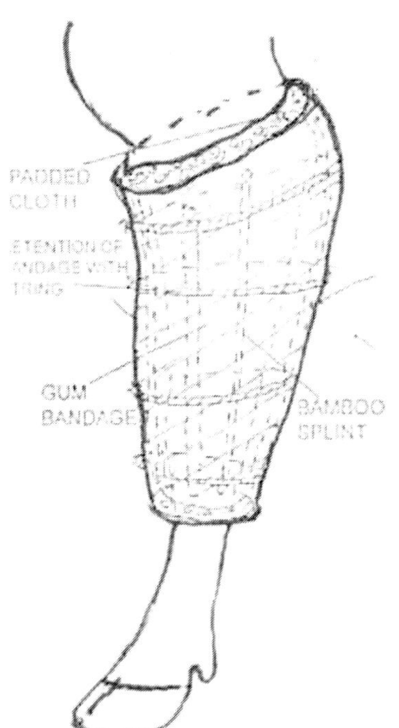

Fig. 5: Immobilization of fracture with gum band

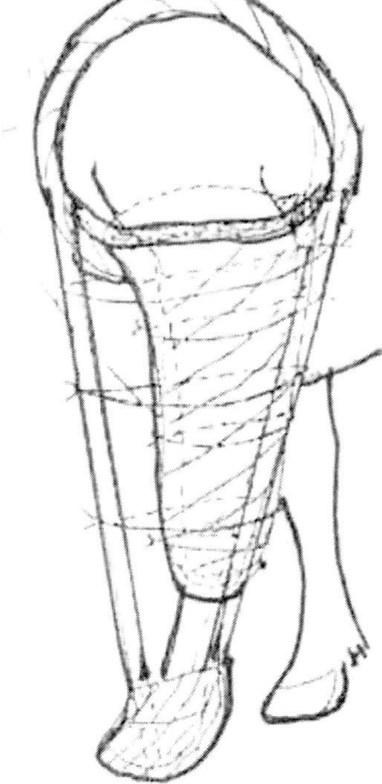

Fig. 6: Immobilization of fracture with gum bandage limb with Thomas Spli

52

Middle Level Fracture

Fracture of radius-ulna & tibia-fibula comes under middle level fracture. Pop caste application or bandage along with Thomas splint has been considered as standard method of repair.

(1) The fracture site is immobilized extending between joint below and joint above level with either gum bandage or pop caste bandage (Fig.1).

(2) Pop caste bandage is generally applied after 7 days. Hence gum bandage is preferred than pop caste bandage because of immediate application after occurrence of fracture (Fig.2).

(3) For gum bandage application, a 8-16 layer thick cloth is wrapped over the fracture region covering the joint above & joint below of the site after liberal application of fevicol gum. The cotton cloth Is placed in position with few cotton thread knots (Fig.3).

(4) 4 bamboo splints are kept on the 4 sites of the limb over cotton padding. The end of bamboo splints kept padded to avoid skin damage. Splints are retained in position by thread with knots (Fig.4).

(5) A 2nd layer fevicol gum is applied over entire bandage & finally the entire bandage cloth is covered with bandage roll (Fig.5).

(6) At the end the immobilized limb is over strengthened with Thomas splint (Fig. 6).

Application of Pop Cast and Thomas Splint in Middle Level Fracture

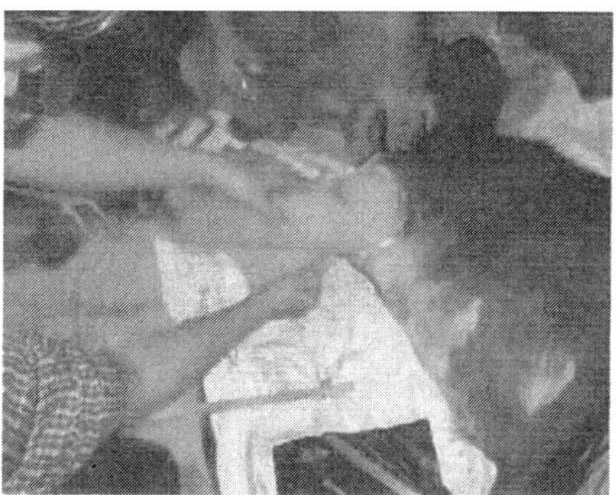

Fig. 1: Photo feature showing immobilization of radius-uina

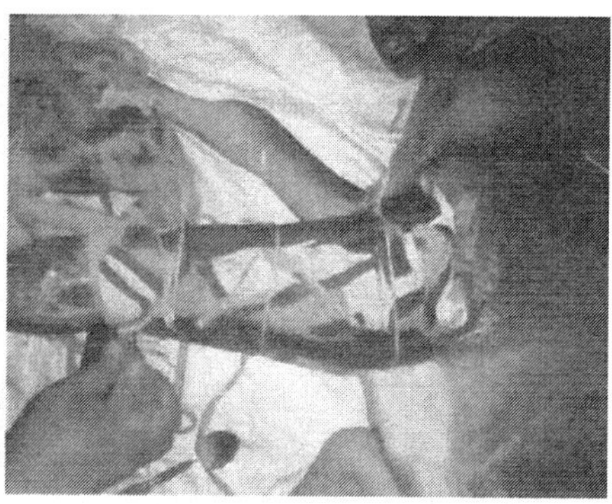

Fig. 2: Photo feature showing gum bandage application of radius-ulna

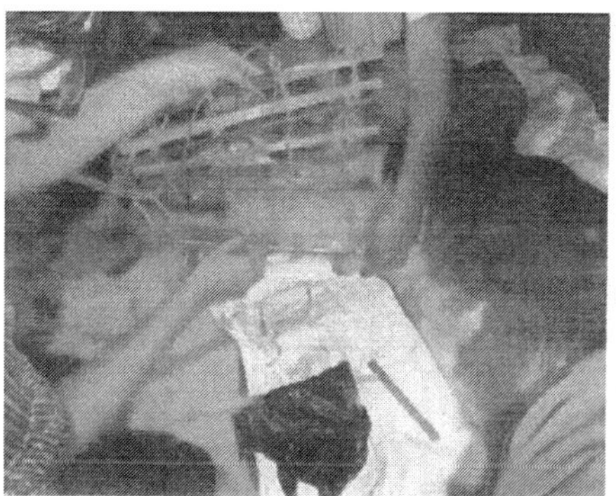

Fig. 3: Photo feature showing thick cloth wrapping in the facture of radius-ulna

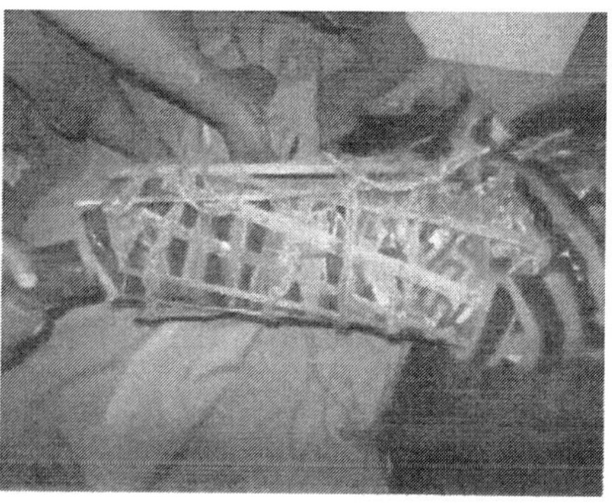

Fig. 4: Photo feature showing bamboo splint application in radius-ulna

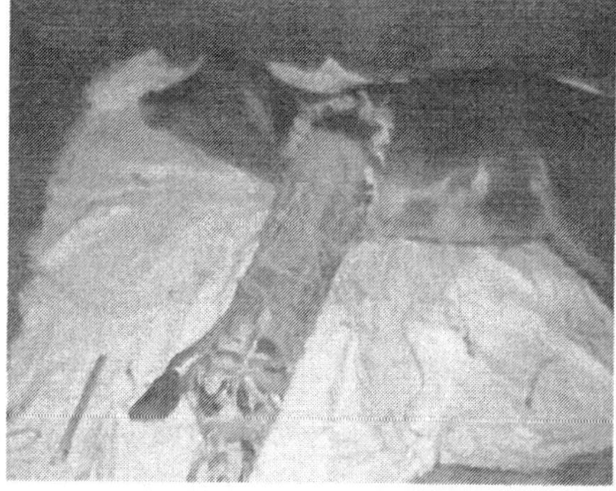

Fig. 5: Photo feature showing 2nd layer gum bandage application in radius-ulna

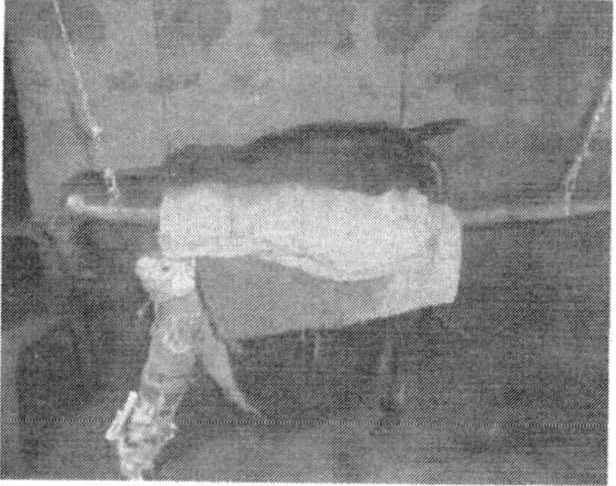

Fig. 6: Photo feature showing limb by application of Thomas splint in radius-ulna

Management of Radius Ulna Fracture by Modified Thomas Splint

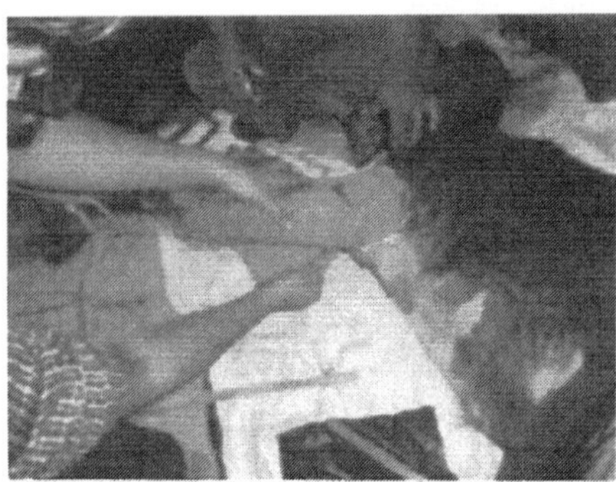

Fig. 7: Application of gum resin and covering of cloth.

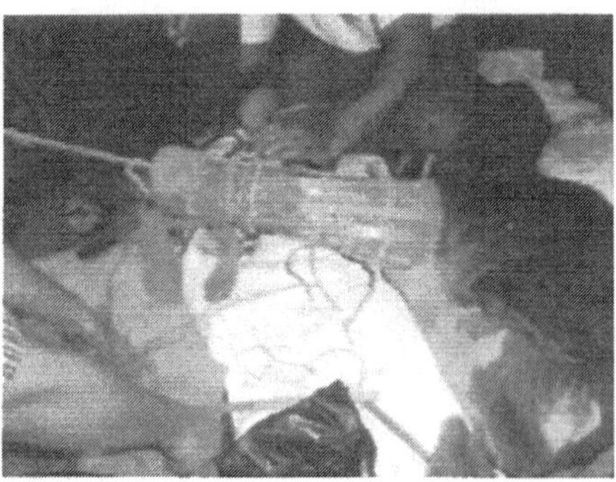

Fig. 8: Re-strengthening of the coapted limb by application of netted bamboo splint.

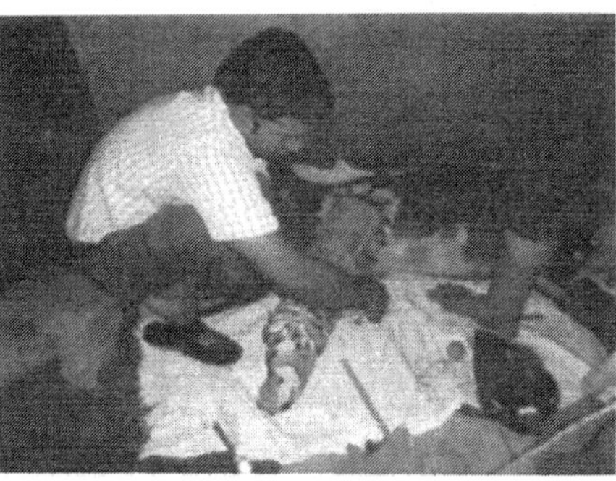

Fig. 9: Fixation of modified Thomas splint.

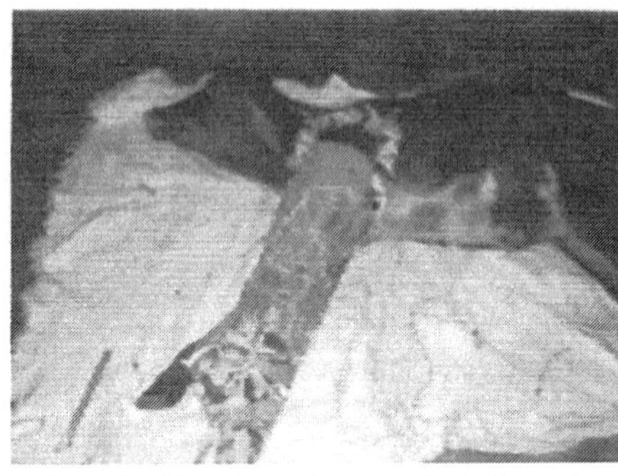

Fig. 10: Fixation of coapted limb to the ring of modified Thomas splint.

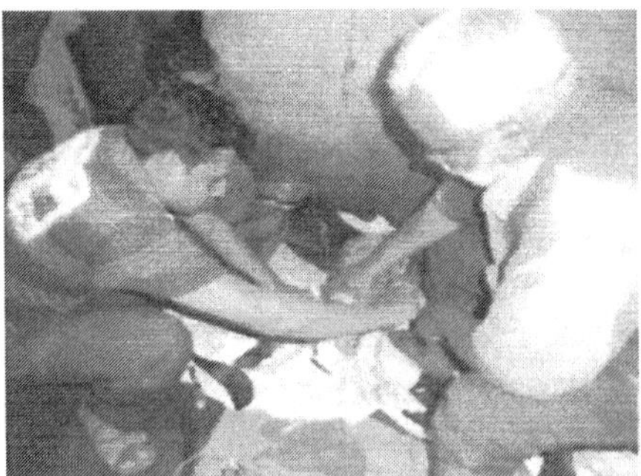

Fig. 11: Fixation of MTS to hoof.

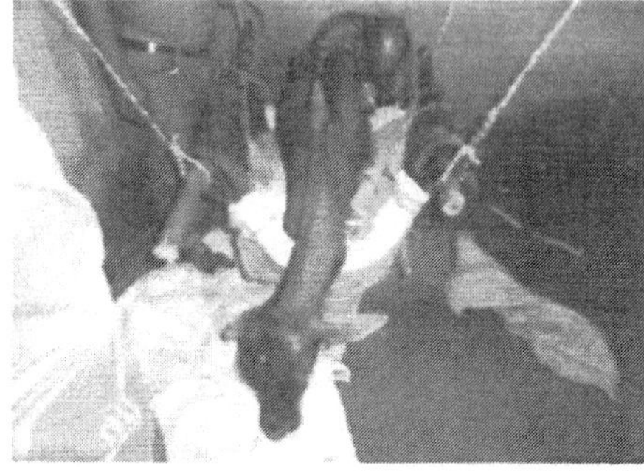

Fig. 12: Rehabilitation of animal within the sling.

Management of Radius Ulna Fracture by Modified Thomas Splint

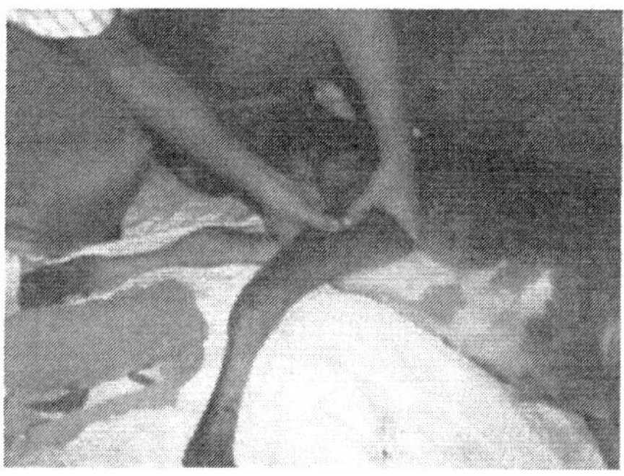

Fig. 1: Casting of animal on lateral recumbency keeping the proximal level fracture limb up.

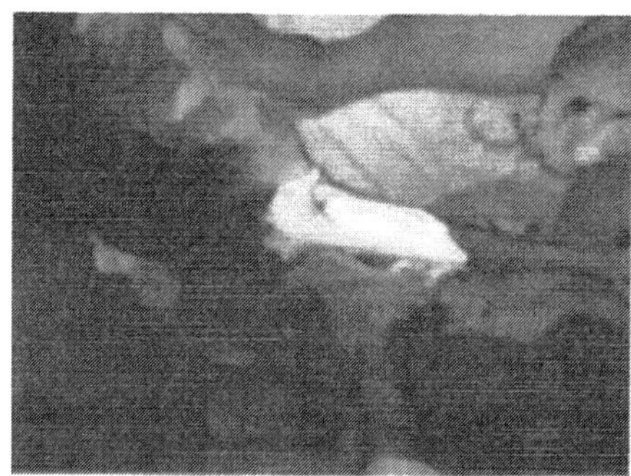

Fig. 2: Application of fevicol gum on the proximal level radial fracture limb.

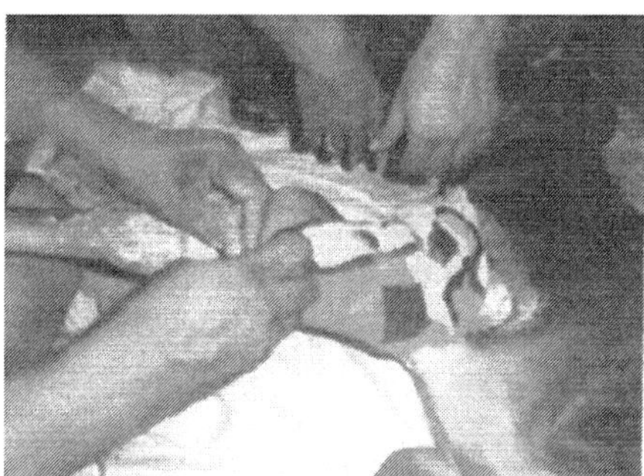

Fig. 3: Application of 16 layer unsterilized clean cotton cloth over the gum.

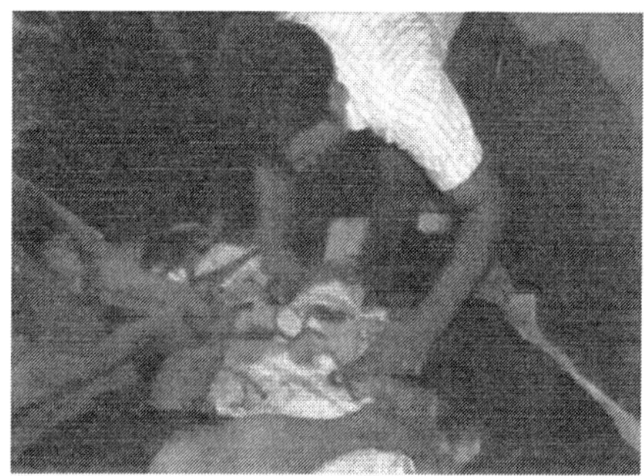

Fig. 4: Application of traction.

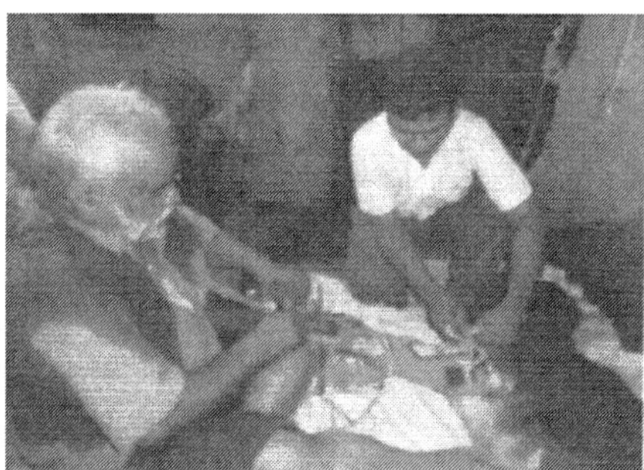

Fig. 5: Application of retention knots.

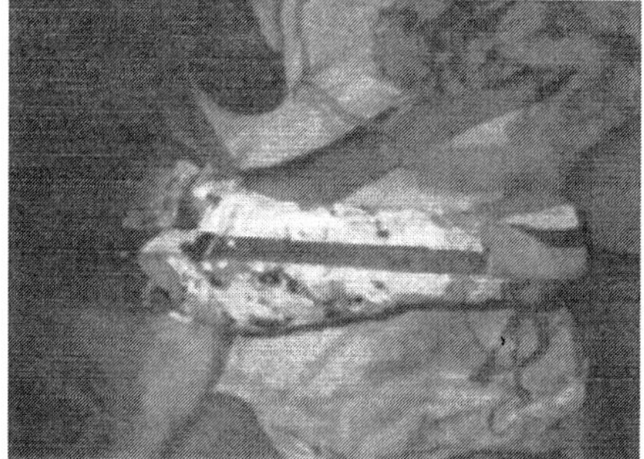

Fig. 6: Placement of four gum impregnated bamboo splint over the cloth.

Tibio-Fibula Fracture Repair in Large Animal

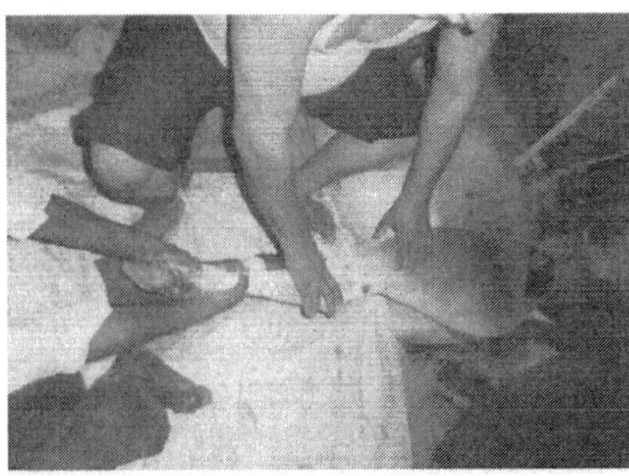

Fig. 1: Correction of fracture site with traction and counter traction before immobilisation.

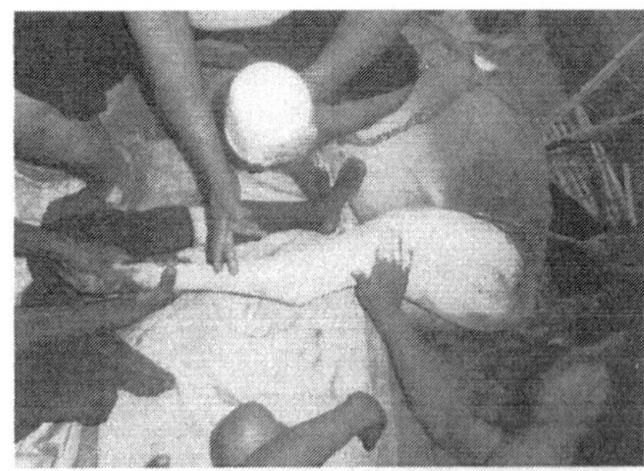

Fig. 2: Liberal application of adhesive gum over the fracture site.

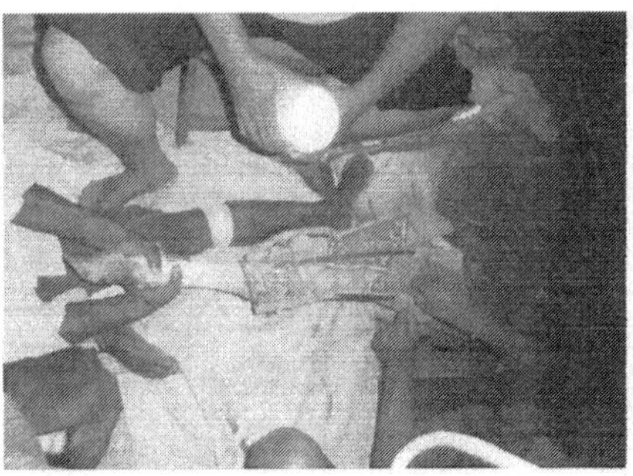

Fig. 3: Application of soft cotton bandage strengthened with bamboo splint.

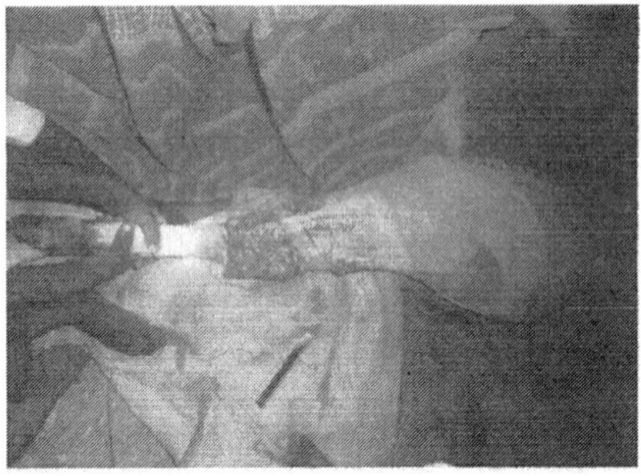

Fig. 4: Over padding of fracture site with gum bandage.

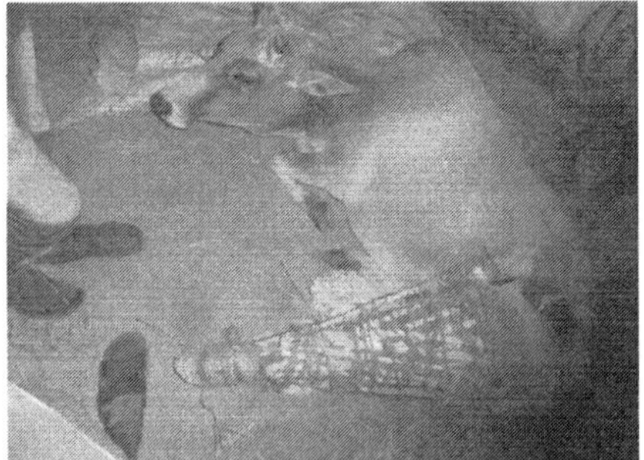

Fig. 5: Covering with netted bamboo splint and Thomas splint.

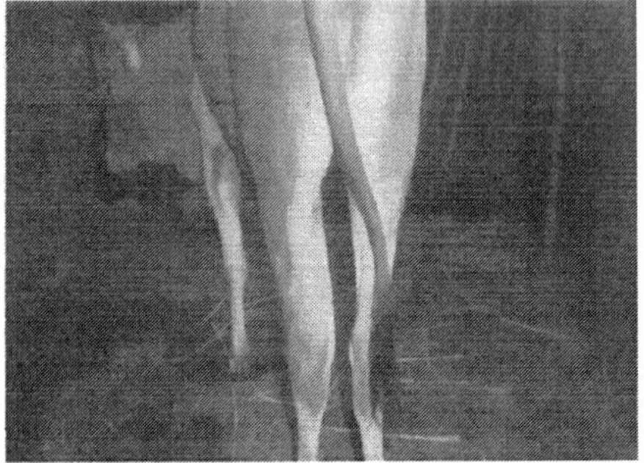

Fig. 6: Recovered animal.

Tibio-Fibula Fracture Repair in Large Animal

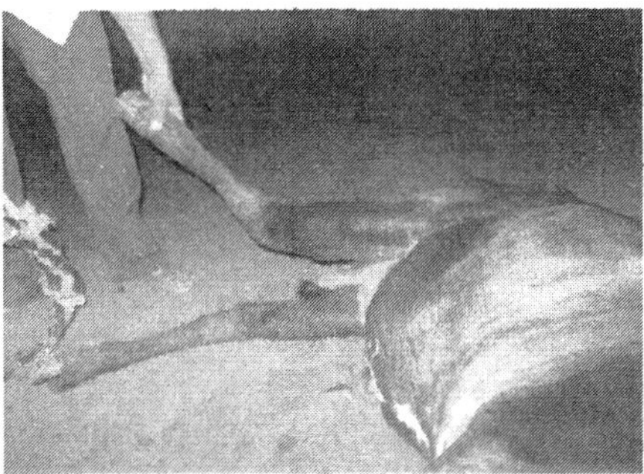

Fig. 1: Overside view of fracture site

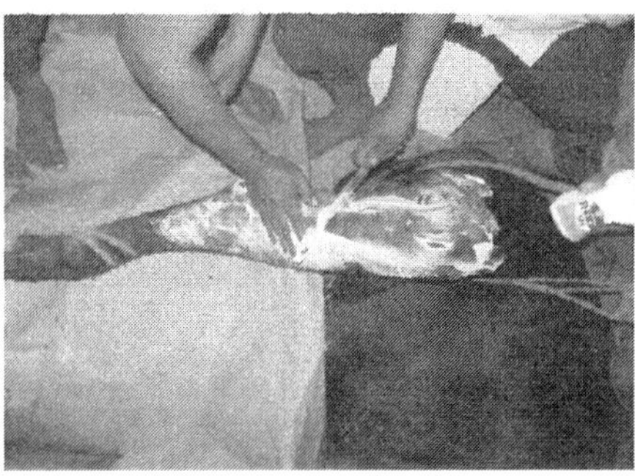

Fig. 2: Liberal application of adhesive gum over the fracture site.

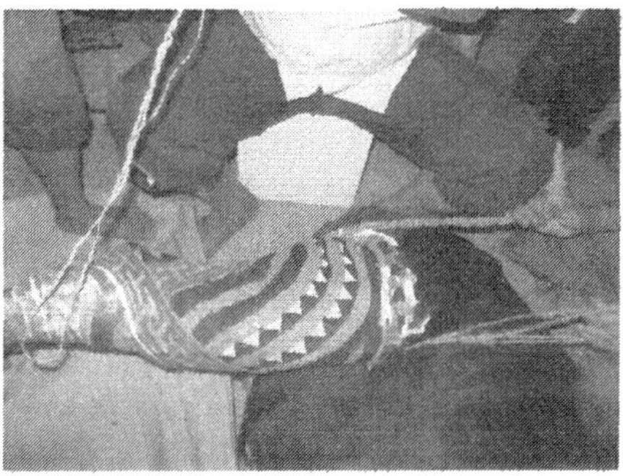

Fig. 3: Covering of fracture site with soft cotton traction and counter traction.

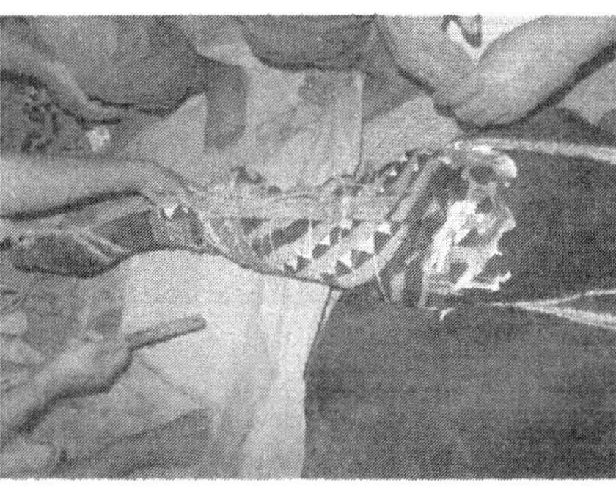

Fig. 4: Strengthening of cotton padding with bandage with green bamboo splint.

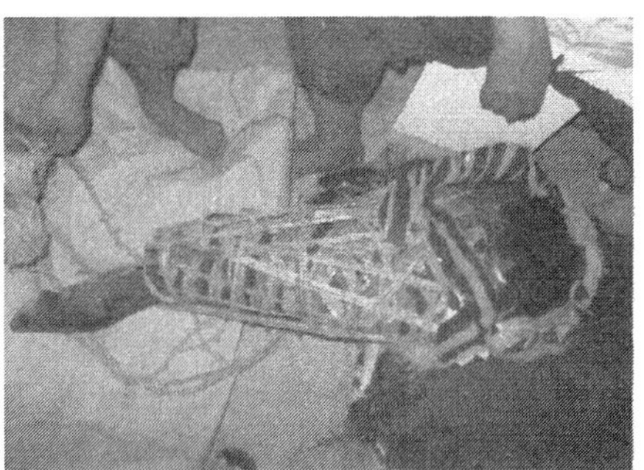

Fig. 5: Over strengthening with netted bamboo Thomas splint.

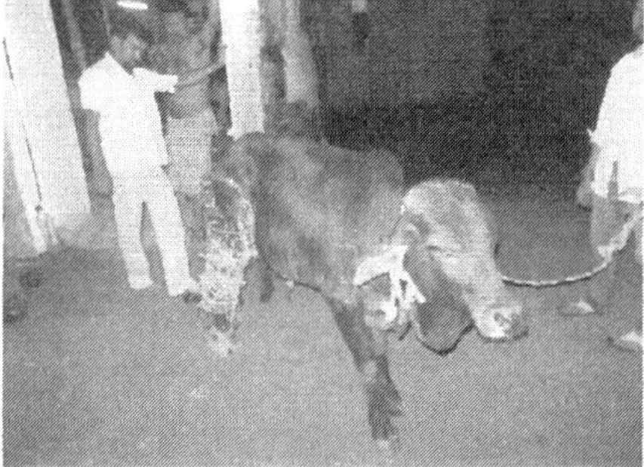

Fig. 6: Complete immobilisation splint

53

Higher Level Fracture Repair

Definition

Fracture of humerus bone and femur bone are generally categorised under higher level fracture.

Methods Used For Fracture Repair

1. These level fractures are repaired appropriately by intramedullary pinning and Thomas splint application.
2. Only pinning or only Thomas splint are not the method for its repair as the distal fragments of bone get tourqed by pinning only and the fracture fragments get distracted by simple Thomas splint application.
3. Hence after pinning a humerus or femur bone, the limbs are kept immobilised perfectly by Thomas splint application.
4. When pinning as well as Thomas splint application are not possible the fractured bones are kept immobilised with fevicol gum bandage only. So for this purpose modification of velpeau sling is generally adopted and animal is restrained within limited space for 21 days.

Procedure For Fracture Repair

1. Gum is applied 3-4" below the elbow in forelimb or stifle in hind limb and upto the hump in forelimb or rump in hind limb. Thick cloths of several layers are pasted over the site covering around the fore arm and leg region as shown in fig 1.
2. Belts of cotton cloths are passed around other side limb and are fixed with the gum bandage (coaptation bandage) with several stitches with strong thread as shown in fig 2.
3. After fracture repair the animal is kept under restricted movement for 21 days within 6’x6’, 8’x8’, or lO’xlO’ size space enclosures. During this period the neck of the animal is not tied with rope.

Modified Velpeau Sling for Management of Higher Level Fracture in Cattle

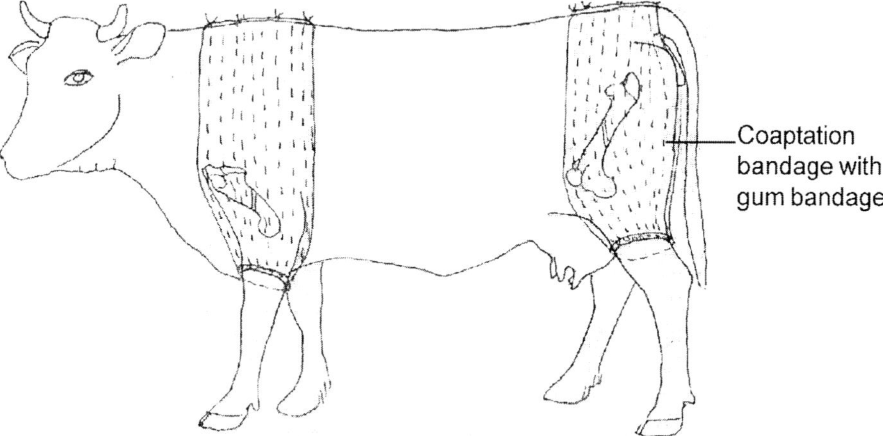

Fig.1: Left side view of cow showing immobilization technique for humerus and femur fracture with gum bandage

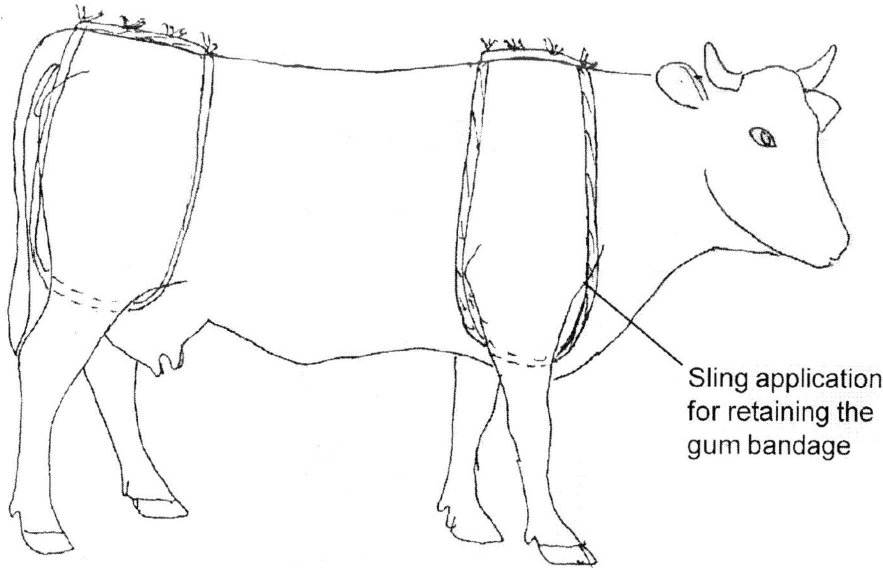

Fig. 2: Right side view of cow showing sling application for retaining the gum bandage in posititicn.

54

Photo Feature of Higher Level Fracture

Definition

Fracture of humerus and femeur bone has been grouped under higher level fracture. Pinning as well as Thomas splint application are considered to be the approved method of immobilization for repair of these bone fracture.

Both method of repair are highly essential. Any one method of repair has been considered dangerous for the animal. Only pinning of the bone makes the limb to be turked where as only Thomas splint application disturbes the bone alignment at fracture site. Hence leaving one method of repair other method is not possible.

When above method of repair is not possible a modification of velpue sling can be attempted.

Modified Valpeau Sling for Management of Higher Level Fracture in Cattle

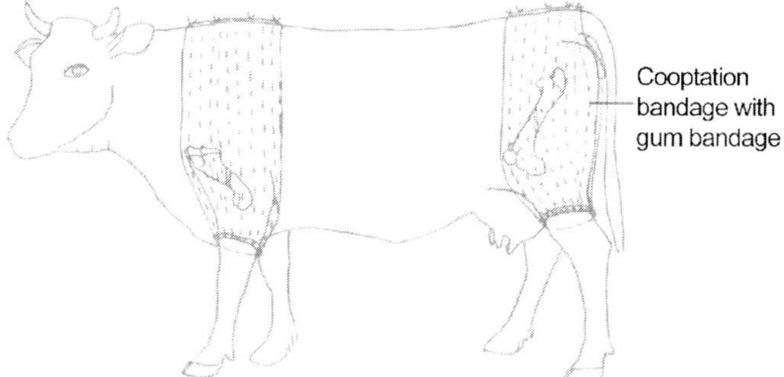

Fig. 1: Left side view of cow showing immobilization technique for humerus and femur fracture with gum bandage

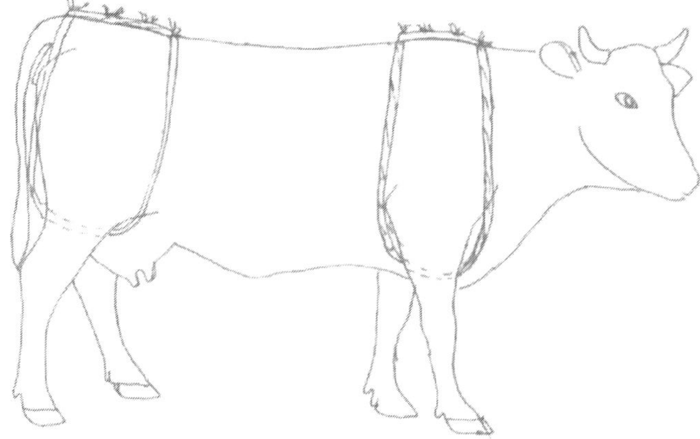

Fig. 2: Right side view of cow showing sling application for retaining the gum bandage in posititiion.

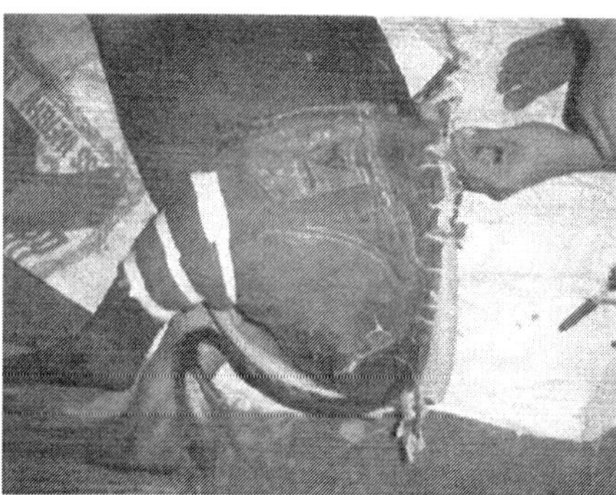

Fig. 3: Photo feature showing gum bandage and sling application at femur

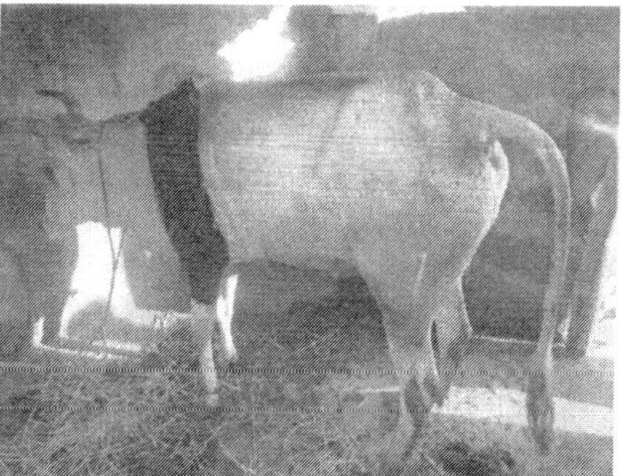

Fig. 4: Photo feature showing gum bandage and sling application at humerus

Humerus Fracture Repair by Modified Velpeu Sling

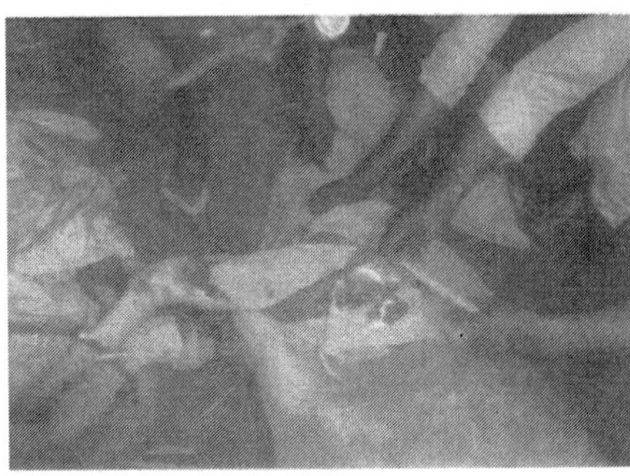

Fig. 1: Application of layer of Gum and Cotton Bandage

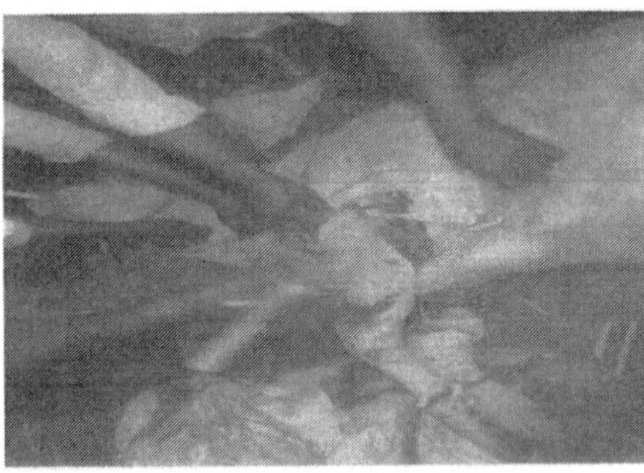

Flg. 2: Application of 2nd layer of Gum and Cotton Bandage

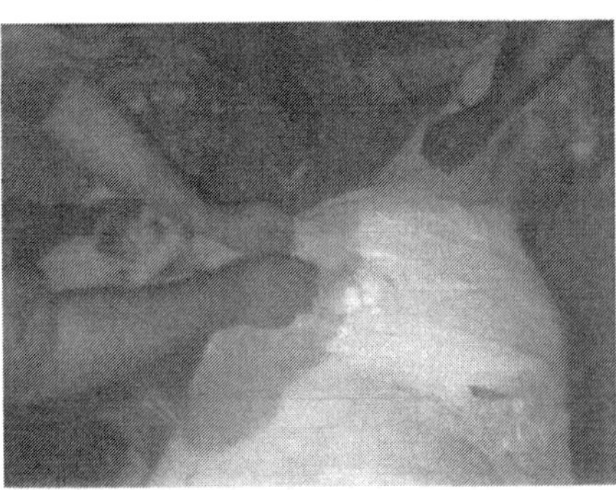

Fig. 3: Application of final layer of Gum and Cotton Bandage

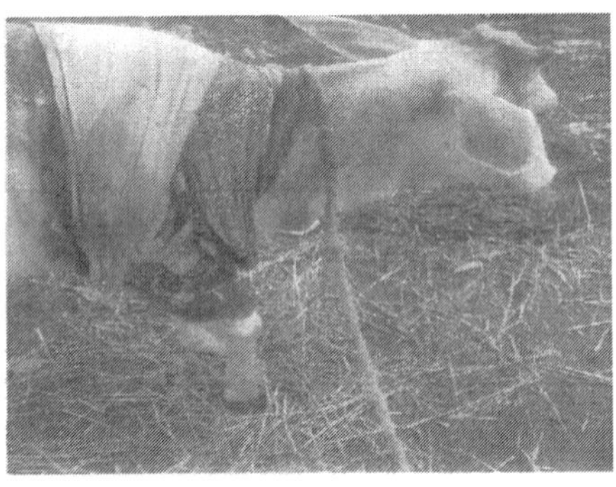

Flg. 4: Right side view of the animal with modified Velpeau sling

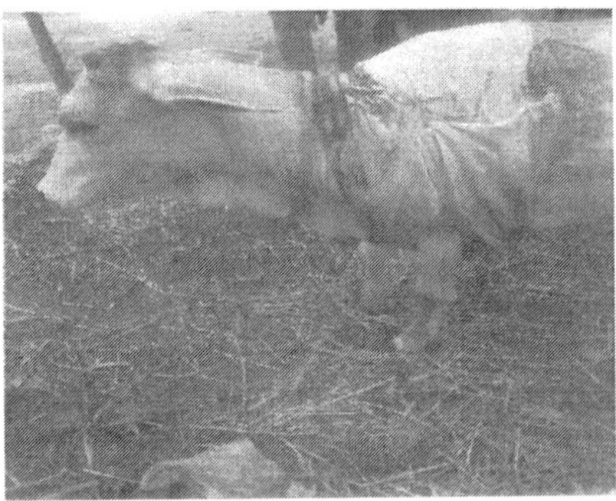

Fig. 5: Left side view of the animal with modified Velpeau sling

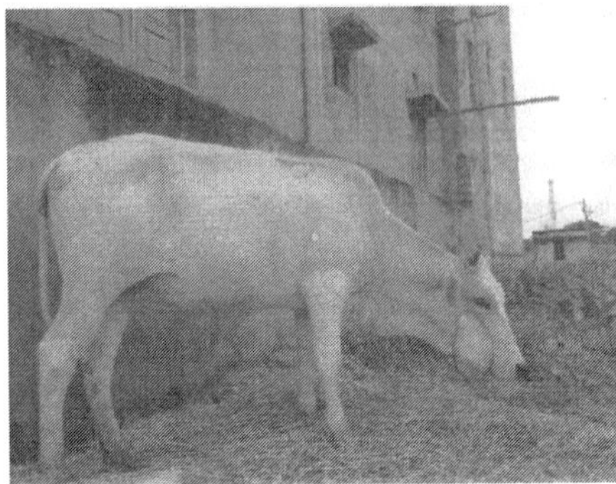

Fig . 6: Animal after recovery

55

Highest Level Fracture (HLF) and its Management

Definition

Any fracture or discontinuity in bony structure like scapula and pelvic girdle present above the shoulder joint and hip joint respectively are called as highest level fracture.

Aim

To know the method of repair of highest level fracture.

Procedure

As there is no satisfactory method of external immobilisation till date, generally animal is kept under restricted movement. Sometimes application of charge (glue bandage) externally may give some satisfactory result.

a. Fracture of scapula: area above shoulder joint upto hump and below on the opposite side is applied with glue (Fevicol gum) and a thick cloth is pasted over the area. Sometimes the thick cloth may be applied upto 2-3 layers for achieving restriction against the movement of fracture fragment (Fig-1).

b. Fracture of pelvic girdle: area above hip joint upto the loin and to some extend below it on other side is applied with fevicol gum liberally. Thick clothes are paste over the gum area upto 2-3 layers to achieve restriction of movement of fractured fragment (Fig-2)

Highest Level Fracture (HLF) and its Management

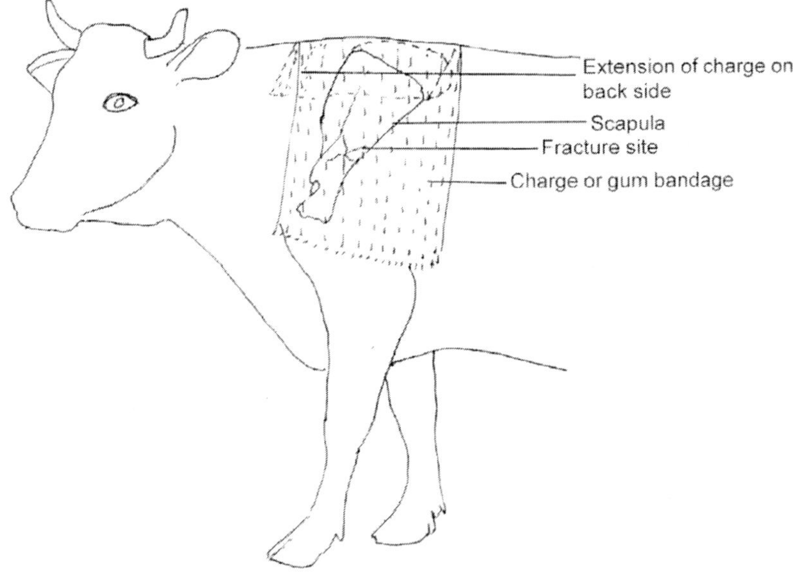

Fig. 1: Showing fracture of Scapula

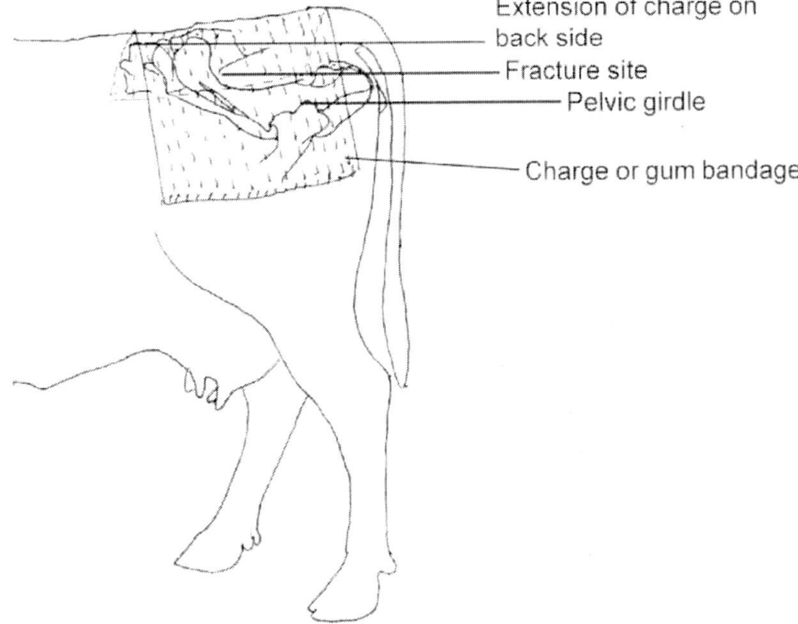

Fig. 2: Showing fracture of Pelvic Girdle

56

Photo Features of Highest Level Fracture

1. Fracture of scapula, shoulder dislocation, fracture of pelvic girdle, hip dislocation have been grouped under highest level fracture.
2. For large animal, immobilization of bone & joint have not been developed satisfactorily/ till date. Hence after correction of dislocation or rearrangement of fractured the site Is kept immobilized with application of gum bandage.

Technique

1. Fevicol gum is applied over the site extending the other side also to retain the bancJage for longer period in position.
2. Site is kept covered with thick layer of cotton bandages by application of gum as well as cloth cover for 3-4 layers.
3. Animal is kept within restricted movement for 15-25 days.

Photo Features of Highest Level Fracture

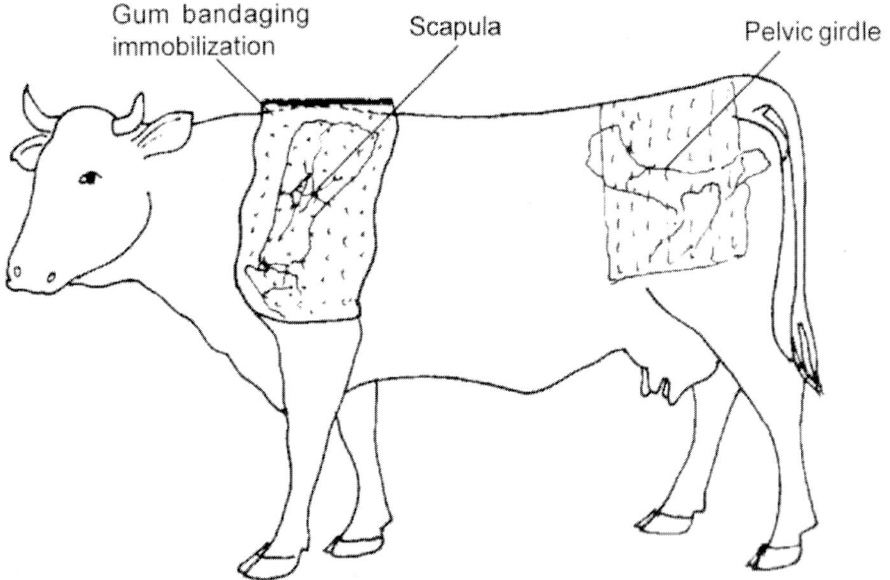

Fig. 1: Showing immobilization technique for highest level fracture of forelimb and hindlimb (Left side).

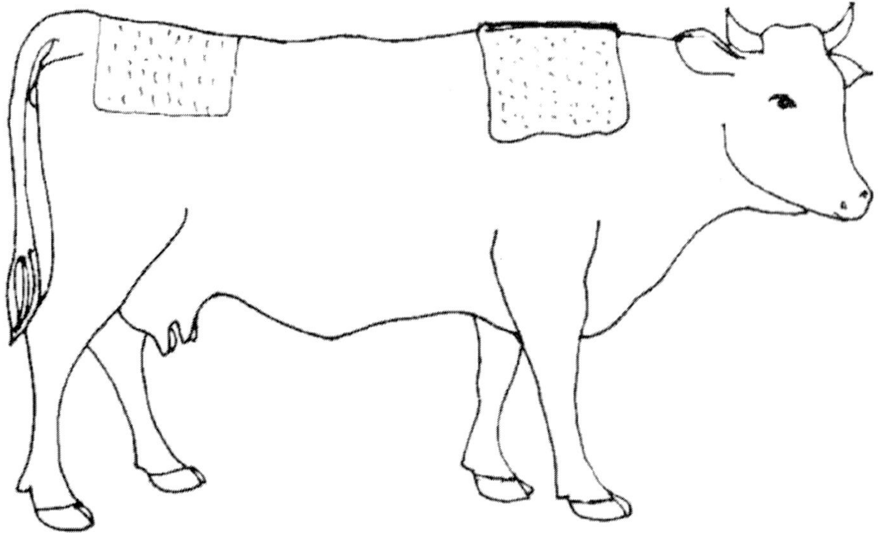

Fig. 2: Showing immobilization technique for highest level fracture, gum bandaging extending upto right side

57

Conjoined 'U' Plate with Ring for Immobilisation of Radius and Ulna Fracture

Aim

To know the use of Conjoined 'U' Plate with Padded ring for fracture side immobilization.

Site to be immobilized

Upper 3rd metacarpus, Carpo - meta carpo joint dislocation, Radio - Carpal Joint dislocation. Lower Radius & Ulna fracture are can also be immobilised with this device

Material Required

6mm Iron rod. Bandage, Cotton.

- Preparation of Conjoined 'U' Plate with ring (Fig 2a)
- Conjoined 'U' Plate with ring is prepared with use of 6mm Iron rod taking the length of entire limb upto axila to foot & a ring off circumference of the axila is welded at the top of the rod (Fig.2a).
- The ring of the Conjoined 'U' Plate is padded with thick cotton bandage (Fig.2b).

Procedure of Immobilisation

The fracture site is immobilized with thick padded cloth cover & padded netted bamboo splint (Fig.3a).

Finally entire immobiliser is kept straight by the use of Conjoined 'U' plate v/ith padded ring. (3b).

Conjoined 'U' Plate with Ring for Immobilisation of Radius Ulna Fracture

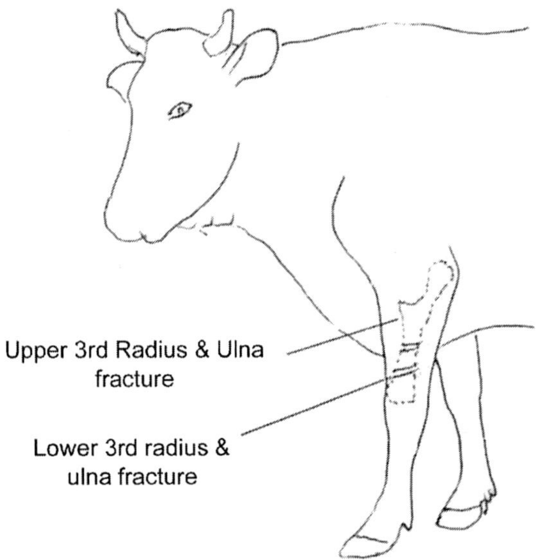

Fig. 1: Upper 3rd R&U fracture

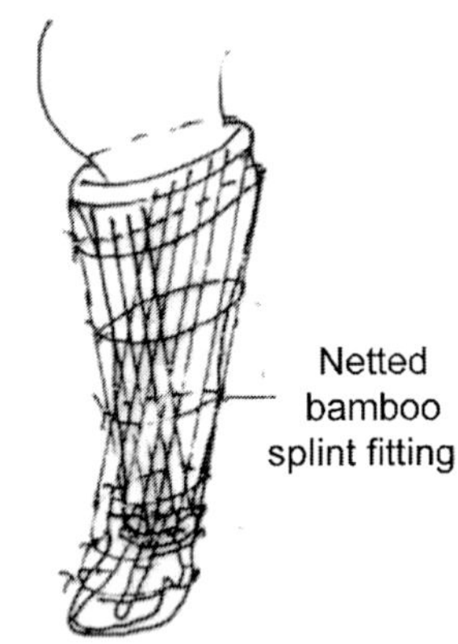

Fig. 3: Immobilise of fracture side with thick padded cloth & netted bamboo splint

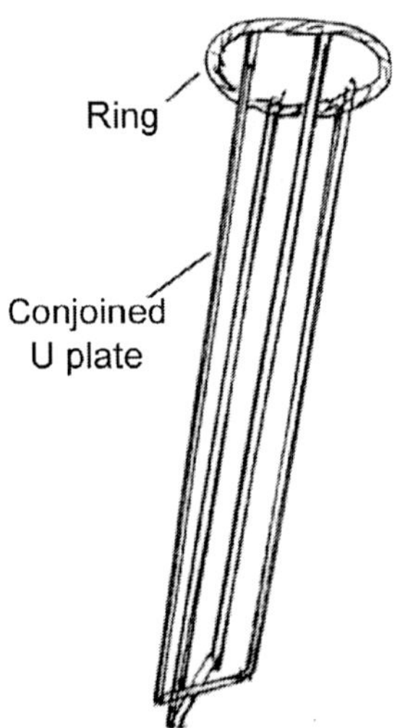

Fig. 2b:

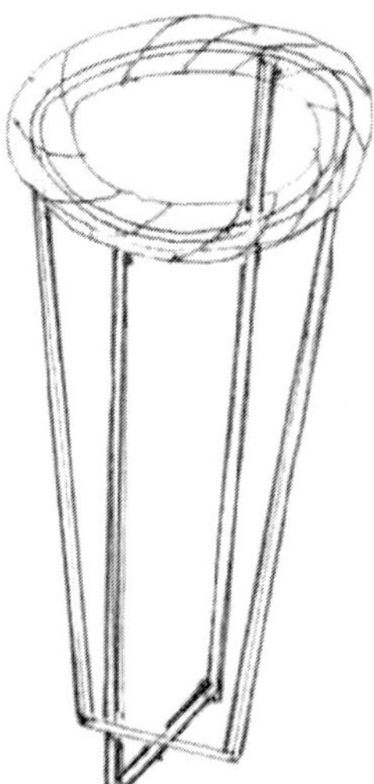

Fig. 2b: Conjoined U plate with thick cotton bandage

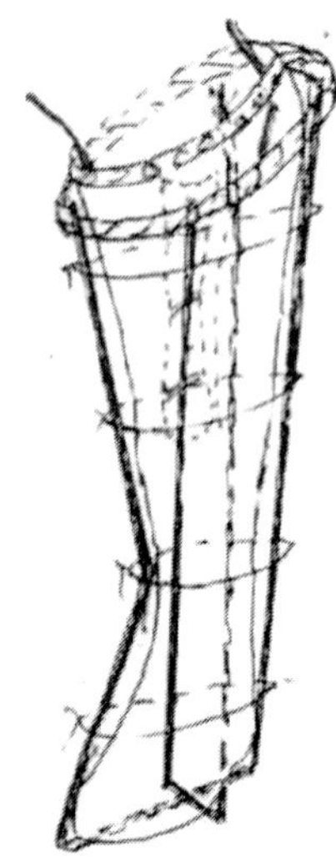

Fig 3a: Immobilisation of Lower 3rd R&U fracture with conjoined U plate with padded ring

58

Hanging Pin Cast

Definition

Handing pin cast is used for management of longbone fracture. Pin which is used for immobilisation of fracture of proximal radial and tibial bones is called hanging pin cast.

Special equipment

Intramedullary pin, hand driven drill, plaster of paris bandage **Procedures :,**

1. One pin is inserted transversely through the proximal fragment.
2. A plaster cast is applied to immobilise entire distal part of limb anchoring the proximal transverse pin.

Advantage

1. It helps in preventing rotational fracture bone and downward slipping of plaster cast.

Note

Fig. 2 (a) Position of pin in radius bone, (b) Position of pin inside tibial bone

1. The principle that, the joints proximal and distal to fracture should be included in piaster cast may not be applicable.
2. ft is not used to immobilise comminuted fracture and also oblique fracture Post operative care:

   A course of antibiotic for 7-10 days.

***Reference**:* Amresh Kumar, (2004) Veterinary Surgical Techniques, Vikas Publishing House, Pvt. Ltd., New Delhi, PP - 375-377.

Hanging Pin Cast

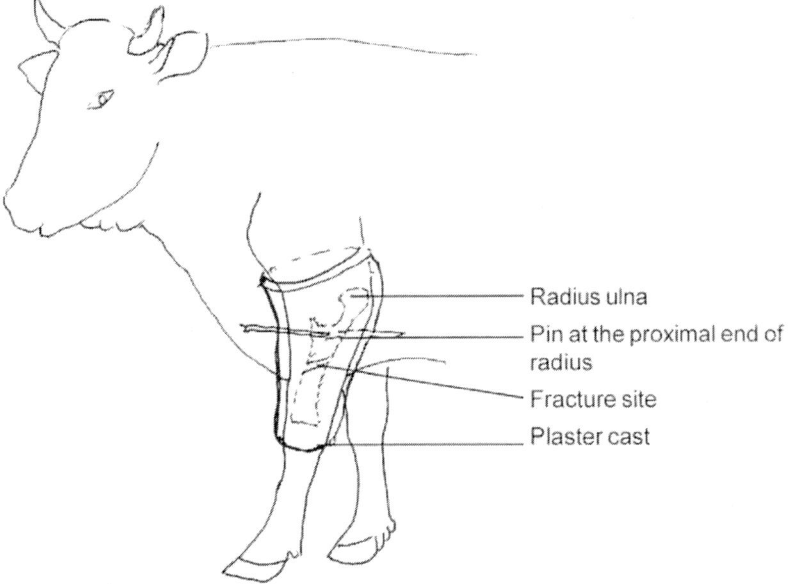

Fig. 1: Position of pin in radius ulna (Forelimb)

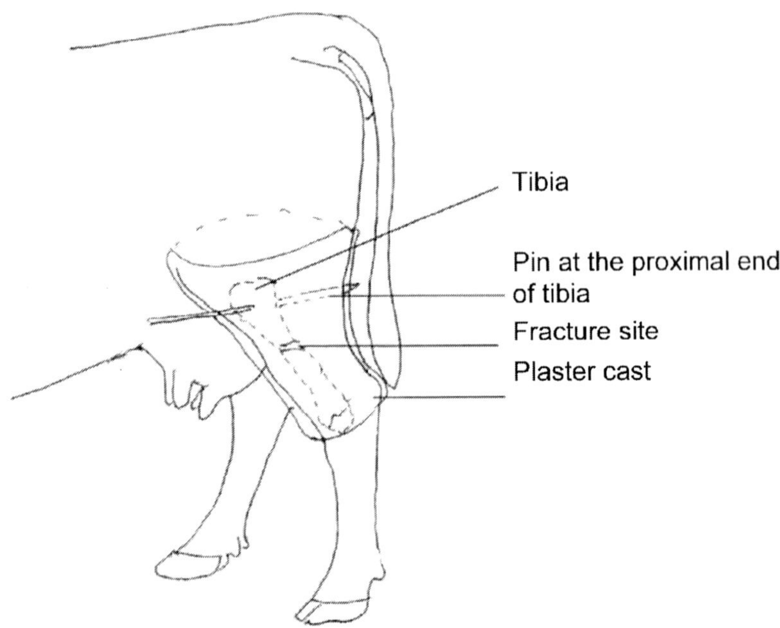

Fig. 2: Position of pin inside tibial bone (Hindlimb)

Reference: Amresh Kumar, (2004) Veterinary Surgical Techniques, Vikas Publishing House, Pvt. Ltd., New Delhi, PP - 375-377.

59

Intramedullary Pinning of Humerus in Large Animal

Definition

Humerus is long selender and has slight spiral twist.

Oblique type of fracture is most common in diaphyseal region .

It come under higher level of fracture.(Fig. No-1)

Appropriate method of fixation is by intramedullary pinning and modified thomas splint.

Requirement

1. Parentral sedative
2. Local anaesthesia
3. 6mm 1 fit long intramedullary pin (Fig.No-3)
4. Electric bone drill
5. Bone hammer
6. Pin cutter

Surgical Anatomy

The detail of humerus be depicted (Fig.No.2)

Procedure

1. Point of the pin is placed open the greater trochanter of humerus
2. Drilling of bone carry out till the pin remain in the medullary cavity of the humerus bone

3. The length of pin is shortest with piun cutter, tip of the pin kept under the skin .
4. Skin is closed with intrarrupted suture (Fig.No-4)

Post Operative Care

1. A course of parentral antibiotic
2. Pain killer
3. Fluid therapy as for the requirement
4. The limb is fruther immobilised Thomas splint application
5. The animal kept under restricted movement for 21 -30 days
6. Thomas splint removed after one month
7. Intramedullary pin removed affer 2-3 months

Intramedullary Pinning of Humerus in Large Animal

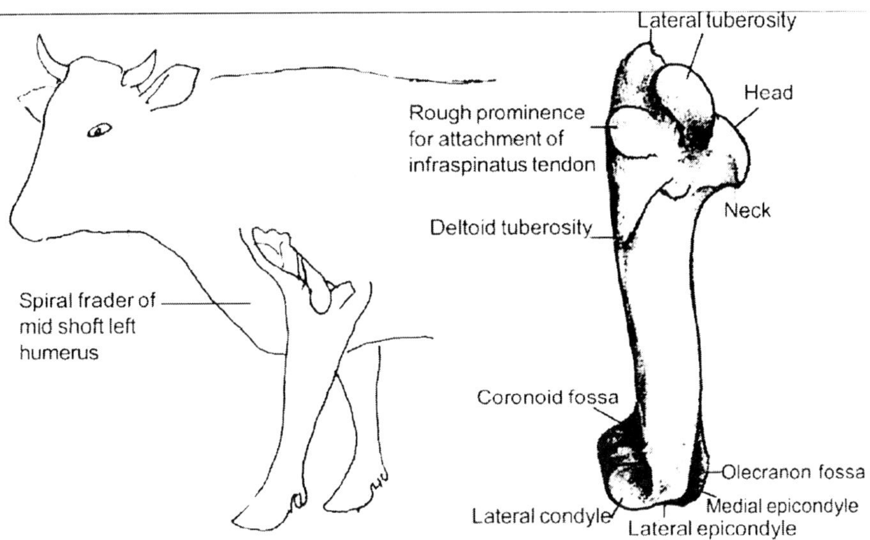

Fig. 1: Fracture of left humerus mid shaft **Fig. 2:** Left humerus of ox lateral view

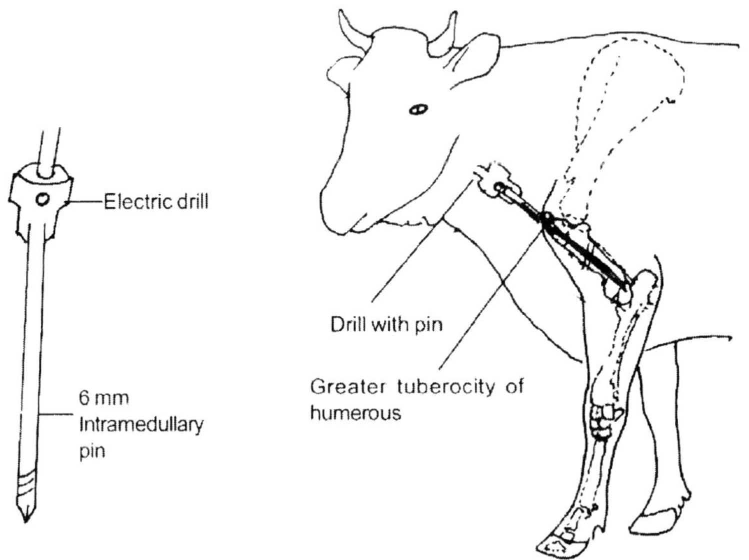

Fig. 3: Intramedullary pin with drill fitter **Fig. 4:** Close pinning of left humerus

Humerus Fracture Repair by Pinning and Thomas Splint

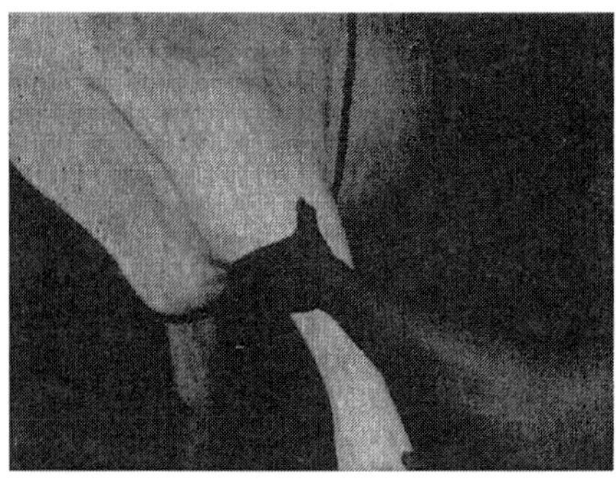

Fig. 1: Showing the fracture site of left humerus

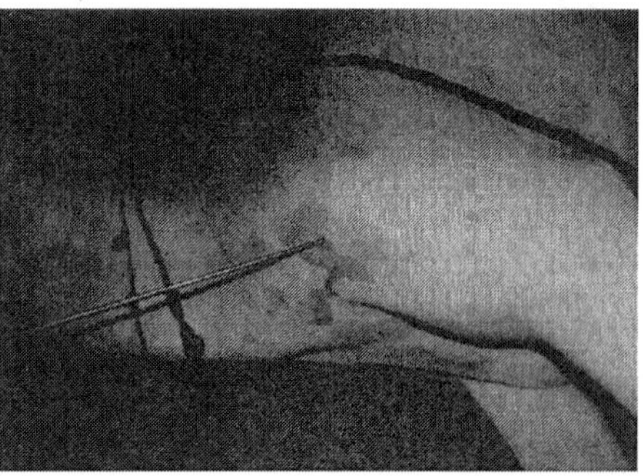

Fig. 2: Close pinning of fractured humerus

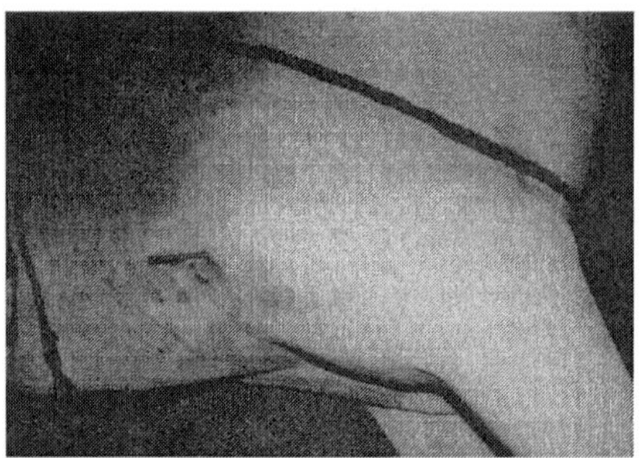

Fig. 3: Close pinning completed

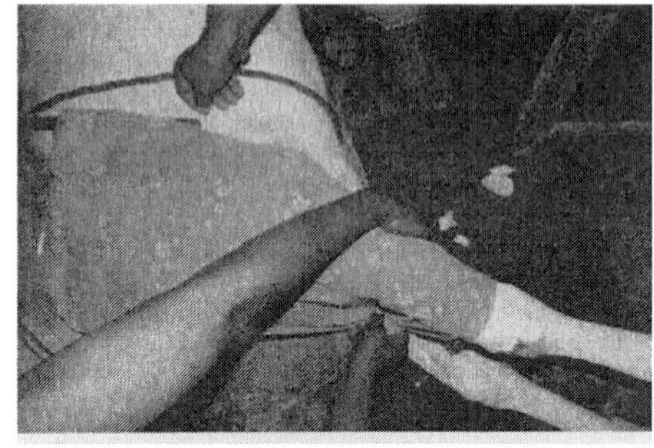

Fig. 4: Application of charge over the fracture site

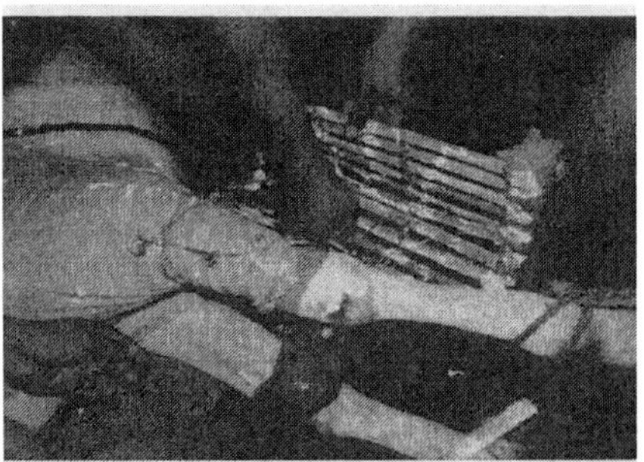

Fig. 5: Self impregnated gum in padded netted bamboo splint

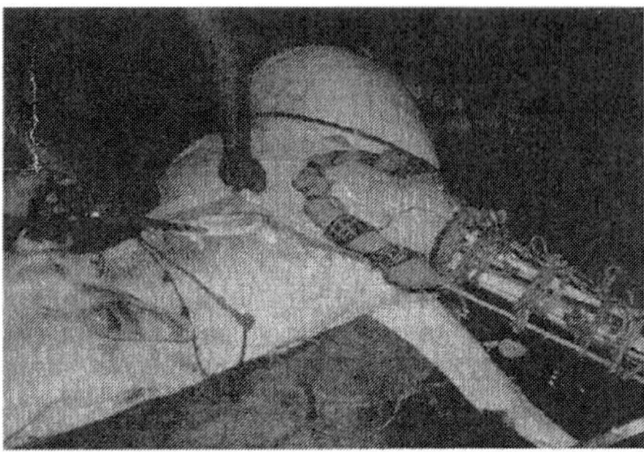

Fig. 6: Application of Thomas splint

60

Intramedullary Pinning of Femur in Large Animal

Definition

Fracture of femur comes under higher level fracture (Fig. 1) where the appropriate treatment is intramedullary pinning and modified Thomas Splint.

Requirement

1. Parentral sedative
2. Local anaesthesia
3. 6mm 1fit long intramedullary pin (Fig.No-3)
4. Electric bone drill
5. Bone hammer
6. Pin cutter

Surgical Anatomy

The detail of femur as be depicted (Fig. No.2)

Procedure

1. Point of the pin is placed open the trochanterin of fossa of femur bone.
2. Drilling of bone carry out till the pin remain in the medullary cavity of the femur bone
3. The length of pin is shortest with pin cutter, tip of the pin kept under the skin.
4. Skin is closed with intrarrupted suture (Fig.No-4)

Post Operative Care

1. A course of parentral antibiotic
2. Pain killer
3. Fluid therapy as for the requirement
4. The limb is fruther immobilised with Thomas splint.
5. The animal kept under restricted movement for 21 -30days
6. Thomas splint removed after one month
7. Intramedullary pin removed after 2-3 months.

Intramedullary Pinning of Femur in Large Animal

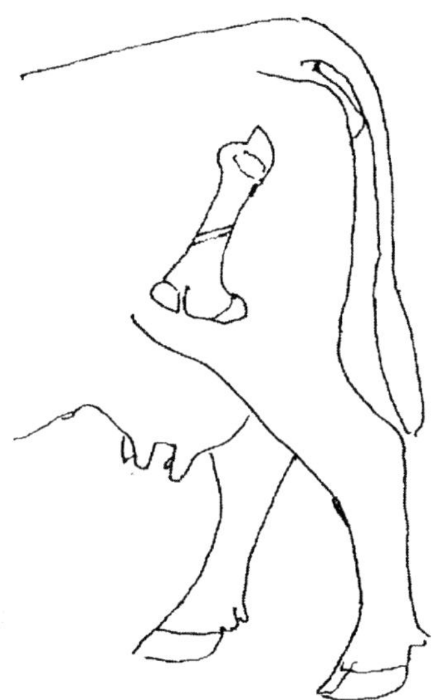

Fig. 1: Mid shaft fracture of left femur

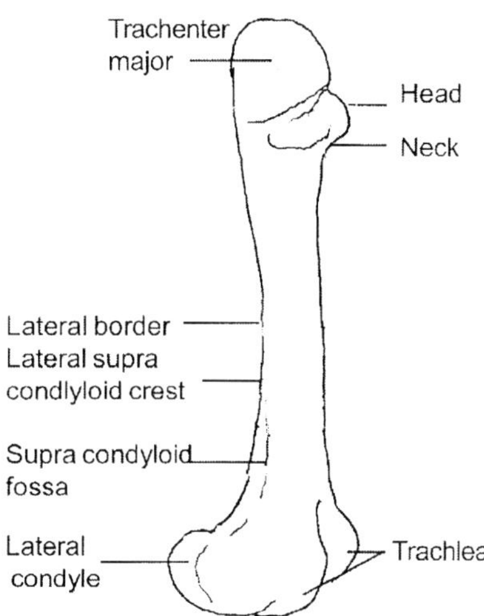

Fig. 2: Left femur of ox lateral view

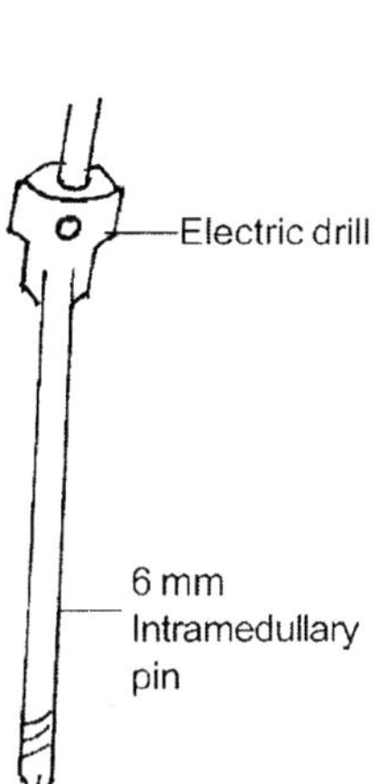

Fig. 3: Intramedullary pin with drill fitter

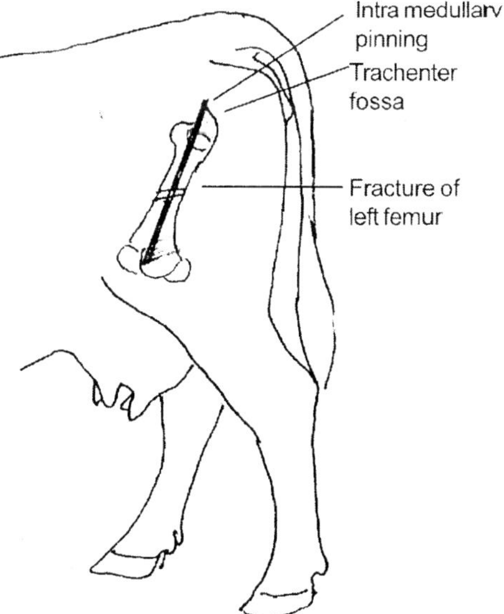

Fig. 4: Close pinning of left femur

Femur Fracture Repair By im Pinning

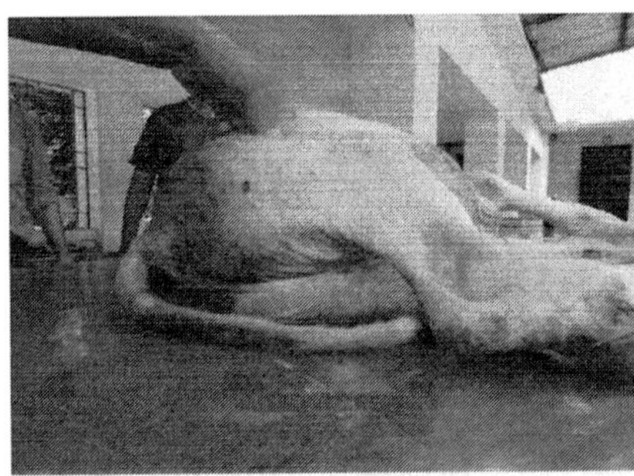

Fig. 1: Diagnosis of fracture by palpation

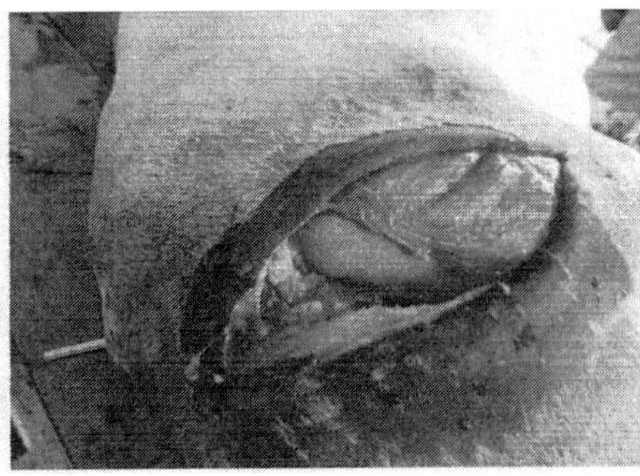

Fig. 2: Insertion of of IM pinning by open method.

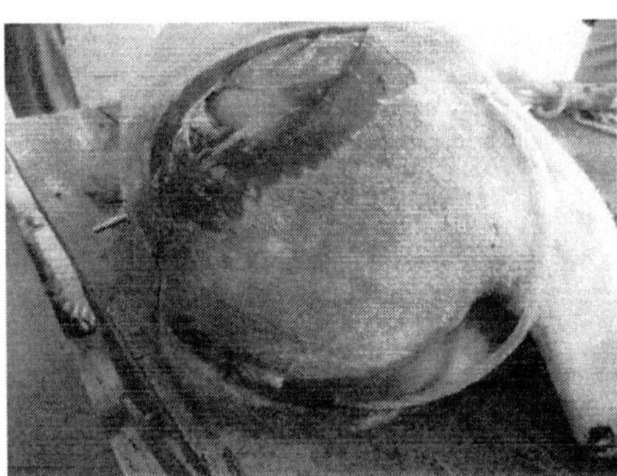

Fig. 3: Insertion of drainage catheter for clear out debrises.

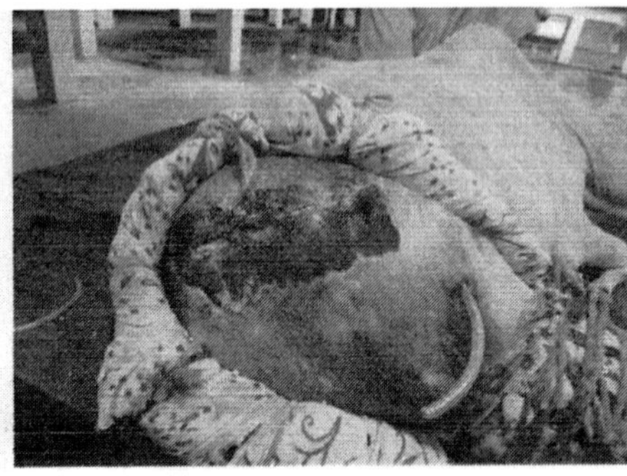

Fig. 4: Closing of skin after successful reduction of fracture fragment

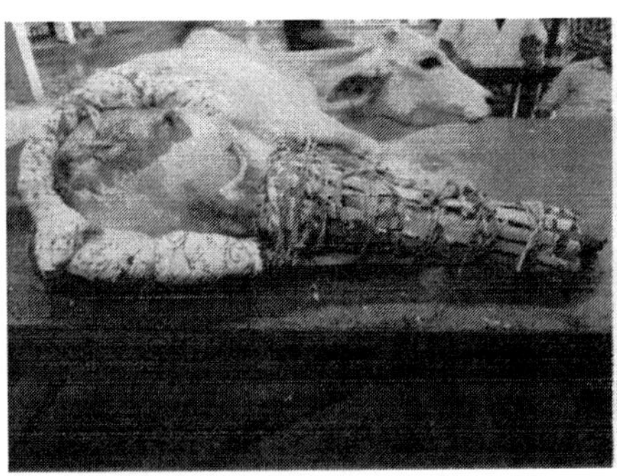

Fig. 5: Application of netted bamboo Thomas splint for immobilisation.

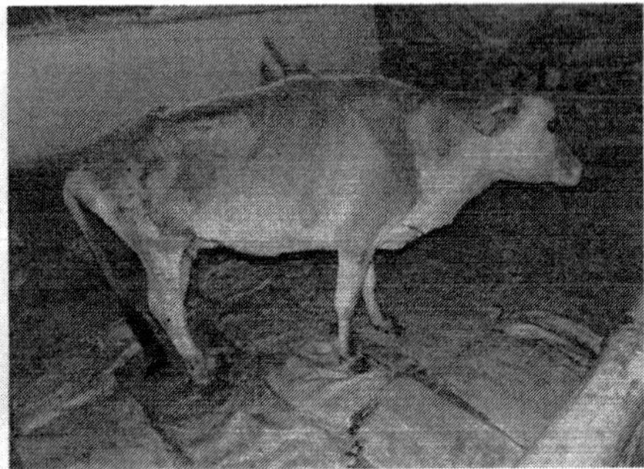

Fig. 6: Recovered animal after one month.

61

Modified Valpeau Sling for Highest Level Fore Limb Fracture

Clsssification

Fracture of upper third humerus, shoulder dislocation and scapula has been grouped under highest level fracture. (Fig.1)

Purpose

To know the method of casting the highest level fracture by modified valeau sling application.

Requirement

Thick 8 layer cotton padding, adhesive gum, 6"-8" long bandage rolls.

Procedure

1. Adhesive gum is applied over the fracture site covering an area below elbow and upto the hump.
2. An 8 layer thick absorbent cotton cloth is spread over the fracture site as well as to the other healthy site over the hump. (Fig.2).
3. The both end of the padded cloth near elbow are kept around the axilla and retained in position with gum. (Fig.2).
4. A long 6"-8" width bandage roll is use to retain the later padded cloth in position by moving it in figure 8 manner around the body including both the axilla. (Fig.3).
5. The bandage cloth rapping is retained in position with adhesive gum with cotton sutures.
6. A cross section of the padding as well as bandage roll rapping technique is shown in fig.4.

Post Operative Care

The animal is kept under restricted movement up to 1 month after which bandage is removed.

Modified Valpeau Sling for Highiest Level Fore Limb Fracture

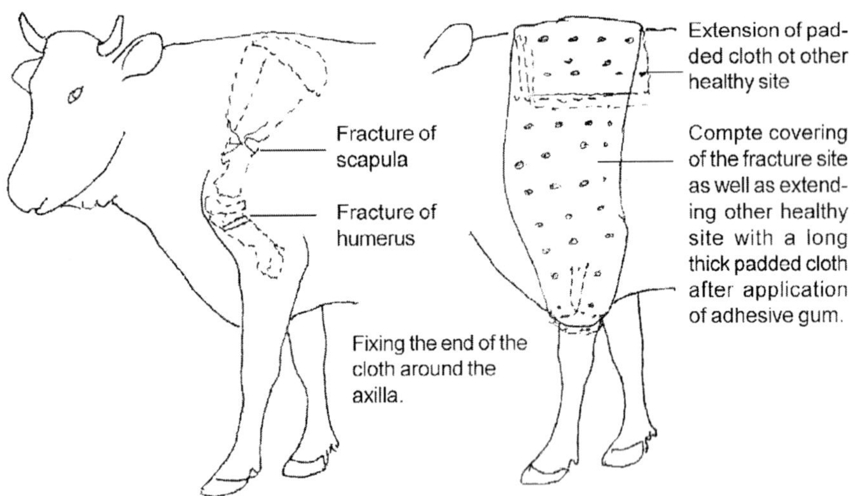

Fig. 1: Fracture of upper 3rd humerus and scapula comes under highest level

Fig. 2: Covering of the fracture site as **well as other healthy site of hte body** with padded cloth.

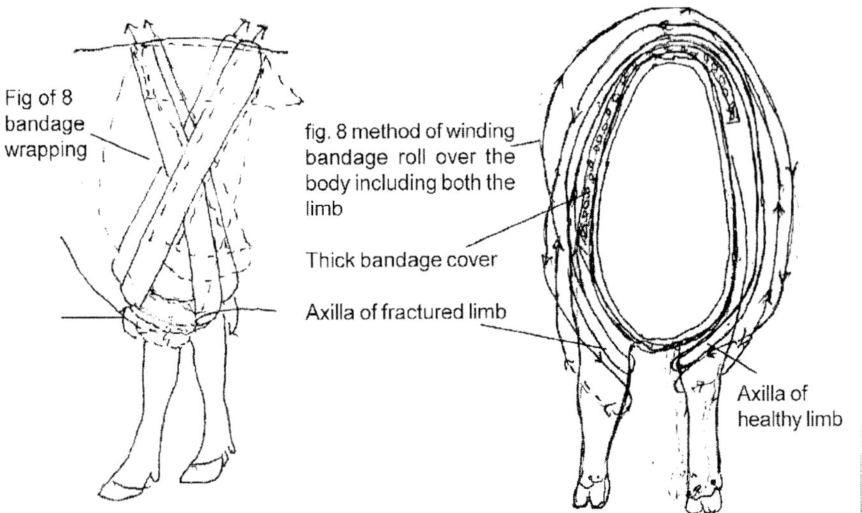

Fig. 3: Fixation of padded cloth over the fractured site with long bandage in a fig. of 8 manner anchoring both the axila.

Fig. 4: A cross section of the body near the therax showing the method of wrapp cotton padding and bandage rolls.

62

Modified Velpeau Sling for Highest Level Fracture of Hind Limb

Indication: Highest level fracture (femur fracture) (Fig. 1)

Treatment: Modified Velpeau Sling application

Requisite

1. Adhesive gum
2. Damage Cloth

Procedure for Velpeau sling application

1. Gum is applied over the thigh region of the fracture site as well as on the healthy opposite side of the thigh.
2. A 4 layer thick cloth is spread over the area in the affected side as well as the healthy side. (Fig. 2)
3. With the help of long 6-8 inch width cotton bandage the prefixed cloth is retained in position by wrapping around the thigh of the affected site as well as including opposite healthy thigh around its groin region for perfect retention of the cooptation bandage. (Fig. 3)
4. A pictorial representation of thick bandage cloth & figure of '8' movement of the gauze bandage has been depicted. (Fig. 4(a) & 4(b))

Post operative care: Animal is kept in restricted movement for 15-21 days.

Modified Velpeau Sling for Highest Level Fracture of Hind Limb

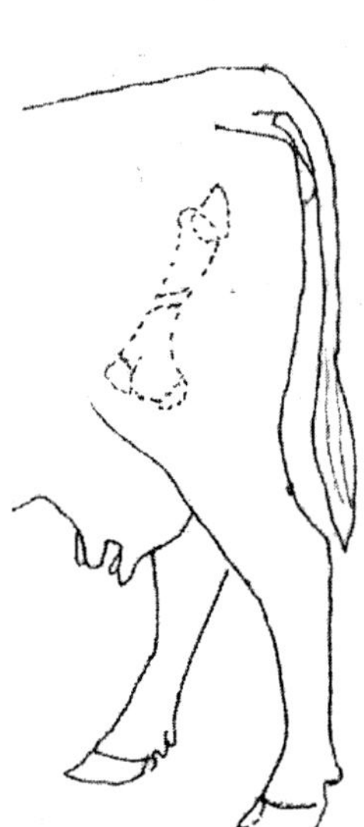

Fig. 1: Highest level fracture (femur fracture)

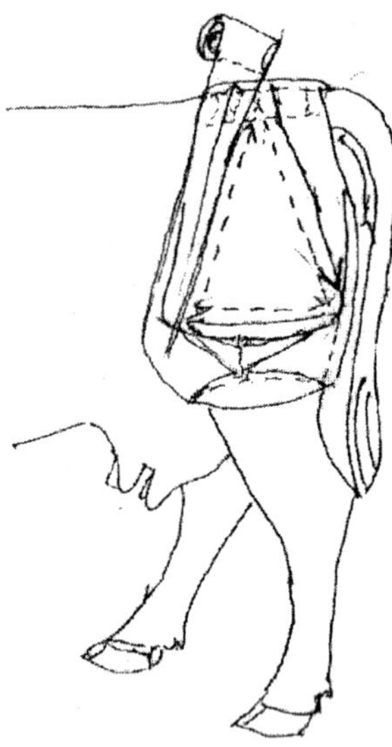

Fig. 2: Application of cloth

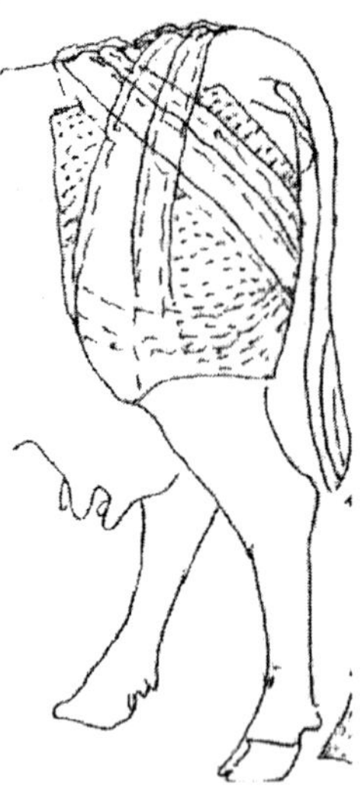

Fig. 3: Application of cooptation bandage

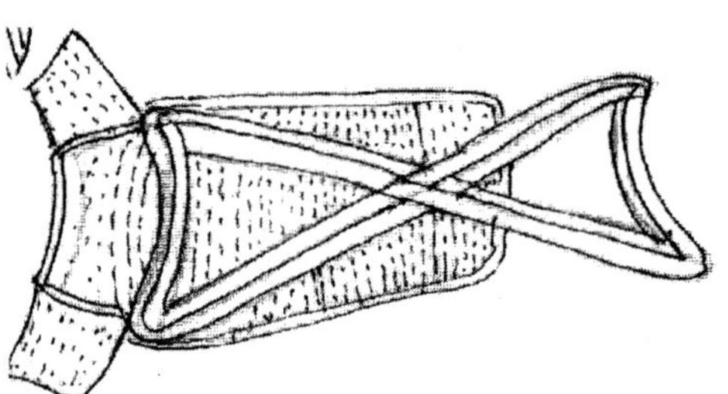

Fig. 4: (a). Thick bandage cloth.

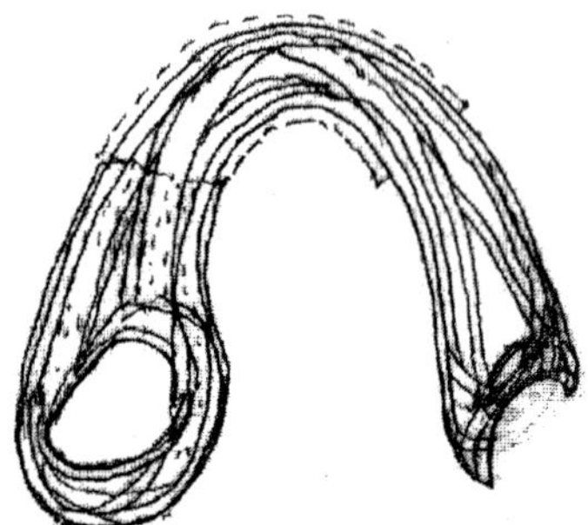

Fig. 4: (b). Figure of '8' gauze bandage

Large Animal Thomas Splint

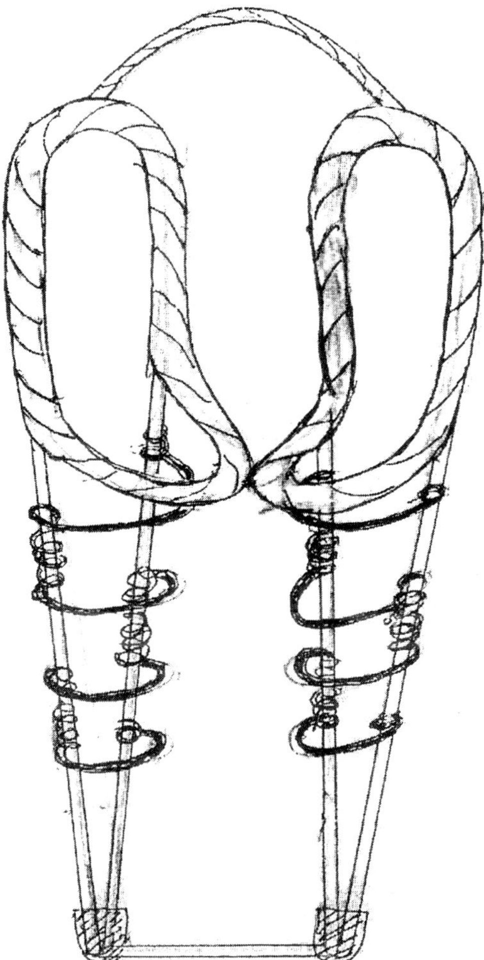

Fig. 5: Conjoint double Thomas splint for pelvic girdle fracture repair

63

Different Types of Thomas Splints

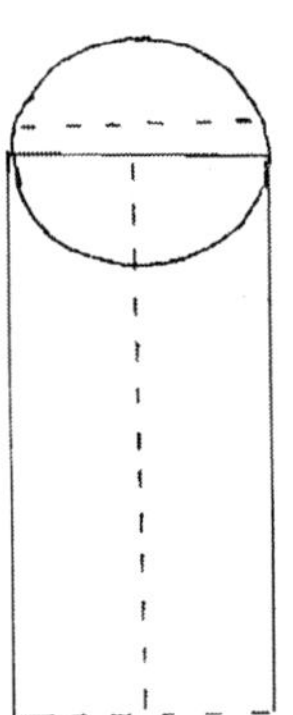

Fig. 1: Fundamental structure of Thomas splint.

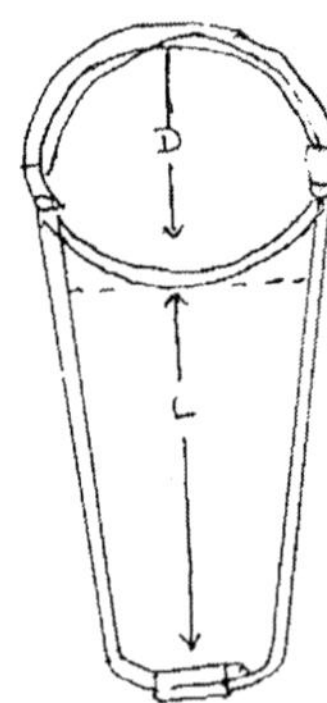

Fig. 2: Diagram of Thomas splint showing dimensions used in formula for etermin-ing rod length.

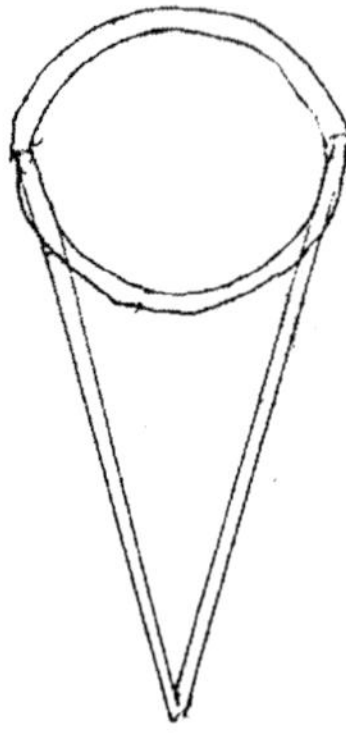

Fig. 3: Simplest model of thomas splint.

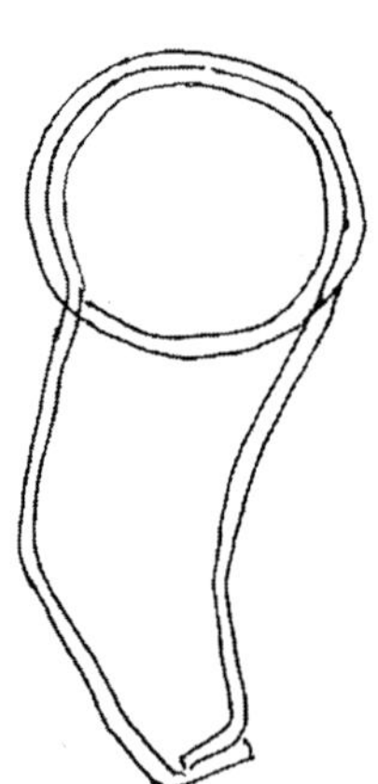

Fig. 4: Thomas splint fashioned with No. 9 wire by J.F. Thomas (1938).

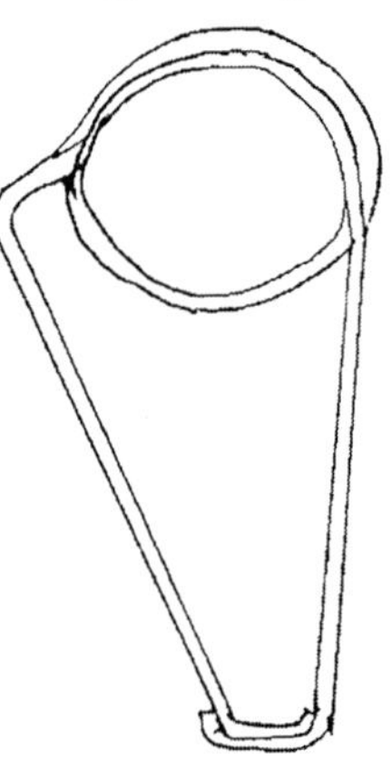

Fig. 5: Thomas splint prepared by W.F. Guard for a Jersey Fleifer (1953).

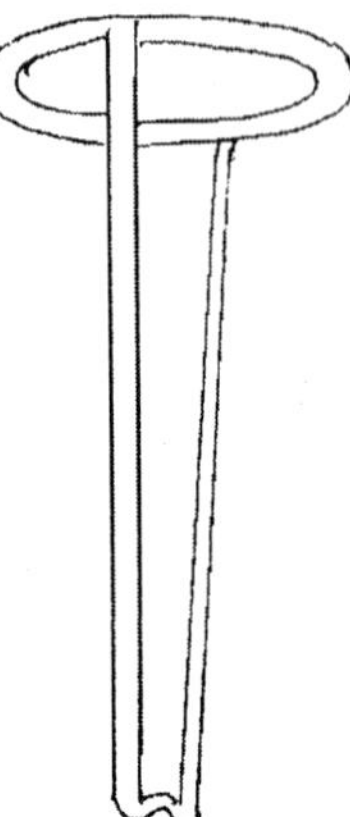

Fig. 6: Thomas splint for man (1957) *Courtesy*- Down Bros. Ltd.).

64

Thomas Splint Used in Animals (For Fore limb)

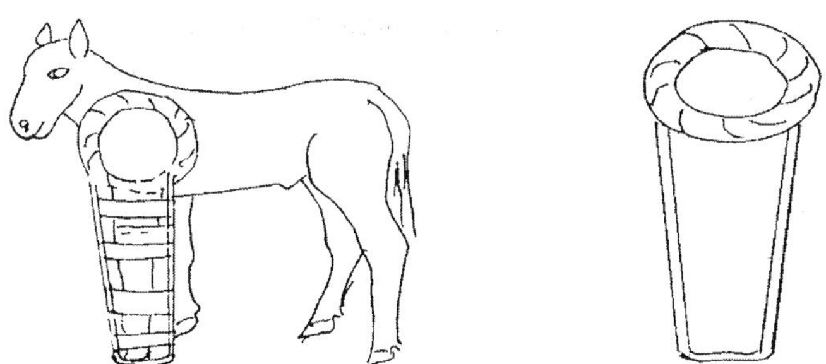

Fig. 1: Thomas splint applied to a horse (Thomas, J.F. 1939)

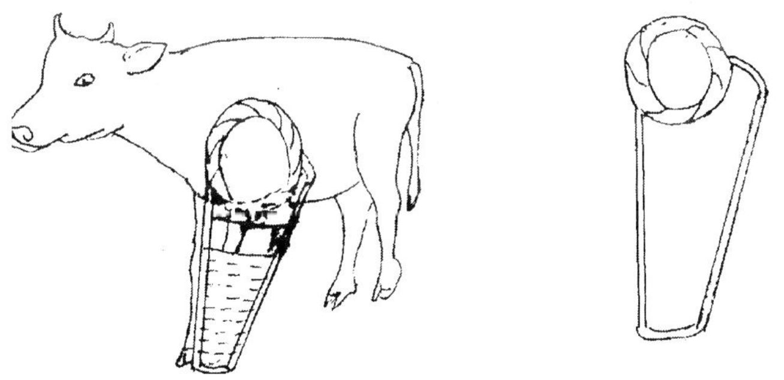

Fig. 2: Thomas splint applied to a buffalo.

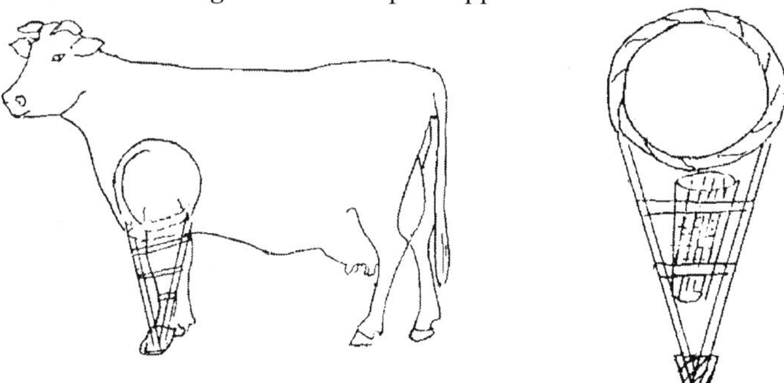

Fig. 3: Conventional method of fixation of Thomas splint using plaster of pans cast.

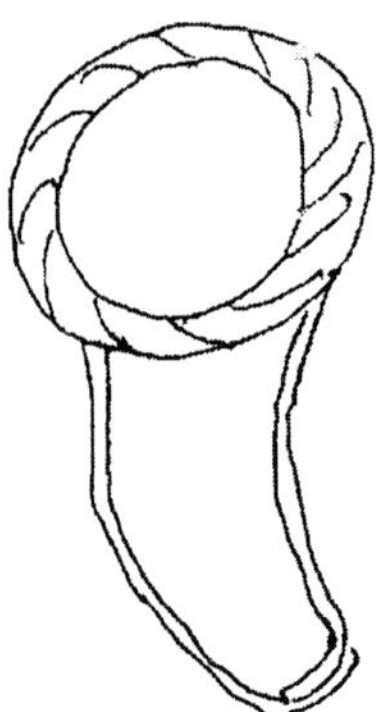

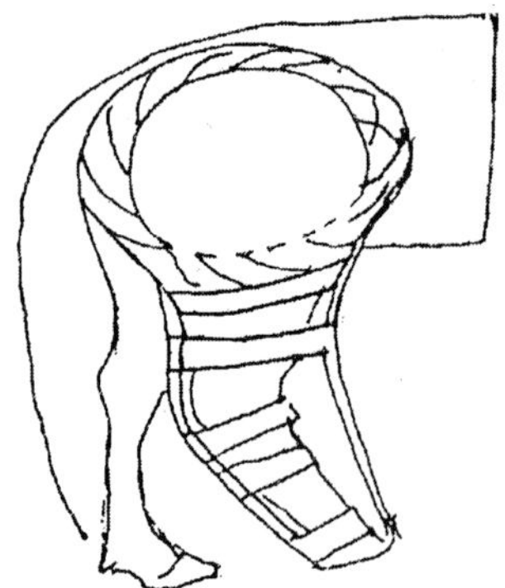

Fig. 4: Thomas splint applied to a horse (J.F., Guard 1939)

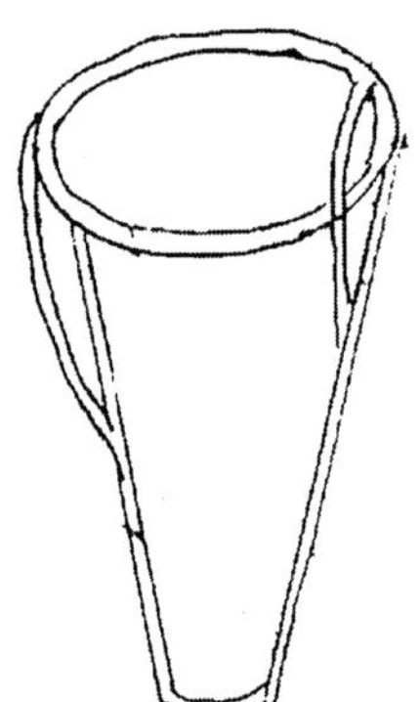

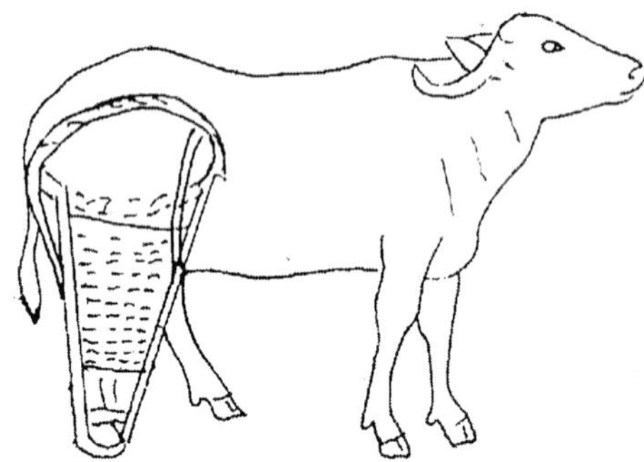

Fig. 5: Thomas splint applied to a buffalo

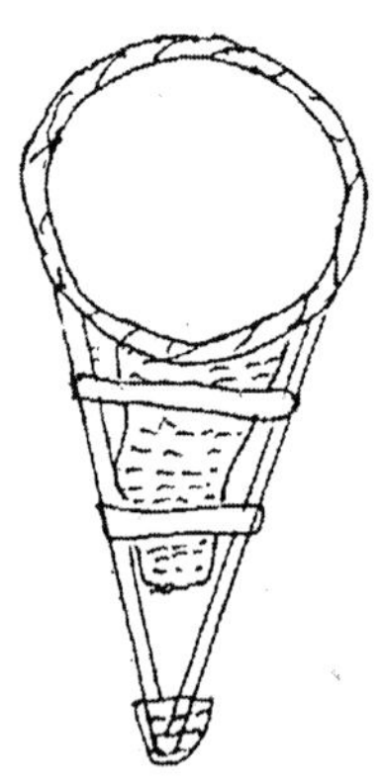

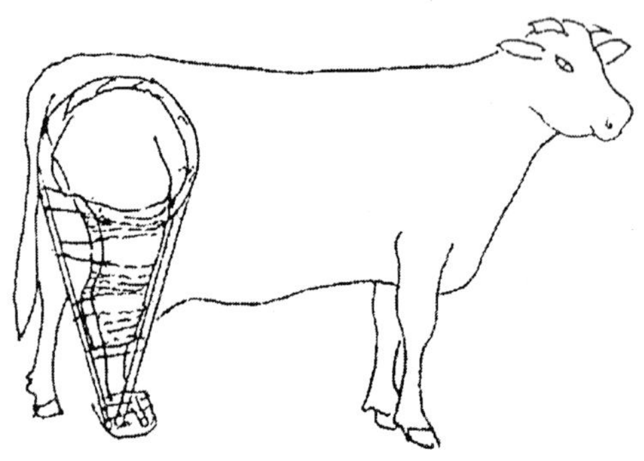

Fig. 6: Conventional method of fixation of Thomas splint using plaster of paris cast.

65

List of Requisite for Preparation of Large Animal Thomas Splint

1. Strong bamboo

   4 feet long of 4 inch diameter
2. Gl.Wire

   6 mm diameter of 34 kg G.l. wire

Approx, age of the animal	Height of the animal	No. of rounds in Thomas Splint Ring	Diameter of Wire
Less than 1 year	10 to 21 inch	1	3 to 6 inch
1 to 3 years	22 to 37 inch	2	7 to 10 inch
3 to 6 years	38 to 39 inch	3	11 to 16 inch
Above 6 years	50 to 57 inch	4	17 to 22 inch

3. Jute / gunny bag- 1/2 kg jute is required.
4. Jute thread- 300gm
5. Cotton bandage roll-6 inch and 4 pieces
6. Bicycle tube 3 feet one

List of Requisite for Preparation of Large Animal Thomas Splint

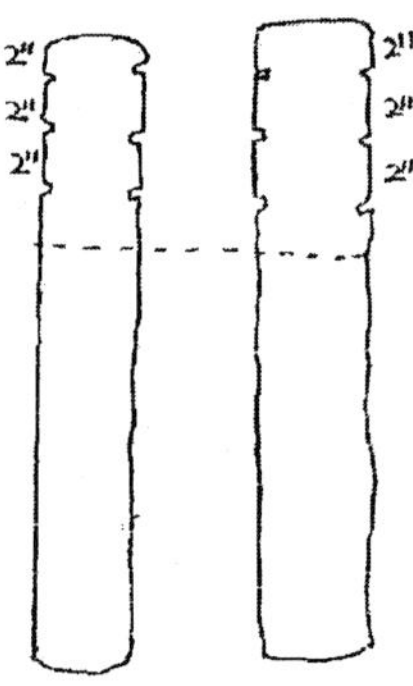

Fig. 1: Bamboo Three nicks 2" apart tying string with ring

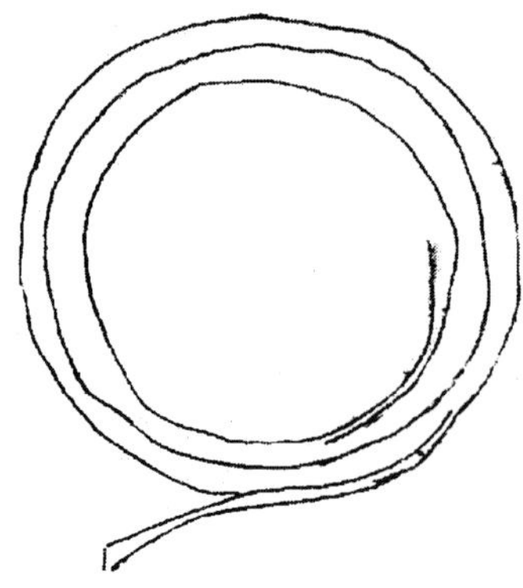

Fig. 2: Selfwinding G.l. wirering.

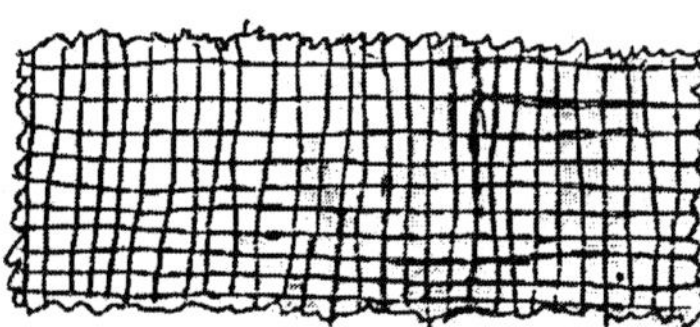

Fig. 3: Jute gunny bag

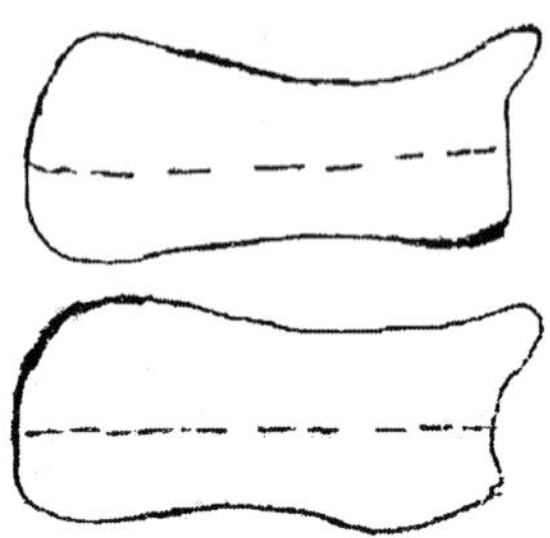

Fig. 4: Cycle tube 1'X2

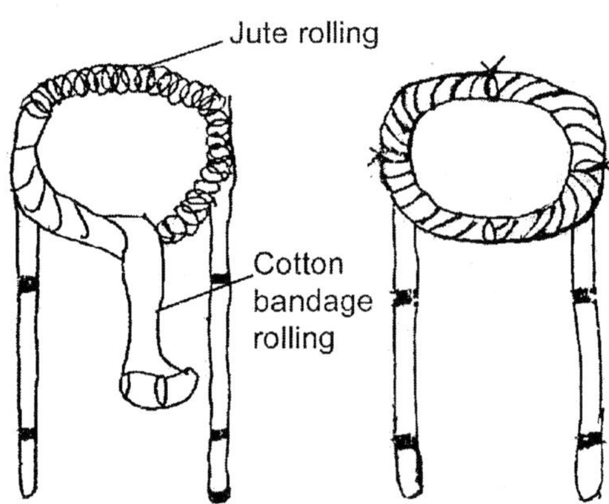

Fig. 5: Starting of cotton bandaging around jute bandaging

Fig. 6: Completion of cotton bandaging

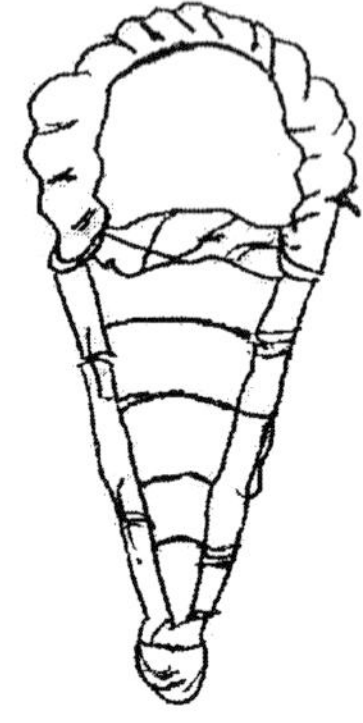

Fig. 7: Complete Thomas splint net fabrication

66

Measurement of Ring of Thomas Splint for Large Animal

Aim:- To know the measurement for preparation of an appropriate size of ring of Thomas splint for a large animal.

Objective: Measurement of an appropriate size Thomas splint essential to avoid complications like tight fitting which may affect bone healing.

Materials required: 6mm G.l. wire, jute thread

Procedure

- Length of humerus or femur bone takenwith help of a jute thread (Fig. 1)
- The measured length is multiplied by 3 times and the length is marked.(Fig. 2)
- A cicular ring is prepared using G. I. wire prepared ring is fitted to limb of animal .the appropriate size of ring is assessed visually by adjusting G.l. wire as well as in considering the reference points for limb. (Fig.1)

• Reference point for fore limb

1) Close to axilla
2) infront of shoulder joint
3) Up to tuberus spine of scapula .

• Reference point for hind limb

1) Close to groin
2) Behind angle of illium
3) Infrontof pin bone

- Length of wire required in circle is marked. (Fig. 3)
- Length of wire is required in circle and 3 $^1/_2$ times length of humerus or femur bone measured in rope are matched . In an ideal measurement both length should match (Fig. 4).

Measurement of Ring of Thomas Splint for Large Animal

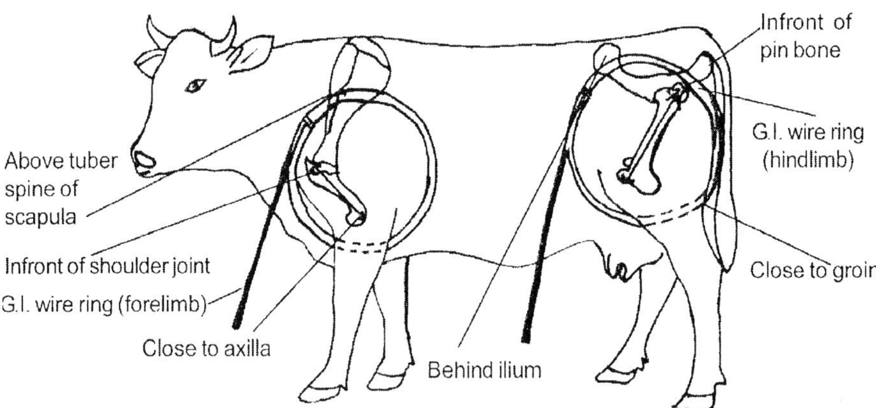

Fig. 1: Showing the reference point on the bone for accurate measurement of wire

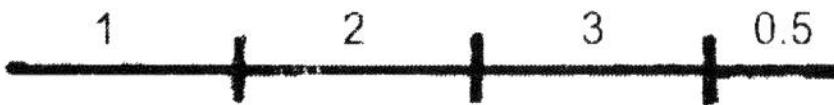

Fig. 2: Three and halftimes the length of humerus and femur.

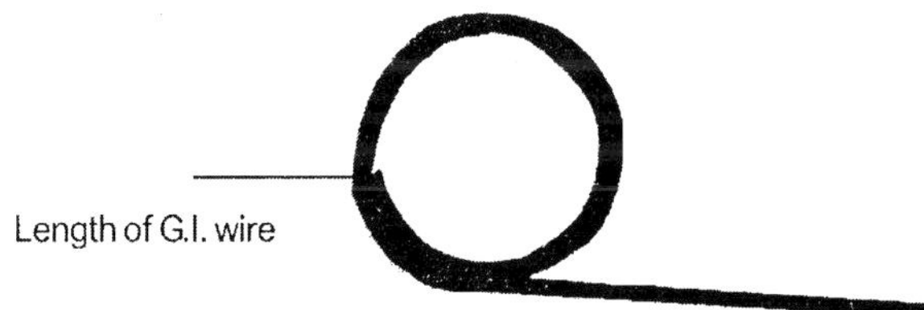

Fig. 3: Measurement of size of ring with the help of G.I. wire

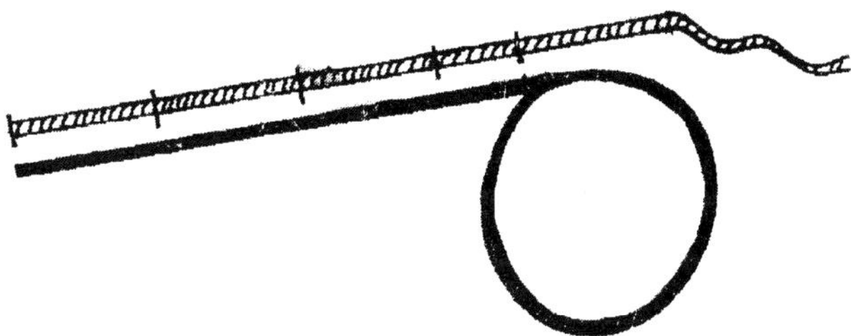

Fig. 4: Matching hte measurement of G.l. wire 3.5 times length of humerus or femur bone (Both measurements should be matched)

67

Wire Rings Required for Different Age Group of Animals

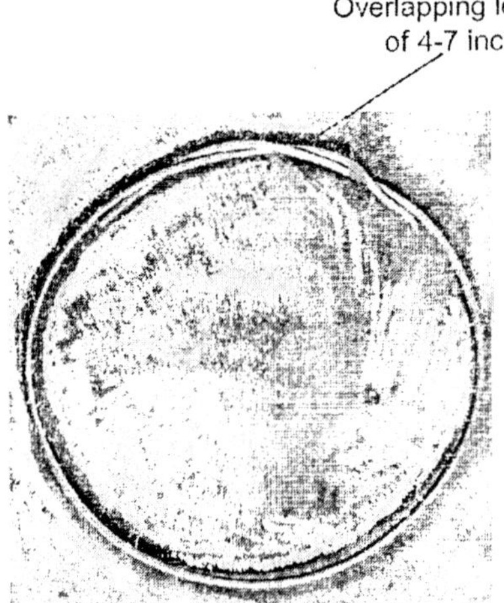

Fig. 1: One round ring for young calf (Age less than 1 year)

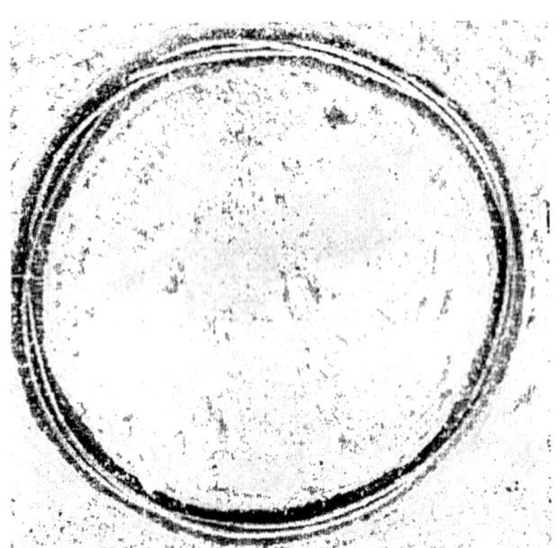

Fig. 2: Two round self-winding fc adult calf (Age 2 years to 4 years)

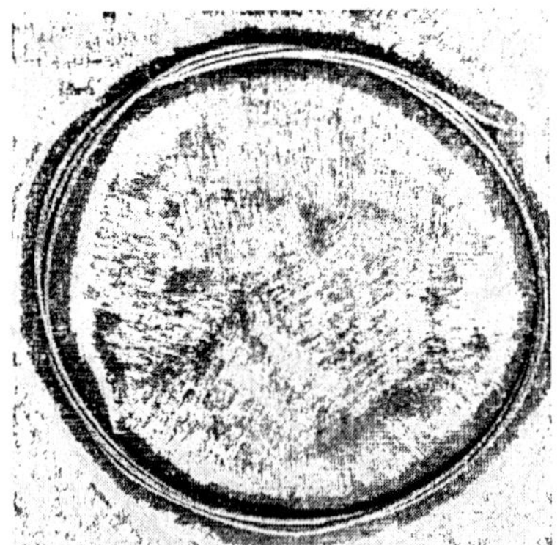

Fig. 3: Three round self-winding ring for middle age cattle (Age 4 years to 6 years)

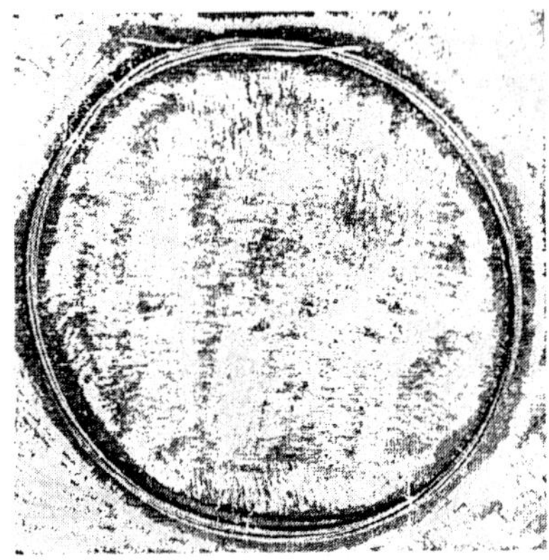

Fig. 4: Four round self-winding ring for old age cattle (Age above 6 years)

68

Preparation of Side Bars of Large Animal Thomas Splint

Aim

To know the methods of preparation of side bars for large animal Thomas splint fabrication

Procedure

I. Two strong dry matured bamboo splints are of more than actual length of Thomas splint are prepared, (figure 1)

II. Three nicks at a distance of 2 inch are grooved on the side of the side of the splint at one end of the splints for keeping the tying end of the ropes in position (figure -2)

III. The bamboo splints at the lateral ends are thinned to some extent. For knob kniiting of splint to the metal ring by making an arc (figures).

IV. All the steps are depicted in figure 1 -4.

V. Before fixing the metal ring with the bamboo extention splint the thinned ends are emersed inside water for easy arching of the bamboo splint.

Preparation of Side Bars of Large Animal Thomas Splint

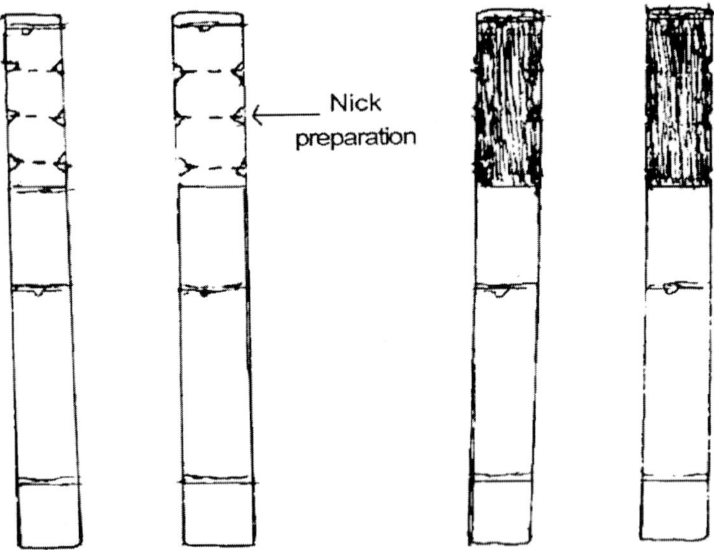

Fig. 1: Two equal size strong bamboo

Fig. 2: Three nicks for tying string

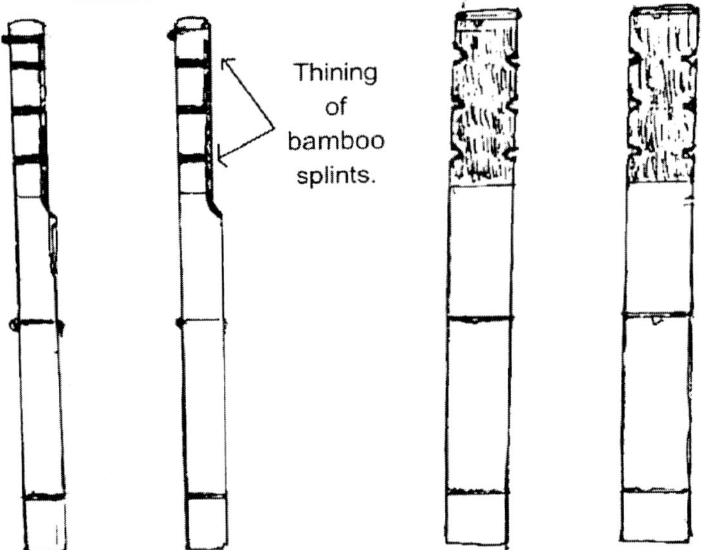

Fig. 3: Ring type area is thinned to make an arc.

Fig. 4: Final bamboo splint

69

Method of Tying Ring with Bamboo Splint and Description

Purpose

Method of tying with bamboo splint with ring is very important because of the following points.

A string fitting with the bamboo splint is required as with loose fitting with it may come up at any stage before actual bone healing.

Method of Tying

1. Overlapped psortion of ring kept upward.
2. Bamboo extension kept parallel to ring.
3. The ring is tied with the middle neck of the prepared bamboo splint with a clove knot using 6" long small rope (Fig -1).
4. The bamboo splint is lifted upward & start tying the upper portion of bamboo splint with ring.
5. First 8-10 circular round followed by 3-4 fig '8' shaped wrappings done.
6. Then tie with small rope of clove knot (Fig -2).
7. The lower half of bamboo splint is pressed to the ring , first 8-10 circular round followed by 3-4 fig '8' round.
8. Then tie with small rope of clove knot (Fig -3).
9. Second bamboo splint is tied with ring in the same manner.
10. After tying ring with bamboo splint, both bamboo splint should remain parallel to each other (Fig -4) so that upper portion of ring will be equal to lower half.

Tying Bamboo Splints with The Ring for Fabrication of Large Animal Thomas Splint

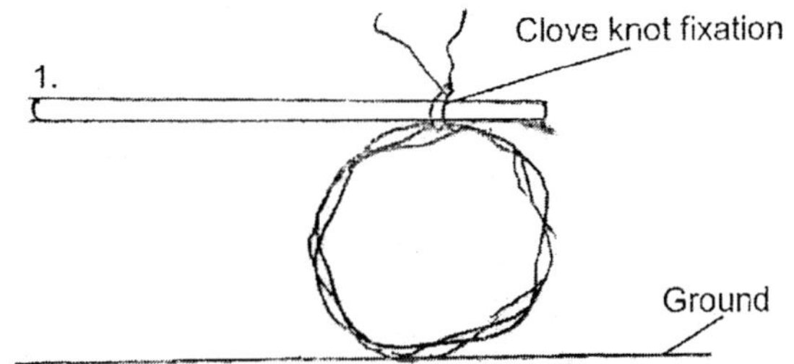

Fig. 1: Fixation of ring with bamboo with clove knot.

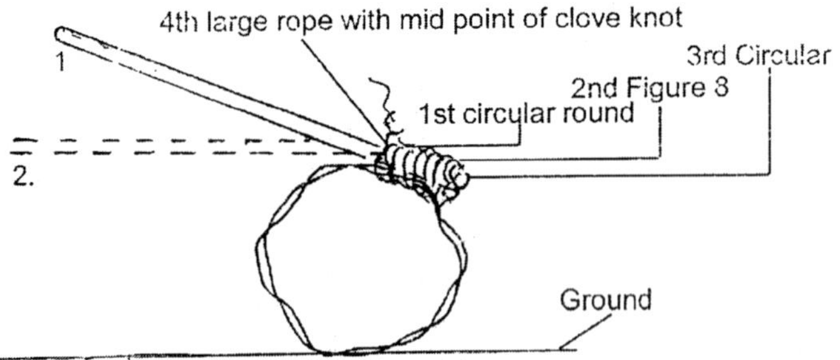

Fig. 2: Upper half tying.

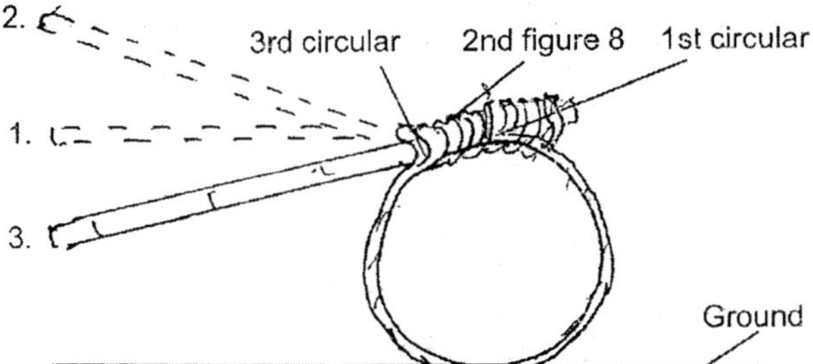

Fig. 3: Lower half tying.

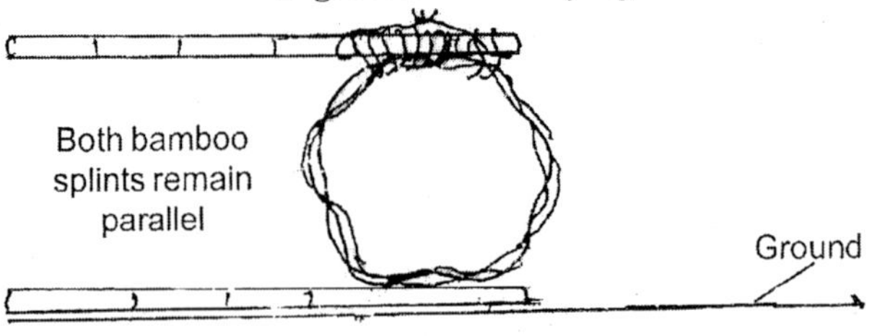

Fig. 4: Final fixation of bamboo split with ring

70

Padding of Thomas Splint Ring with Jute & Cotton Bandage

Aim

To knw the method of softening the ring of the perpendicular Thomas splint to avoid direct trauma of the metal wire with the skin.

Materials required

Jute /thin gunny bag,bandage roll,cotton threads

Procedure

The jute/gunny bags are rolled over the rings of the Thomas splint in a systematic manner from one end to other end.(fig; 1,2)

The lower half of the ring is padded more than of upper half

After complete covering of jute retention of jute wrapping are made with knots of cotton threads at several places(fig;3)

Cotton bandages are wrapped to cover the jute padding(fig;4)

Finally the cotton bandase wrapping are held in position with knots of cotton threads of several places

Padding of Thomas Splint Ring with Jute and Cotton Bandage

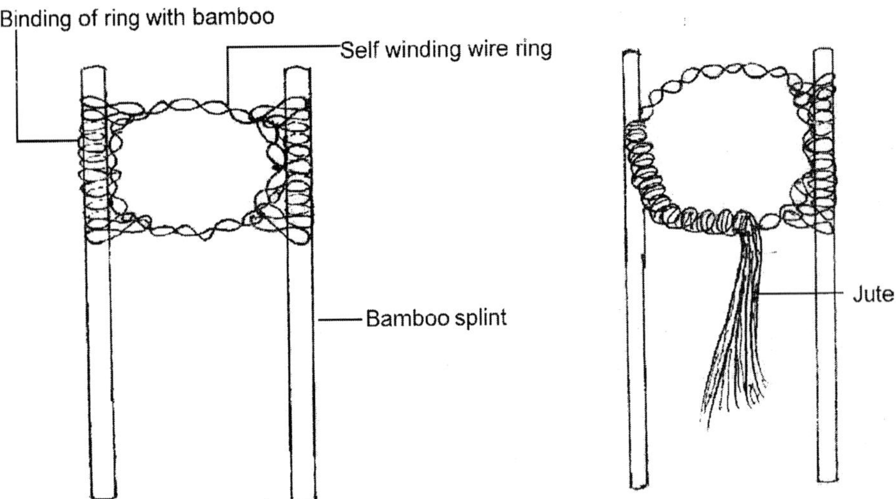

Fig. 1: Fixation of bamboo splint with ring

Fig. 2: Starting of bandaging of jute on ring.

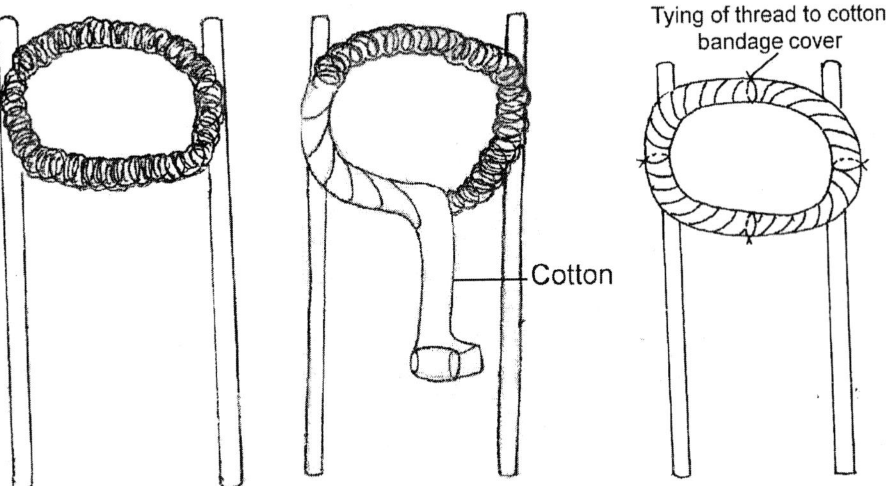

Fig. 3: Completion of covering of jute padding

Fig. 4: Starting of cotton bandaging around jute bandaging

Fig. 5: Completion of cotton bandaging

71

Medial Bending of Lower Half of Thomas Splint

Aim: Bending of the lower half of the ring of Thomas splint to an angle 45-60degree to comfort the limb and to provide free circulation.

Importance

After tieing the ring with bamboo splint and padding the ring with jute and cotton .bending the lower half of the ring upto more than 45 degree angle is highly essential because of placement of the fractured limb within the ring of Thomas splint comfortably, so as to the flow of blood circulation in fractured limb uninterruptedly.

Method

- The padded Thomas splint is kept upon a border of a barandah. Both the bamboo splint close to the ring are held strongly .the lower half of ring pressed downward with the help of an attendant.
- After bending the lower half of the ring both the lower end of bamboo splint will close together.

Medial Bending of Lower Half of Thomas Splint

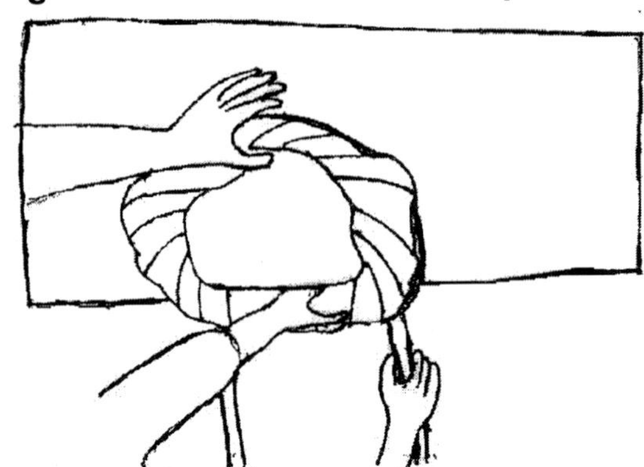

Fig. 1: Bending of lower half of ring of Thomas splint

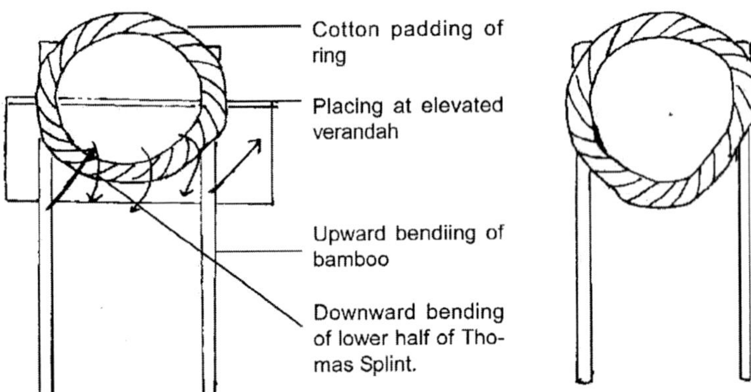

Fig. 2: Bending of lower half of ring of Thomas splint

Fig. 3: Front view.

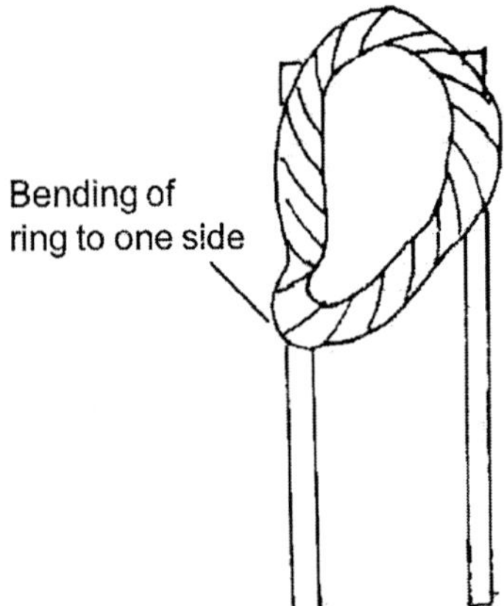

Fig. 4: Side view.

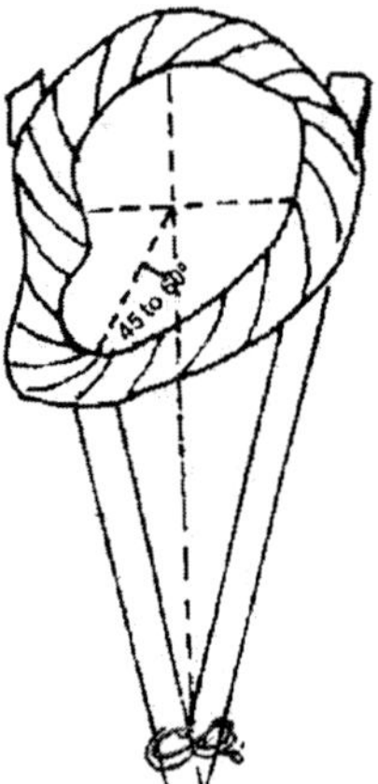

Fig. 5: Complete Thomas splint

72

Measurement of Length of Thomas Splint, Shortening of Length & Padding of Distal End

Aim: To know the actual length of a Thomas splint & measurement for an animal.

Procedure

1. Animal is kept in lateral recumbancy with affected limb upward.
2. After padding & medical bending of Thomas splint, it is fitted upon the fractured limb.
3. At the time of measurement, the limb should be kept vertical to body for accurate measurement, otherwise the length of Thomas splint may be shorteror longer if the limb is kept forward or backward respectively.
4. The ring of the Thomas splint is kept close to the axilla (forelimb), groin (hind limb).
5. Limb is put downward & Thomas splint is pushed upward keeping both the extension bamboo of Thomas splint in crossed manner, measurement of length of Thomas splint is taken up to the bulb of the heel & mark is recorded.
6. The excess length is trimmed short (figure-1). Two nicks are made on the distal end for retaining the thread in position.
7. Both the distal ends are tied together with thread, soft padding is placed at the site where hoof is to be kept & retained in position with bandage (figure-3).

Measurement of Length of Thomas Splint in Large Animal

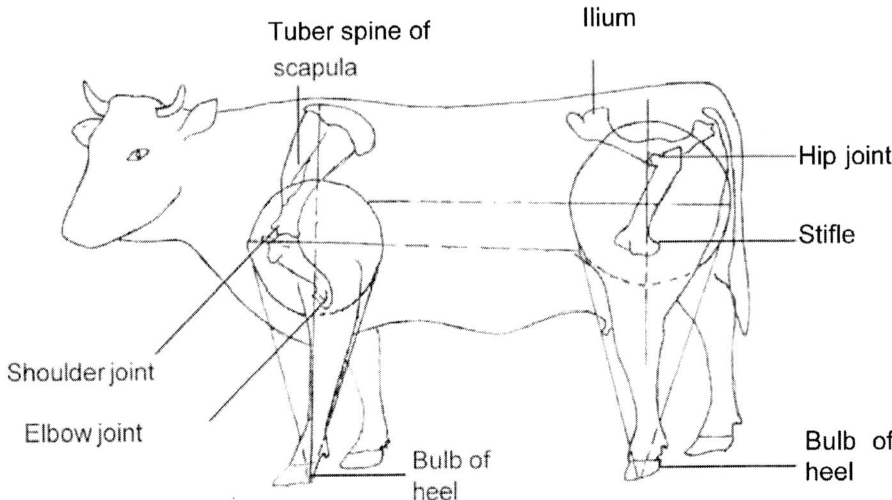

Fig. 1: Showing correct method of taking measurement of thomas splint by positioning the leg in 90° angle to the body

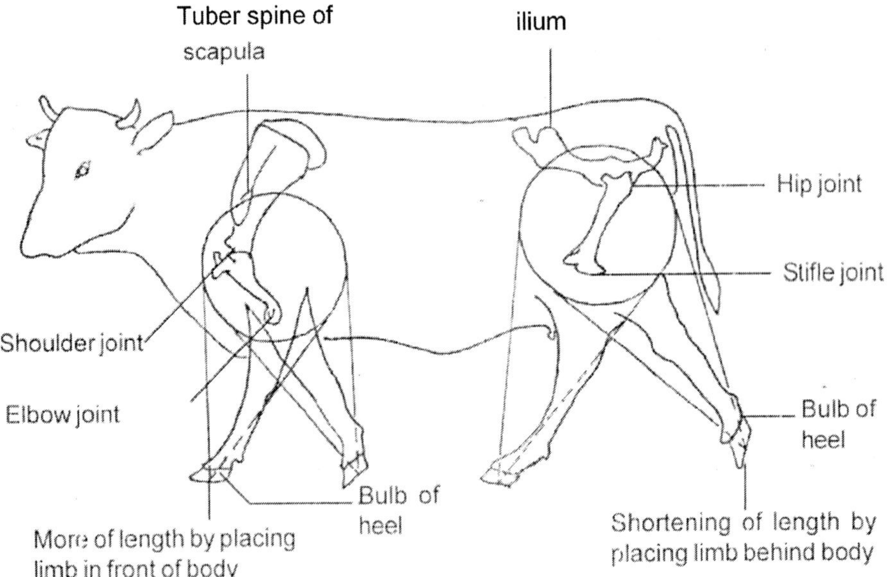

Fig. 2: Showing incorrect method of taking measurement of thomas splint

73

Net Fabrication in Large Animals Thomas Splint

Indicaion

To know the importance and method of net fabrication in large animals thomas splint. Objective;

1. To make the application of thomas splint lightest.
2. To avoid use of plaser of pahs bandage.
3. To prevent possible all direction of the immobilised limb in thomas splint.

Method

1. Afterfabricationofthomas splint as per required measurement against the animal finally net fabrication is made.
2. For net fabrication, 6 mm Gl wire is necessary.
3. The main technique is the wire is moved in such a manner that the bend of netting always remain towards the ring bending of thomas splint so that immobilised limb can be placed within the medial bend of groove and wire netting. (.Fig.1)
4. In another method wire netting can be given through the drill hole on the extension splint of thomas splint. Fig. 2(a) and 2 (b).

Measurement of Length of Thomas Splint, Shortening of Length & Padding of Distal and

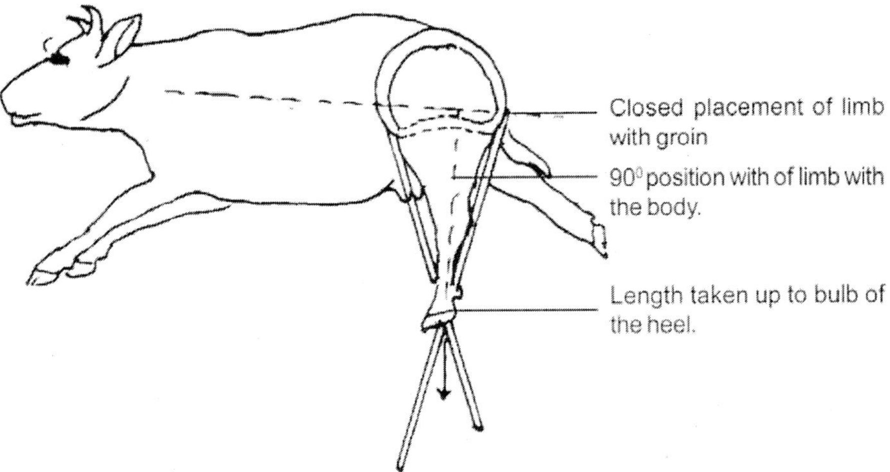

Fig. 1: Position of animal for length measurement of Thomas splint

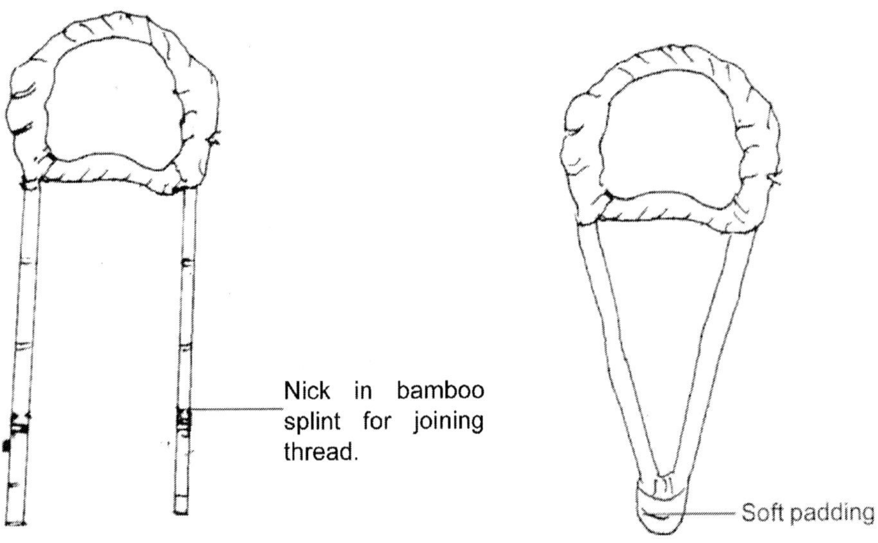

Fig. 2: Shortening level or trimming of extra length.

Fig. 3: Soft padding to avoid pressure injury to foot.

Net Fabrication of Thomas Splint

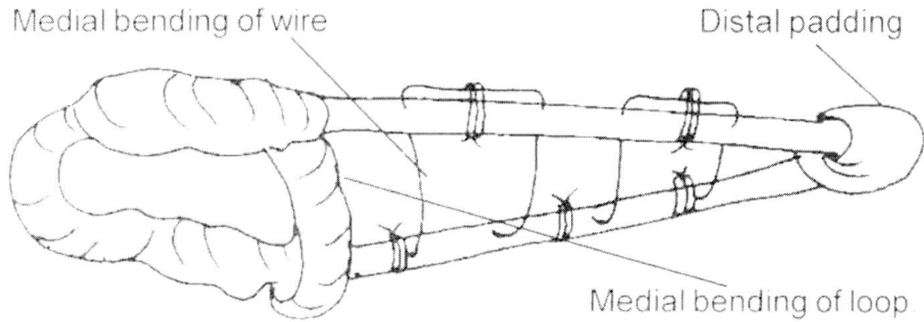

Fig. 1: Longitudinal

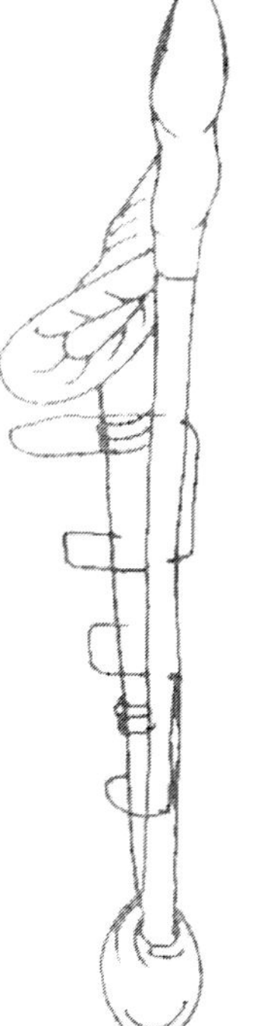

Fig. 2: Side view

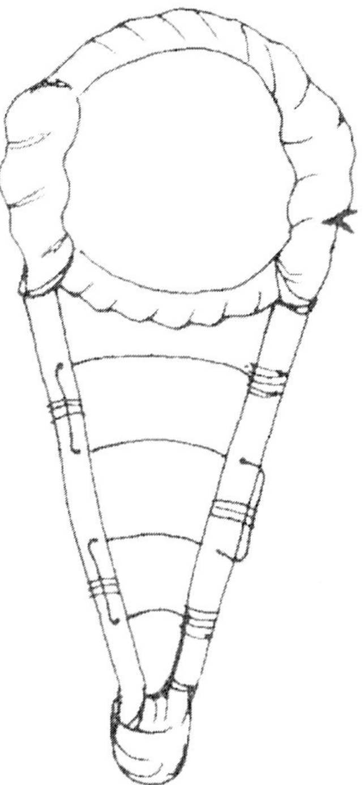

Fig. 3: Front view

74

Fitting Thomas Splint and Its Retention Over Gum Bandage

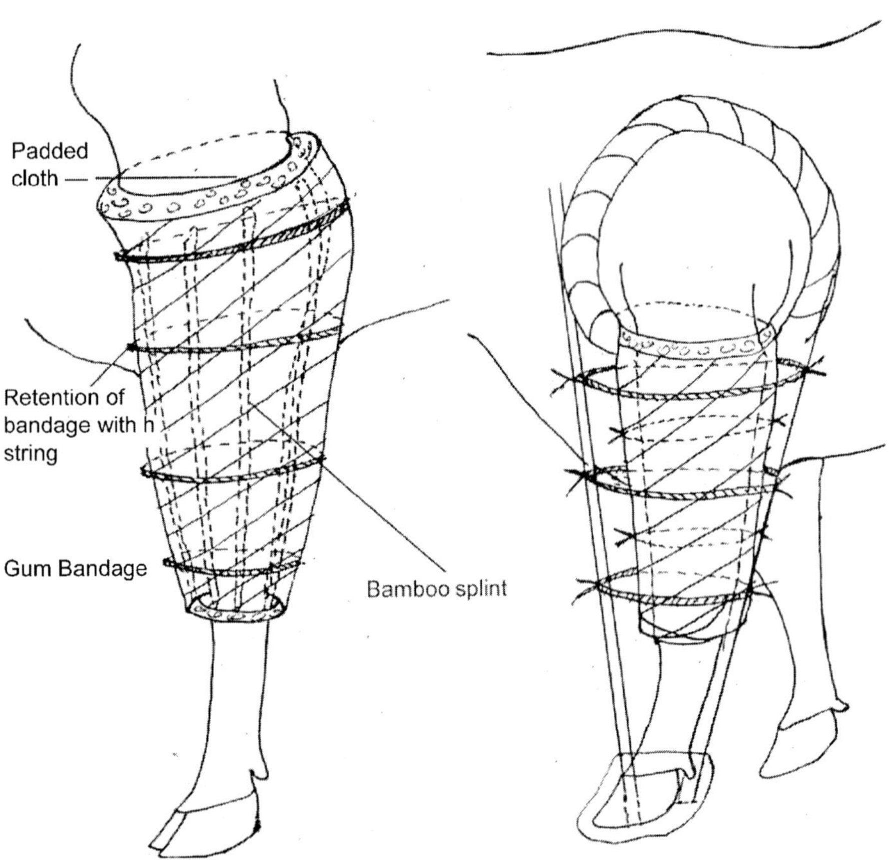

Fig. 1: Immobilisation of fracture with Gum bandage

Fig. 2: Immobilisation of fracture with Gum

75

Fitting of Thomas Splint in Forelimb of Large Animal

Aim: To know the method of securing thomas splint, in the forelimb.

Description

1. After immobilising the fracture site covering the distal as well as proximal end properly the thomas splint is fitted over the forelimb.
2. The foot is immobilised to the distal end of Thomas splint.
3. The immobilised forelimb kept closed and straight with the posterior extension of bamboo of the thomas splint. The limb is fixed with posterior bamboo splint with bandage roll at several place to avoid anterior, posterior movement of the limb.
4. At the time of fixing the limb with posterior extension bamboo of the Thomas splint, bandage are rapped along with the netting of thomas splint, to avoid medullary lateral movement of the immobilised limb.
5. Finally the immobilised forelimb is rapped along with the bandage roll including both the anterior and posterior extension of bamboo splint.

   To avoid outside movement of the immobilised limb, the method of immobilisation of fracture of forelimb has been shown in fig-1.

Fitting of Thomas Splint in forelimb and its Retention

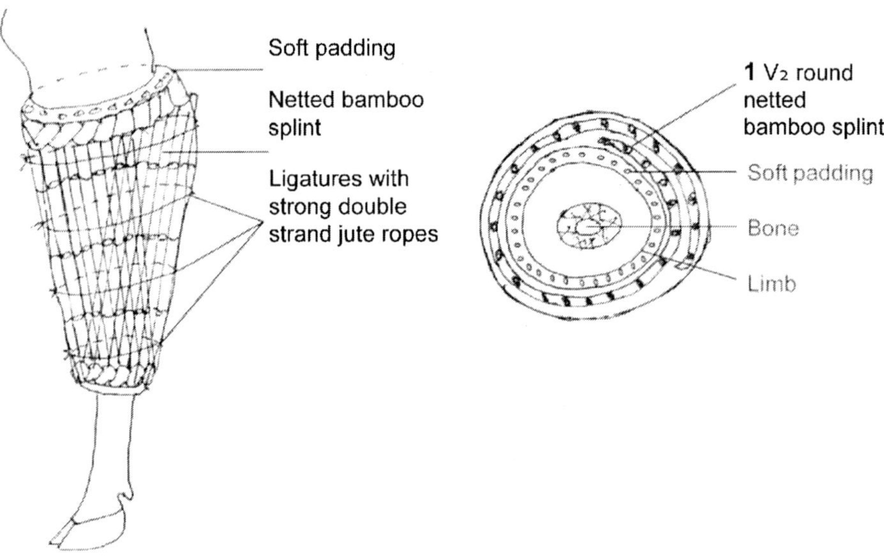

Fig. 1: Immobilization of fracture site with soft padding and netted bamboo splint.

Fig. 2: Cross section of gum bandage immobilisers.

Fig. 4: (a) Cross section of immobilised forelimb with thomas splint.

Fig. 3: Thomas splint fixation over gum bandage.

Fig. 4 (b): Cross section of immobilised hind limb with thomas splint.

76

Method of Fitting of Thomas Splint in Hind Limb of Large Animal

Purpose:- To know the method of fitting the immobilised fractured hind limb in Thomas splint.

Description

1. The fractured site is immobilised properly covering the area joint below and joint above from the fractured site.
2. The immobilised limb is kept within the prepared Thomas splint.
3. The immobilised limb is kept straight and come close with the front extension bamboo of the Thomas splint.
4. The foot is fixed to the distal end of the Thomas splint with bandage roll.
5. In the first attempt the immobilised limb is secured with the front bamboo splint with bandage roll at several places to avoid posterior movement of the immobilised limb.
6. At the time of fixing the immobilised limb with anterior extension bamboo of Thomas splint, the limb is fixed with the netting of Thomas splint to avoid medial movement of immobilised limb.
7. Finally the immobilised limb is covered with bandage roll wrapping around both the anterior and posterior extension bamboo of the Thomas splint to avoid outer movement of the immobilised limb.
8. The method of immobilisation of the hind limb with Thomas splint has been shown in the figure.

Method of Fitting of Thomas Splint in Hind Limb of Large Animal

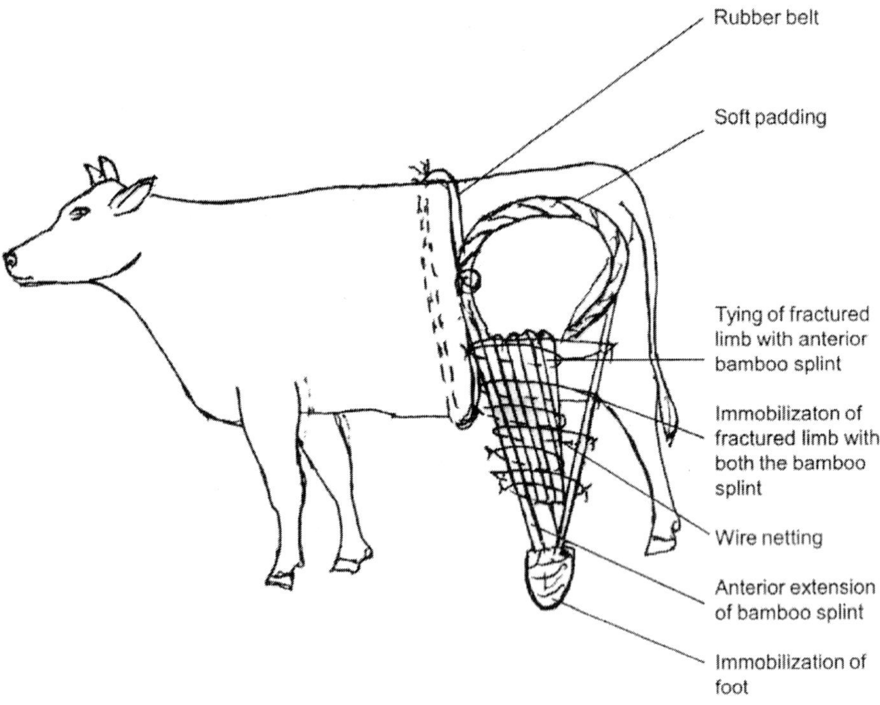

Fig. 1: Immobillization of fractured hindlimb with thomas splint

77

Method of Securing Thomas Splint

Definition : These are the splints made out of light metal rods or bamboo for correction and immobilization of middle and higher level fracture in animals.

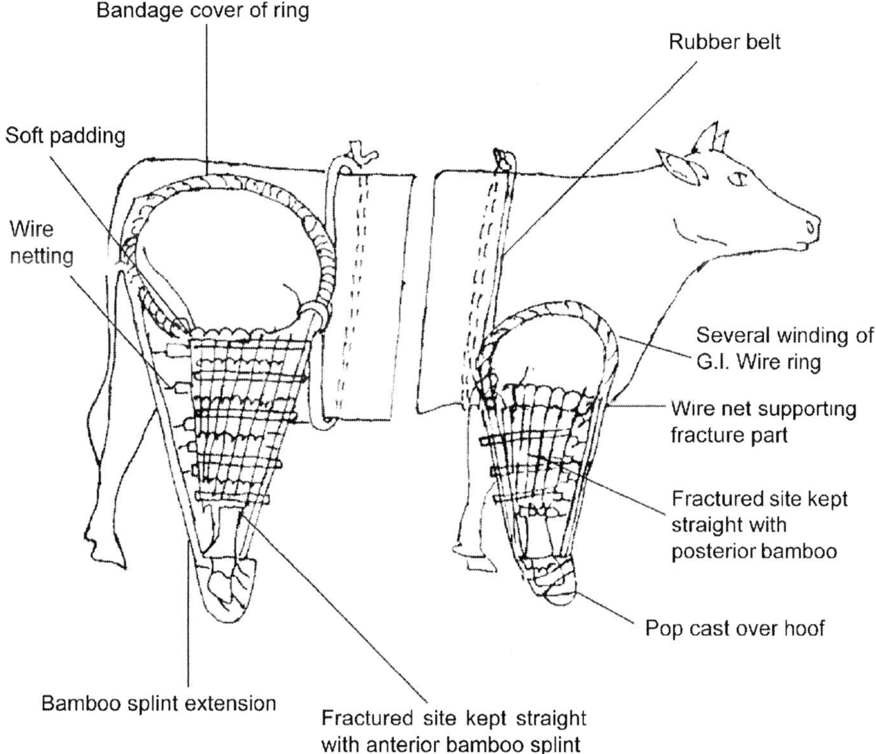

Fig. 1: Method of application of thomas splint in limbs.

78

Method of Fixation of Hoof With the Distal End of Thomas Splint

Aim: To secure the foot on the distal end of Thomas splint.

Procedure

1. Foot is placed upon the distal end of Thomas splint.
2. The foot of the animal is wrapped *V'*- two round with bandage cloth.(Fig.1)
3. 2nd round of bandage cloth is wrapped around the distal end of Thomas splint.(Fig.2)
4. In 3rd attempt, the bandage roll is taken from the ground level of the foot & including the distal end of foot.(Fig.3)
5. The bandage roll is taken through the gap between anterior end of Thomas splint.(Fig.3)
6. In 4th attempt, the bandage roll is taken from the volar or plantar aspect of the limb and passed upon the ground level of foot as well as the distal end of Thomas splint.(Fig.4)
7. Final 2 rounds of bandage cloth is wrapped through entire surface of foot.

Reference: Tyagi R.P.S. and Singh J, (2013), Ruminant Surgery, CBS Publishers, New Delhi, pp-353,354

Method of Fixation of Hoof With the Distal End of Thomas Splint

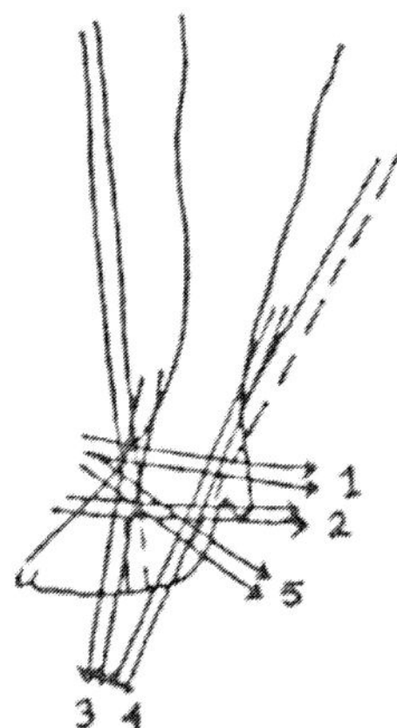

Fig. 1: Showing direction of bandage to be winded

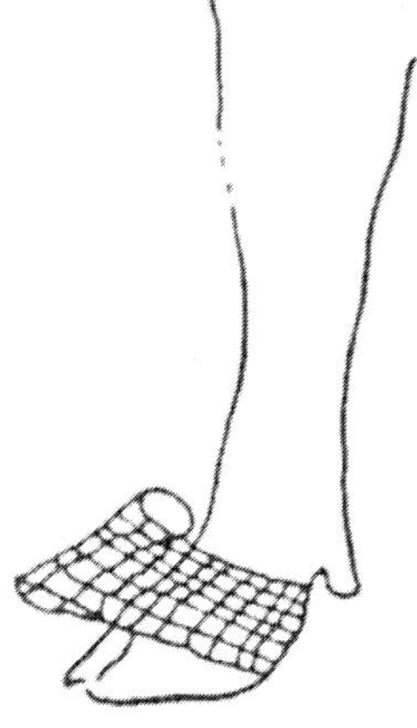

Fig. 2: 1st 2 round of bandage around hoof

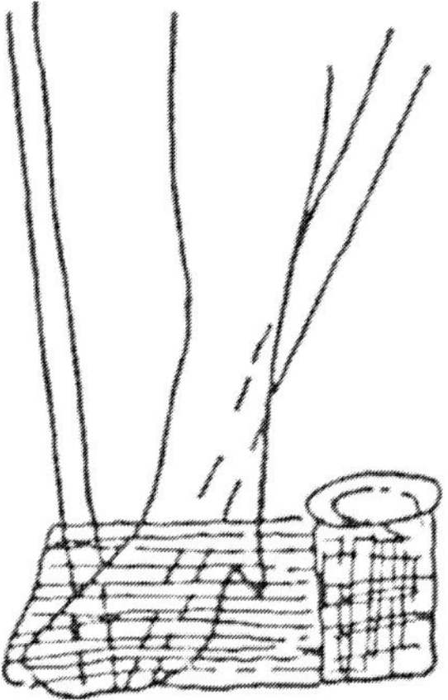

Fig. 3: 2nd round of bandage with distal end of Thomas splint & hoof

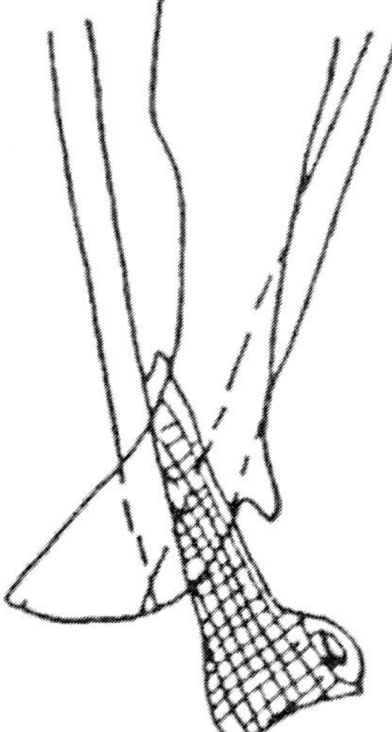

Fig. 4: 3rd 2 round of bandage around front bamboo splint gap & downwards covering the foo

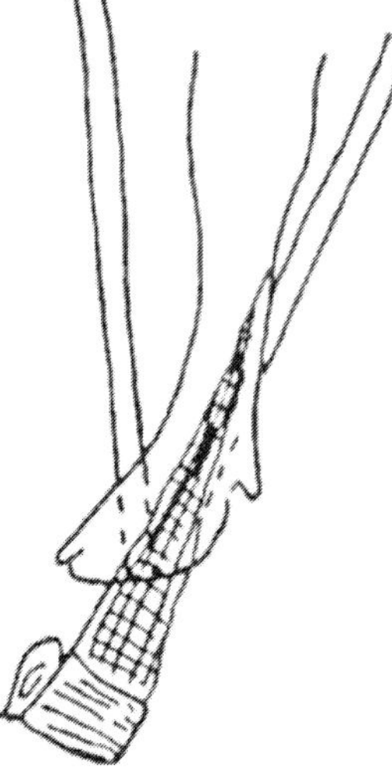

Fig. 5: 4th 2 round of bandage around posterior bamboo splint gap downwards covering the foot.

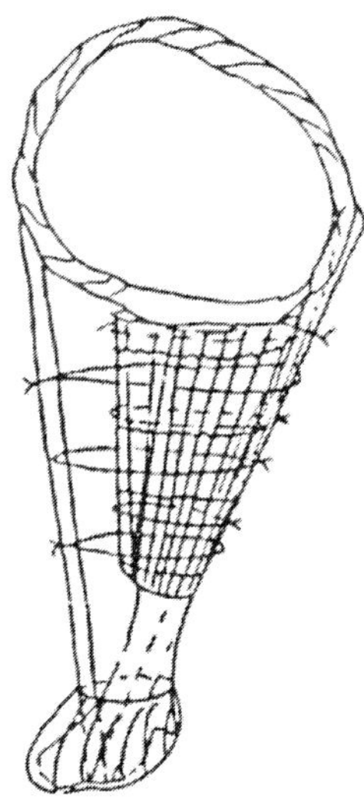

Fig. 6: Method of winding the bandage to include the distal end of Thomas splint with foot. Last 2 rounds covers the entire hoof.

79

Post Operative Care of Patients on Modified Thomas Splint

Large animal orthopedic patients are often managed with modified Thomas splints and to achieve an acceptable outcome with this device the following points should be kept in mind.

- Animals initially find discomfort with the splint and try to reject it by kicking and often show violent movements. Hence initial acclimatization with the device by close observation and supervision of the patient is essential.
- Recumbent animals should be supported in standing position by a sling and they should be managed with the principle "12 hrs on sling and 12 hours on floor".
- Movement of the animal should be restricted.
- The straps and knots on the splinted leg should be tied periodically on loosening.
- The animal should be placed on the floor with the immobilized limb uppermost. In bilateral application of Thomas splint, the sides should be changed daily.
- The floor should be soft and well bedded with sand, straw, gunny bags or other soft materials.
- Close observation of the covered limb should be done particularly at friction points. Any development of myiasis should be immediately treated with naphthalene balls.
- Animals should be given soft diet, grass and good nursing care.
- Open wounds of compound fractures should be dressed regularly till healing.

80

Recommendation of Confinement Space and Time for Fracture Immobilised Patient

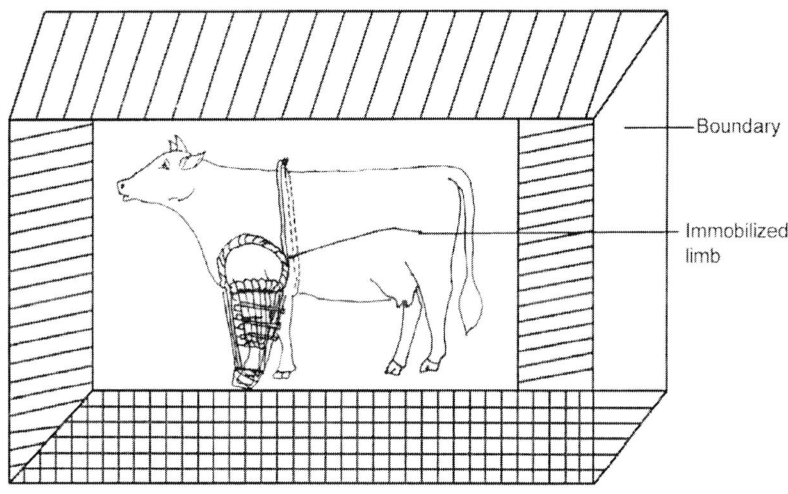

Fig. 1: Provision of bounded confinement space for rehabilitated immobilized patient

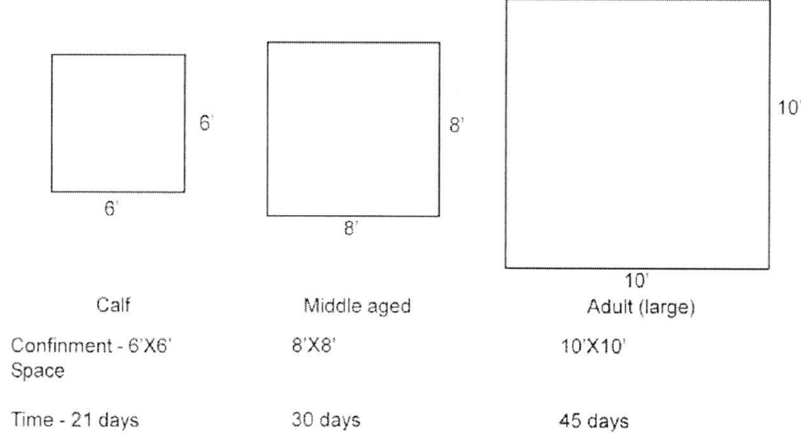

81*

Some of the Measurements for Commercial Fabrication of Thomas Splint and Netted Bamboo Splint for Large Animal (In Inches)

*Table starts from next page.

SI.No.	Total Height of animal	Length of Humerus bone	Length of netted bamboo splint for Radius & Ulna fracture repair	Length of netted bamboo splint for Metacarpal For Fracture repair	Total Length bamboo splint side bar	Length of Femur bone	Length of netted bamboo splint for Tibia & Fibula for fracture repair	Length of netted bamboo splint for Metatarsal forfracture repair	Total length of hind limb Thomas splint side bar
1	2	3	4	5	6	7	8	9	10
1	10	3.5	6	6	11	4	6	6	12
2	11	3.5	6	6	11.5	4	6	6	12
3	12	4	6	6	12	4.5	6	6	13
4	13	4	6	6	12	4.5	6	6	13
5	13	3.5	6	6	12	4	6	6	13
6	13	4	10	9	17	6	12	11	23
7	14	4.5	6.5	7	13.25	5	7	7.5	14.50
8	15	4.5	6.5	7	14.0	5	7	7.5	14.5
9	16	5	6.5	7	15.5	5.5	7	7.5	15
10	18	5.5	6.5	7	15	6	7	8	15.5
11	18	5	7	6.5	12.5	5	8	7.5	14
12	19	5.5	7	6	13	6	7	6	14
13	20	6	7	8	16.5	6.5	7	8	17.5
14	20	4.5	7	8	14	5	8	7	17
15	21	6	8	7	15	6.5	8	7	16
16	22	6.5	10	9	17.5	7	11	10	19
17	23	6.5	10	9	20	6.5	11	10	21
18	24	7	10	9	18	7.5	13	12	19.5
19	25	7.5	10	9	19	8	13	12	20
20	26	7.5	10	9	20	8	13	12	21.5
21	26	6.5	10	9	23	5.5	13	12	24
22	26.5	5	9	10	21.5	6	6	13	22
	26.5	5	7	6.5	12.5	5	8	7.5	14
23	27	8	10	9	20.5	7.5	13	12	22
24	28	8	10	9	21.5	8.5	12	11	23
25	28	5.5	10	11	22	7	15	14	24
26	28	5.5	10	11	22	7	12	14	24

82

Fabrication of Durable Thomas Splint

Aim

Purpose: As there is no institution for preparation ofthomassplintfor large animal till date for which physician are preparing thomas splint hear the patient at the time of need.

These thomas splint are generally prepared with useof bamboo, Gl wire, jute of cottonbandages. These thomas splint are generally weak. These thomas splint work for (2-3) month.

For this reason there is necessity of fabrication of large animal thomas splint with us e of other strong and lightest material for long time stonage and use.

Materials required:

Hollow plastic, cane, G.I. wiere, cotton bandage, plastic foam, insulating

Some of The Measurements for Commercial Fabrication of Thomas Splint and Netted Bamboo Splint for Large Animal (In Inches)

1	2	3	4	5	6	7	8	9	10
27	29	7	13	12	18	7.5	14	13	19
28	29	6.5	9.5	11.5	20.5	7	12	14	24
29	29	6	12	11	34	7	14	13	26
30	29	6	11	10	20	7	13	12	23
31	30	8.5	11	10	22	9	13	12	23.5
32	31	9	12	11	23	9.5	13	12	24
33	32	9	13	12	24	9.5	13	12	26
34	33	7	13	13	25	7.5	15	16	24
35	33	7	11	13	21	7.5	15	17	24
36	34	9.5	13	12	25.5	10	14	13	27.5
37	34	8	11	12	24	10	14	15	30
38	34	8	15	12	28	11	16	15	30
39	35	9	11	16	37	11.5	18	17	39
40	35	9	15	13	35	11	18	16	41
41	36	10	12	10	27	11	12	11	29
42	37	10	12	10	27	11	12	11	29
43	38	11	13	12	28.25	12	13	12	30
44	39	9	13	12	32	10	17	16	35
45	39	7.5	14	13	30	9	15	14	33
46	39	10	12	10	29	11	18	1614	33
47	40	12	15	12	30	13	15	14	32
48	40	9	14	13	33	10	16	14	33
49	40	12	14	12	32	11	16	13	36
50	41	9	15	13	32	10.5	14	13	36
51	42	13	13	12	30.5	14	14	13	32.5
52	43	14.5	13	12	30.5	14	14	13	34
53	44	14	14	13	33	15	14	13	35
54	44	9.5	13	12	34	11	14	14	37
55	44	7	12	12	28	8	14	14	34
56	46	15	14	13	34.5	16	15	14	37
57	46	9.5	15	13	31	11	17	15	37
58	46	10	16	15	33	13	18	16	36
59	47	11	16	15	35	14	17	16	37
60	48	12	17	16	35.5	17	17	16	37.5

Aim : To prepare Thomas splint for long term & repeated use.

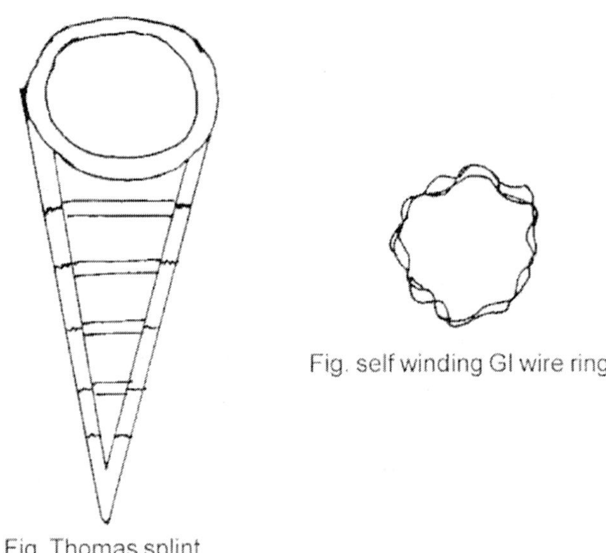

Durable materials for the extension of Thomas Splint :-

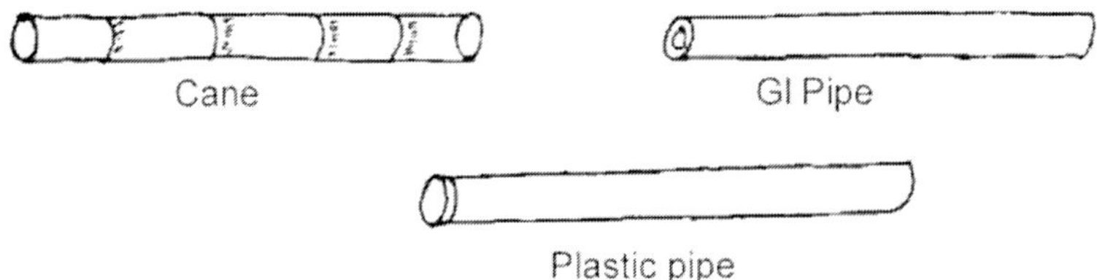

Durable materials for softening of ring are :-

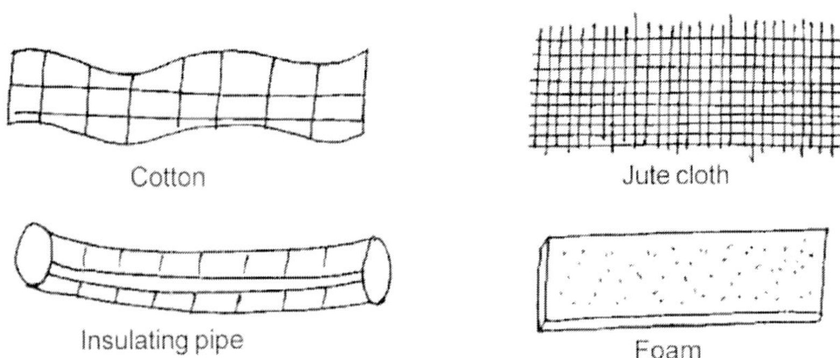

Fig. 1: Fabrication of Durable Thomas Splint

83

Recommendation of Forelimb Thomas Splint for Hind Limb or Vice Versa

AIM: For recommending forelimb Thomas Splint for hind limb and vice versa when use in commercial purpose.

Sub-Group	Height Range(Inch)	Species	Size of standardized Thomas splint				Actual size			
			Fore limb		Hind limb		Fore limb		Hind limb	
			Ring diameter	Length of side bar	Ring diameter	Length of side bar	Ring diameter	Length of side bar	Ring diameter	Length of side bar
1	2	3	4	5	6	7	8	9	10	11
1	10	Caprine	3.5	11.00	4	1200	3.5	11.00	4	12.00
2	12	Caprine	4	12.00	4.5	13.16	4	12.00	4.5	13.00
3	14	Ovine	4.5	13.00	5	14.33	4.5	13.25	5	14.50
4	16	Ovine	5	14.16	55	15.50	5	14.25	5.5	15.50
5	18	Caprine	5.5	15.33	6	16.16	5.5	15.00	6	16.50
6	20	Ovine	6	16.50	65	17.83	6	16 50	6.5	17.50
7	22	Caprine	6.5	17.66	7	19.16	6.5	17.50	7	19.00
8	24	Caprine	7	18.83	75	2050	7	18.00	7.5	19.00
9	26	Ovine	7.5	20.16	8	21.83	7.5	20 00	8	21.50
10	28	Bovine	8.	21.50	8.5	23.16	8	21.50	8.5	23.00
11	30	Bovine	8.5	22.83	9	2450	8.5	22.00	9	23.50
12	32	Bovine	9	24.16	95	2583	9	24.00	9.5	26.00
13	34	Bovine	9.5	25.50	10	27 33	9.5	25.50	10	27.50
14	36	Bovine	10	27.00	11	2883	10	27.00	11	29.00
15	38	Bovine	11	28.50	12	30 33	11	28.25	12	3000
16	40	Bovine	12	30.00	13	31.83	12	30.00	13	32.00
17	42	Bovine	13	31.50	14	33 50	13	30.50	14	32.50
18	44	Bovine	14	33.00	15	35.16	14	3300	15	35.00
19	46	Bovine	15	34.66	16	3683	15	34.50	16	37.00
20	48	Bovine	16	36.33	17	3850	16	35.50	17	37.50
21	50	Bovine	17	38.00	18	4016	17	38 00	18	40.50
22	52	Bovine	18	39.66	19	4200	18	39.50	19	42 00
23	54	Bovine	19	41.33	20	43.83	19	41.50	20	44.00
24	56	Bovine	20	43.00	21	4566	20	42.00	21	44.50

84

Immobilisation of Proximal 1/3rd Metacarpal and Metatarsal Bone

Defination

Dislocation of carpometarcarpus and tarso metatauses along with upper fracture of MC and MT bone (Fig. 1 and Fig.2). It is considered as difficult fracture and may not be healed appropriately by the usual procedure of lower level fracture repair method. Due to constant movement of fracture ends its treatment should be similar to middle level fracture repair method.

Materials Required

1. Thick padded cloth
2. Adhesive gum (fevicol)
3. Netted bamboo splint
4. Thomas splint

Procedure

- The facture site is immobilised by extending padded cloth from elbow to fetlock joint or stifle to fetlock joint
- The limb is further strengthen with netted bamboo splint of above said length.

Lastly the limb is immobilised with modified thomas splint. (Fig.1(b) and Fig.2(b

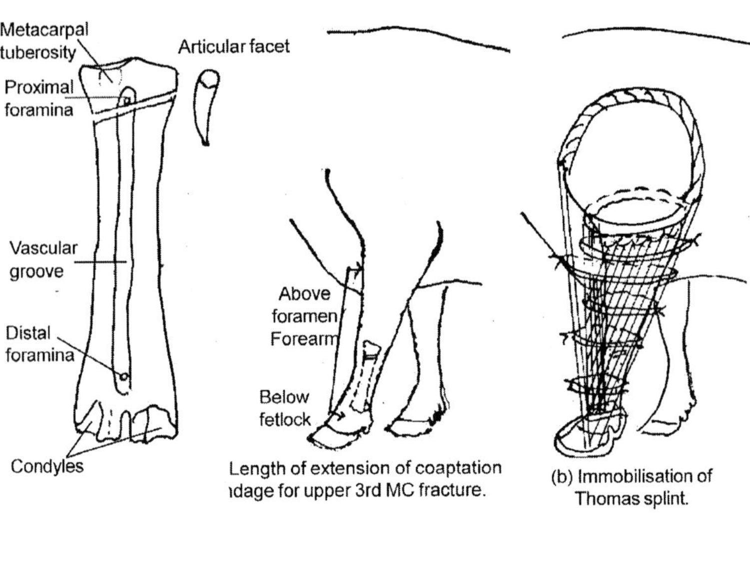

(a) Length of extension of coaptation bandage for upper 3rd MC fracture.

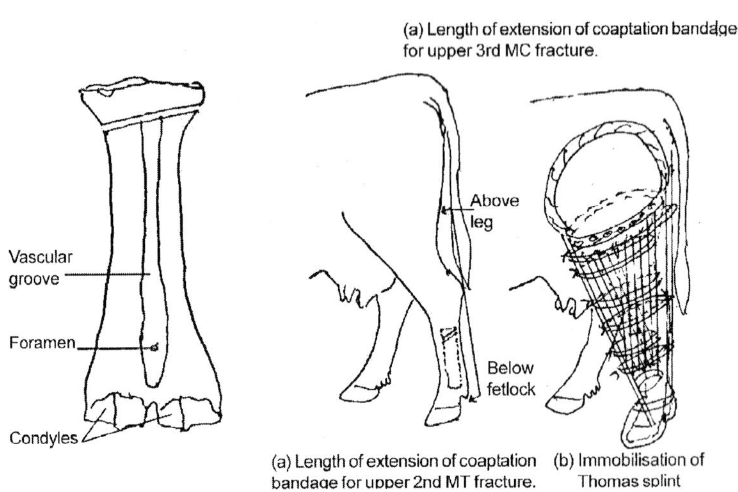

Fig. 1: Metatarsal bone of Ox.

85

Technique of Immobilization of Carpometacarpal and Tarsometa Tarsal or Joint Dislocation

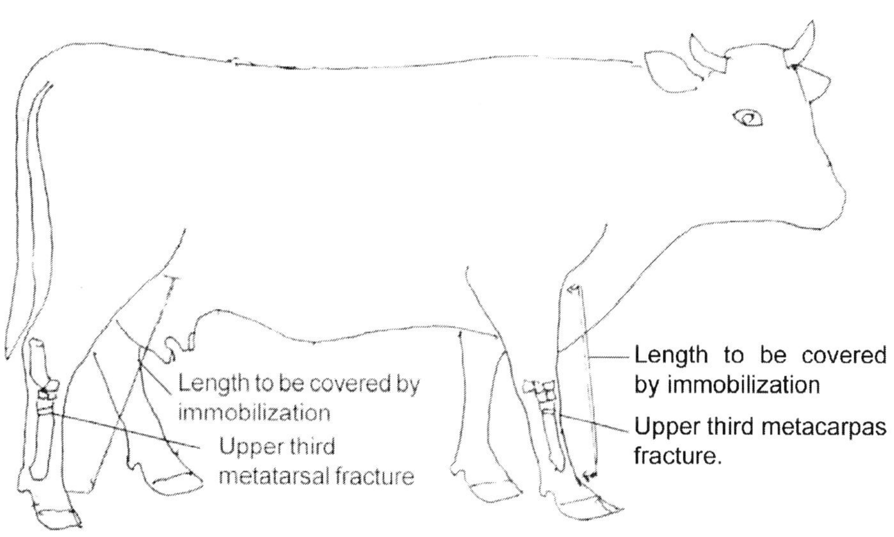

Fig. 1 (a): Fracture of upper third metatarsal and dislocation of

Fig. 1 (b): Fracture of upper third metacarpal and dislocation of carpometacarpal joint.

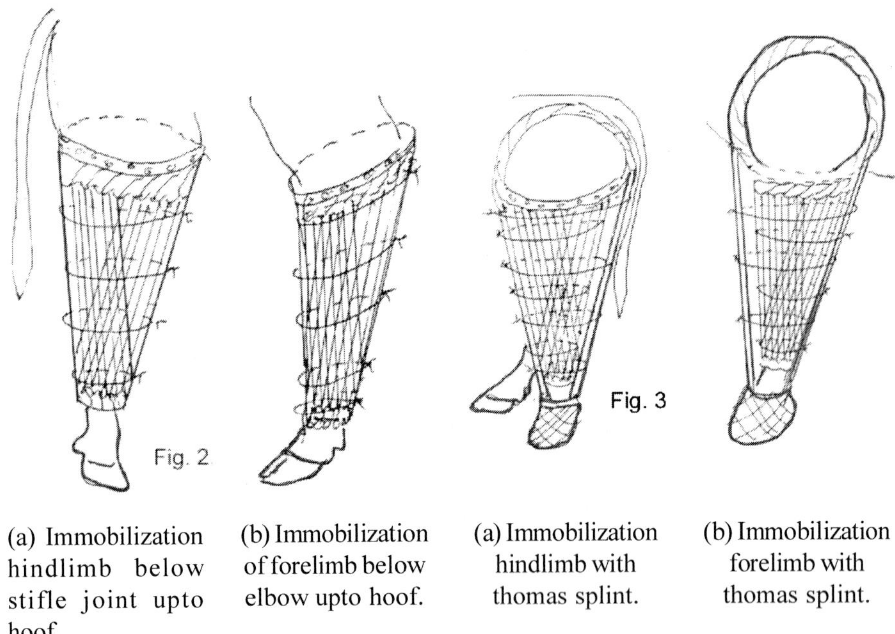

(a) Immobilization hindlimb below stifle joint upto hoof.

(b) Immobilization of forelimb below elbow upto hoof.

(a) Immobilization hindlimb with thomas splint.

(b) Immobilization forelimb with thomas splint.

Fig. 2: 1, 2 and 3 showing fracture of upper third metacarpal and metatarsal bone and dislocation of carpometacarpal and tarsometatarsal joint.

86

Immobilisation Technique for Upper Third Radius-Ulna Fracture

Purpose

As the immobilisation of upper third part of radius ulna is very difficult ,the purpose of the immobilisation tech. Is to fix the upper third of radius-ulna with the posterior half of ring of Thomas splint with bandages are very important for achieving no movement of fracture fragment during healing.

Indication

Correction of upper third fracture of radius-ulna by Thomas splint application indicated in higher level fracture.

Procedure of Fitting

The fracture site is immobilised by the application of coaptation bandage (Fig;3 a) extending from joint above and joint below (Fig. 2)

Thomas splint is fitted. (Fig. 3 c)

The hoof is fixed with Thomas splint. (Fig. 4)

The fracture site is kept straight with the bamboo splint (Fig. 2) of Thomas splint. (posterior bamboo splint)

Fore arm (fracture radius ulna) is fixed by tieing upper part with the posterior side ring of Thomas splint with cotton bandages, wrapping several time fixing with the ring. (Fig. 4)

Post Operative Care

First three days animal should be assisted during sleeping &standing. Animal should be housed in a dry shed/stable.

The moment of the animal is restricted.

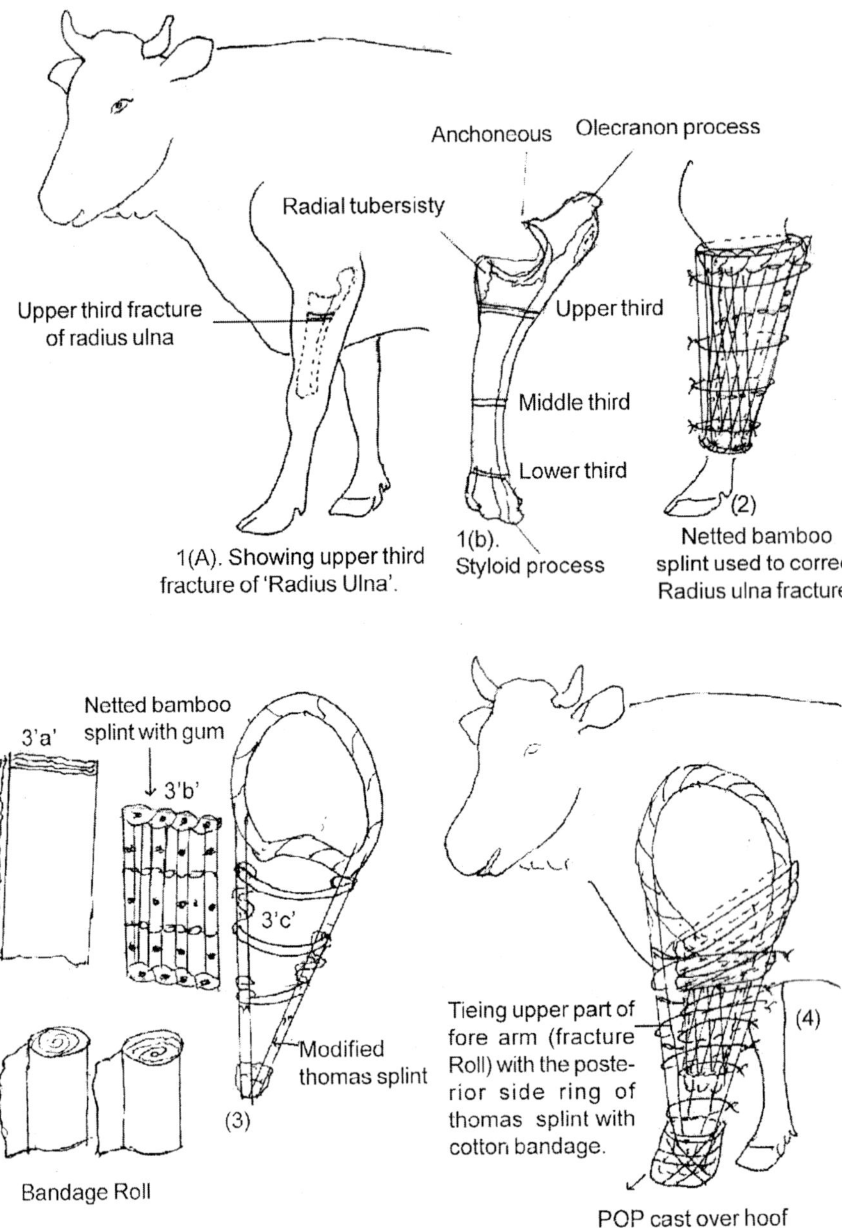

Fig. 1: Immobilisation Technique for Upper Third Radius-Ulna Fracture

87

Technique of Immobilization of Upper 3rd Tibia Fibula Fracture

Definition

Fracture of Upper 3rd of tibio-fibula Presence as a difficult Problem for the Surgeon to immobilise it Perfectly. As the fracture site generally moves within the imobiliser. Its healing becomes difficult. The aim of immobilisation technique of upper 3rd tibio-fibula fracture is to fix the upper 3rd of tibio-fibula with the anterior half of ring of thomas splint with bandages. This is an important step for achieving no movement of fracture fragment during healing.

Indication

Correction of upper 3rd fracture of tibio-fibula (Fig.1) by thomas splint application.

Procedure of Fitting

- The fracture site is immobilised by application of coaptation bandage extending from joint above and beiow fracture site (Fig 2).
- Thomas splint fitted (Fig 2).
- The fracture site kept straight with anterior bamboo splint of thomas splint.
- Leg is fixed by tieing its upper part with anterior ring site of thomas splint with cotton bandage, wrapping several time (Fig 4).

Post-operative Care

- First 3 day animal shoud be assisted during sleeping and standing.
- Animal shoud be housed in dry shed.
- The movement of animal restricted.

Technique of Immobilization of Upper 3rd Tibia Fibula Fracture

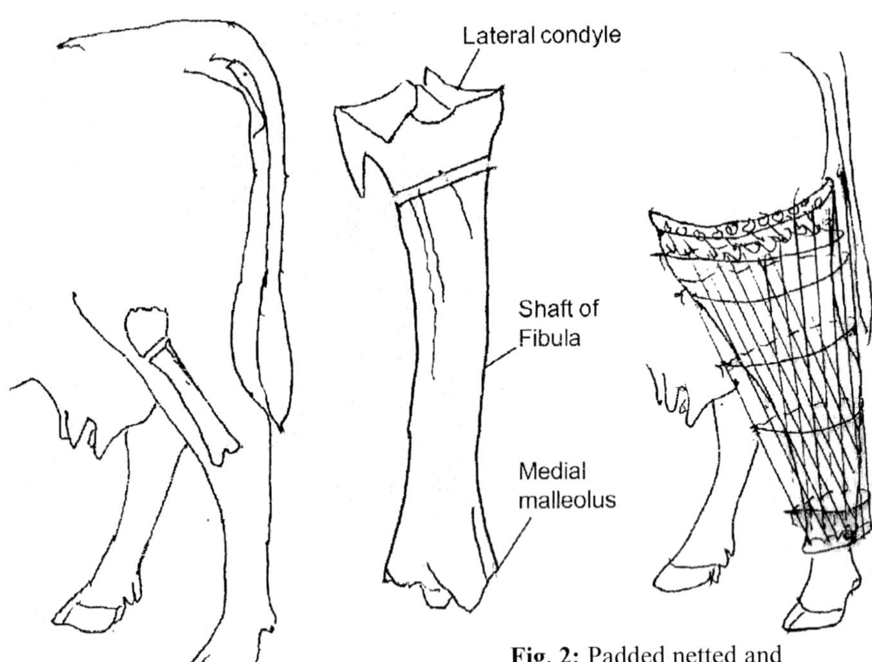

Fig. 1: Length of the limb at the fracture site to be covered with computational bandage.

Fig. 2: Padded netted and Conjoined bamboo splint

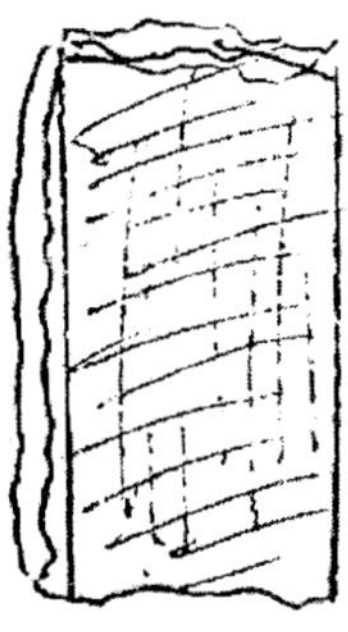

Fig. 3a : Thick padded cloth

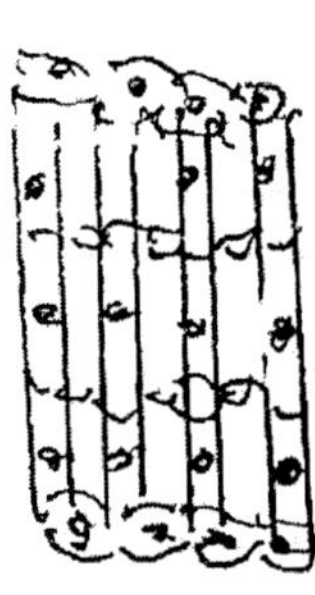

Fig. 3b: Netted bamboo splint with gum

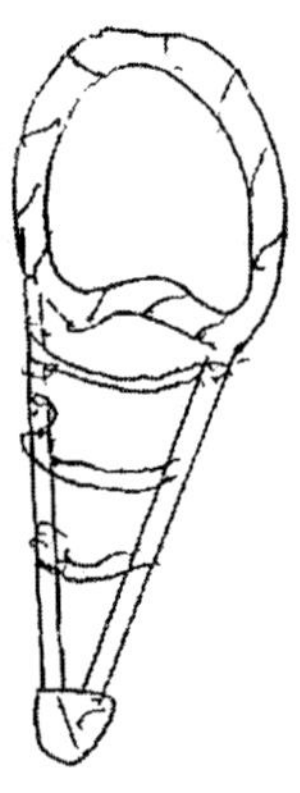

Fig. 3c: Modified thomas splint

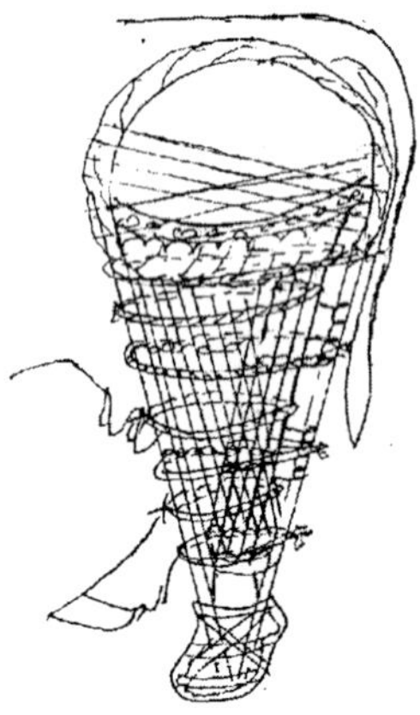

Fig. 4: Tieing upper part of leg region with Anterior site ring of thomas splint with cotton bandage

88

Conjoined Double Thomas Splint for Both Tibia Fibula - Fracture Repair

Use of conjoined Thomas splint for bilateral tibia fibula fracture for large animal.

Aim

To know the immobilization technique for both tibia-fibula fracture in large animal practice.

Instruments

Conjoined Thomas splint (Fig 1).

Procedure

- Both the fracture limbs are immobilsed by co-apted bandage thick padded cotton cloth and netted bamboo splint.
- Both co-apted limbs are further immobilized with the use of conjoined Thomas splint (Fig. 2).

Post-operative Care

- The animal is kept within restricted movement and optimum care.
- Changing of side of the animal frequently 3-4 times a day to avoid bed-sore.
- Animal is kept in standing position within sling to facilitate free-breathing and feeding.
- B The immobilization is removed after 21 days.

Conjoined Double Thomas Splint For Both Tibia Fibula - Fracture Repair

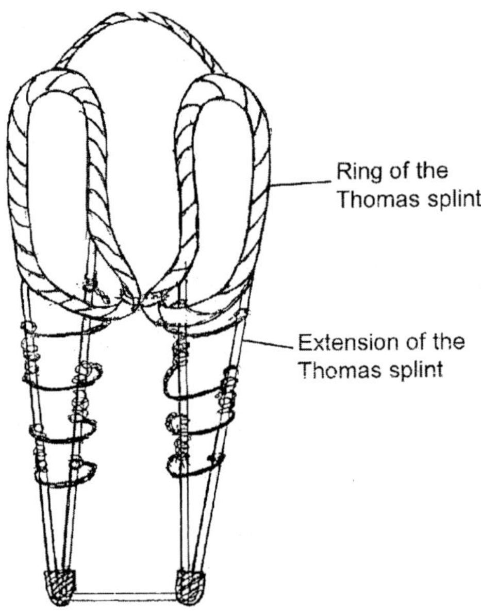

Fig. 1: Conjoined double Thomas splint for both tibia-fibula fracture repair

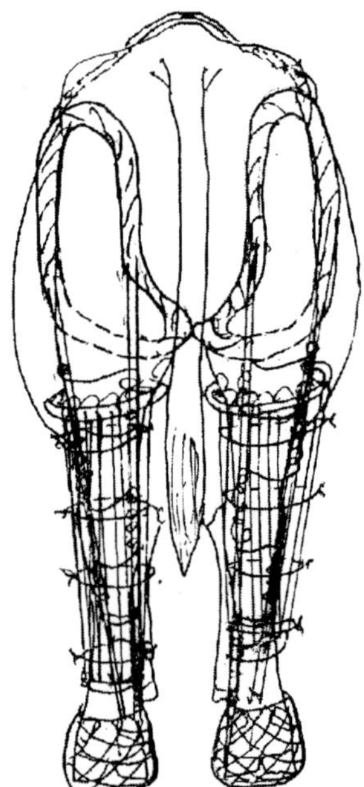

Fig. 2: Fitting of Thomas splint having both Tibia-fibula fracture

89

Immobilization of Symphysial Fractured Mandible in Large Animals

Definition: Mandible forms the skeleton of lower jaw and comprises of a body and two rami. The two halves of this bone fuse incompletely at the mandibular symphysis, situated at the midline within the body.

Indication: Immobilization of fractured mandible, minimally or non displaced fractures with an intact opposite hemimandible, vertical ramus fracture.

Anasthesia: Local anaesthesia for large animals. A20 gauze 2.5 cm needle is used to deposit 5-1 Omi of lidocaine at the exit site and into the canal.

Technique

1. After aseptic preparation of the site ,animal was anaesthesized and operation can be done in standing condition.
2. Bring a single 10 inch long, 20 gauze stainless steel wire.
3. Make a small incision on the skin over the lower jaw and insert a guide needle so that it travels under the skin below the mandible and pierces through the other side. A stainless steel wire is inserted through the guide needle to the other side.
4. The guide needle is removed from the previous position and pierced on the same side (side of exit of wire) through the skin on the lov;er gingiva.
5. The exit end of wire is again guided through this needle and then needle is removed. The two ends of wire are twisted and tightened.
6. Care should be taken so that during insertion of wire any blood vessels and nerves should not be damaged.

Post Operative Care

1. Antibiotics may be continued for 4-5 days.
2. Provide soft and liquid diet.

3. Check wires daily, remove if broken.
4. Remove wires after 4-5 weeks.

Reference : Tyagi R.P.S. and Singh J (2013), Ruminant Surgery, CBS Publishers, New Delhi, PP: 369-371.

Immobilization of Symphysial Fractured Mandible in Large Animals

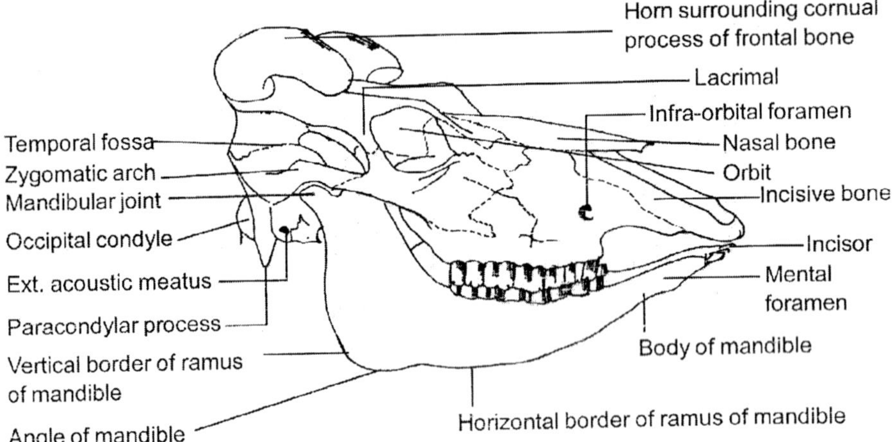

Fig. 1: Bovine Skull with mandible

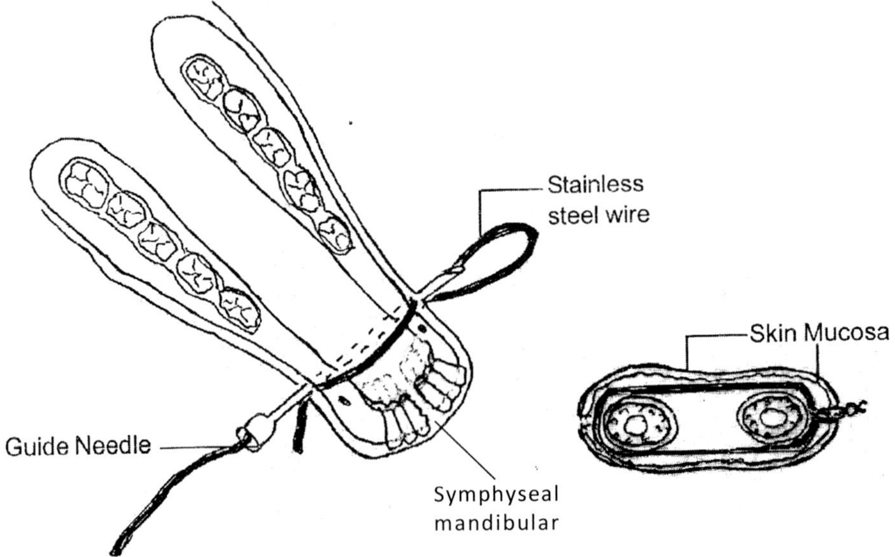

Fig. 2: Wiring technique for symphyseal fracture

Fig. 3: Cross-section of mandible

90

Immobilization of Fracture of Ramus of Mandible

Objectives

Immobilization of fracture of mandible.

Requirements

'U' Plate 4 Pins Electric drill Orthopaedic hammer Pin cutter

Procedure

- Under local infiltration of an anesthetic & parenteral sedatives the 4 pins are drilled 2 on either side of the fracture site from one side mandible to other side mandible. During drilling the pin, the holes, importance should be given for the passage of the pin through prefix of the drill hole in metal frame
- The fracture end should come accurate apposition during pinning procedure & the symmetry of the fractured mandible should be as norma! as possible.
- Sterilised antiseptic gauge bandages are covered, the pin between frame and the body. The pins are retained in position either with nut-bolt or by passing a plastic tube after which the hole of the plastic tube is filled with resin.

Post operative care

- Administration of course of parenteral antibiotic for 5 or 7 days.
- Pin hole should be applied with antiseptic regularly.
- Fluid therapy as per requirement
- Care should be taken to maintain the pin position undisturbed through filling procedure.

Immobilization of Fracture of Ramus of Mandible

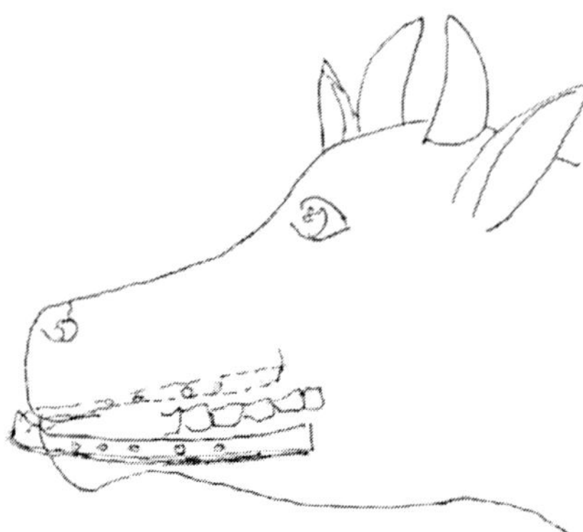

Fig. 1: Immobilization of fracture of mandibie with external 'U' plate and pinning.

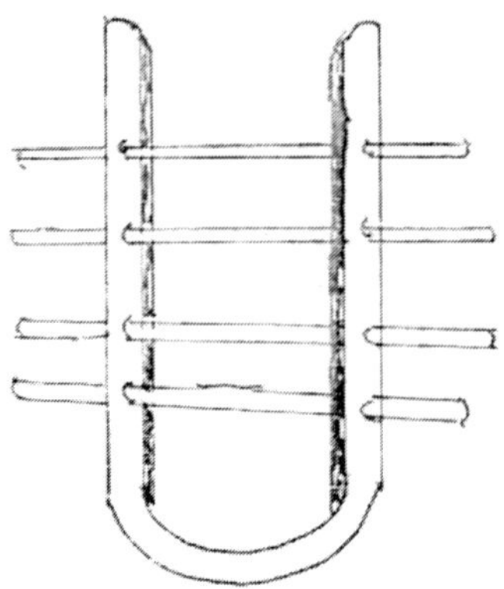

Fig. 2: 'U' plate frame with pinning device for immobilization of mandible fracture.

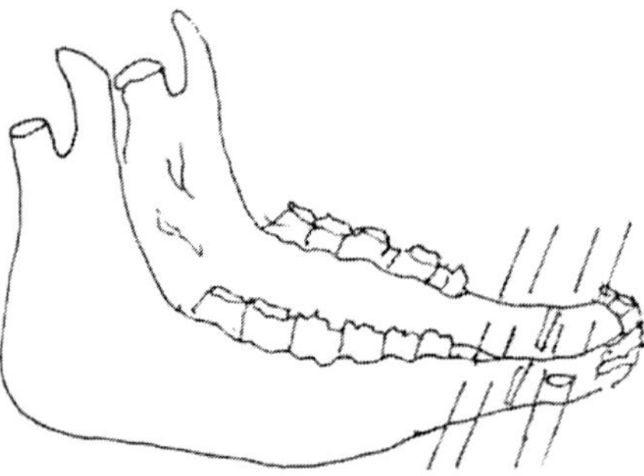

Fig. 3: Pinning sites, either sides of the fracture - lateral view.

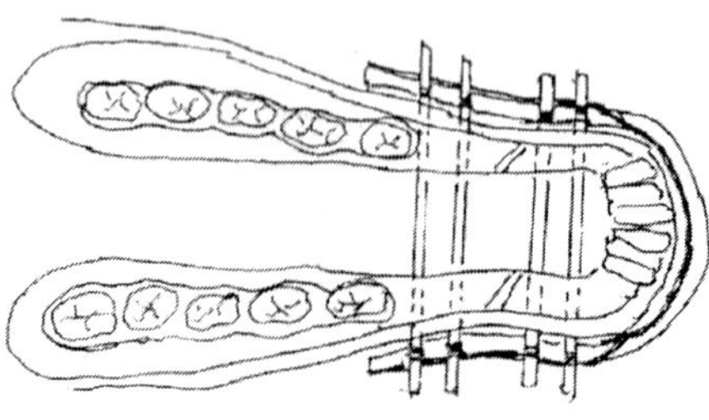

Fig. 4: Pinning sites, either sides of the fracture - dorsal view.

91

Immobilization of Limb for Flexor Tendon Repair

Aim: To know the method of immobilization of the limb after repair of the flexor tendon.

Procedure

The immobilization procedure of limb after flexor tendon repair is done in 2 stages.

1st Stage

1. Immobilization of limb for avoiding movement at tendon suture site.
2. It is done by placing the sutured area within a pre- fabricated metal frame so as to keep the limb undisturbed at the suture site.
3. The frame is given in Figure - 1.
4. The purpose of addition of the metal frame is to immobilize the limb keeping the fetlock and foot away from in a flexed manner to avoid weight bearing during healing period.
5. The limb is immobilized with netted bamboo splint (Fig. 2).
6. The immobilized limb is placed within the metal frame keeping the fetlock and foot in a flexed manner.

2nd Stage

1. After immobilization of the limb within netted bamboo splint and metal frame the limb is further kept immobilized within a Thomas splint. (Fig. 4).

POST OPERATIVE CARE

1. The animal is kept with restricted movement for a period of 2-3 months.
2. Naphthalene is sprinkled.
3. Wound care is taken of as per the requirement.

Immobilization of Limb for Flexor Tendon Repair

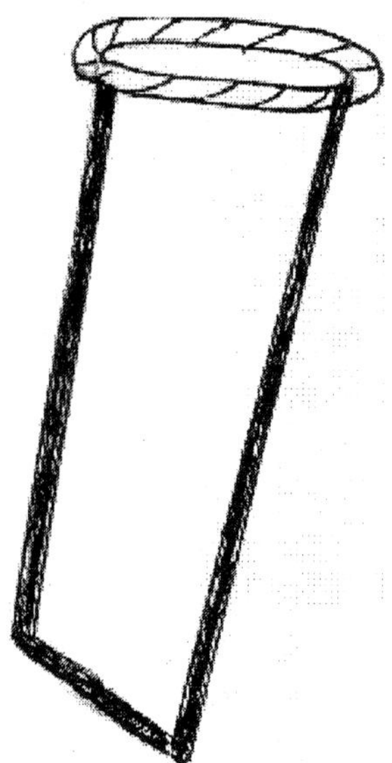

Fig.1: Metal Frame

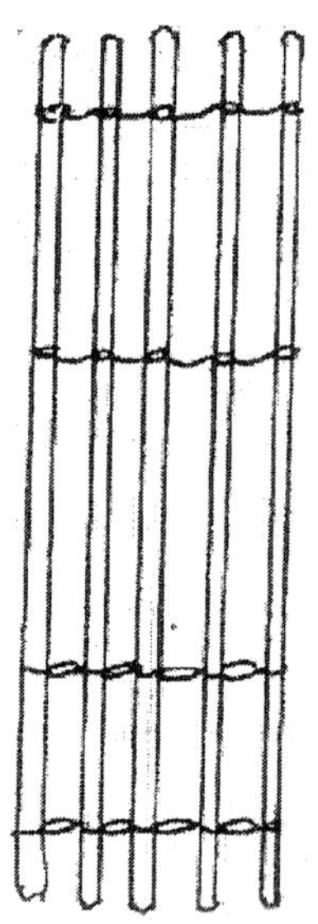

Fig. 2: Netted bamboo splint

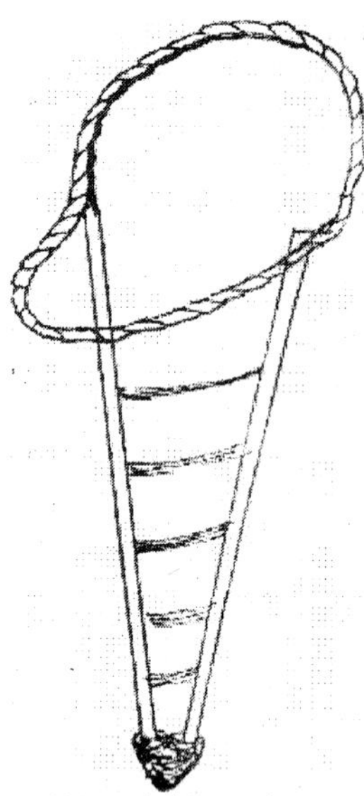

Fig. 3: Thomas splint

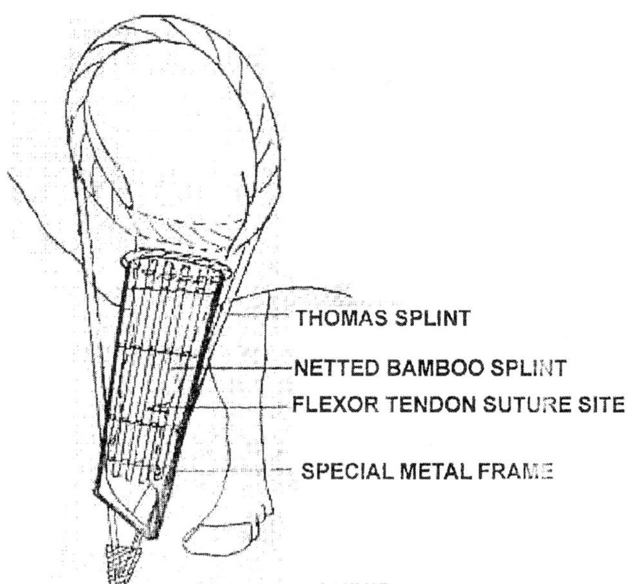

Fig. 4: Immobilization of limb for flexor tendon repair

92

Digital Tendon Repair

Definition

Digital tender include superficial digital flexor, DDF & suspensory ligament which is situated in volar & plantar upset of metacarpus and metatarsus. These tendons are generally transected during ploughing or intensional approach (Fig.1).

Sign

After cutting of these tendon the foot became flat and animal bears weight on fetlock is can't able to walk freely.

Pre-operative Requisite

1) Local Anesthesia
2) Parenteral sedative
3) Suturing material
4) An Iron frame for keeping fetlock in flexed position during healing period.
5) Netted bamboo splint/Thomas splint.

Procedure

1) The cut end of tendons are exposed cleaned thoroughly and apposed with suture.
2) A flushing catheter is anchored within wound. The wound is kept covered with a thick layer, dry, absorbed cotton padding.
3) The limb is kept within a prepared a metal frame, keeping the fetlock In a flexed position (Fig.4). And the limb is immobilized with help of a netted bamboo splint.
4) Finally, the limb is kept immobilized with Thomas splint (Fig.5).

Post operative care

1. Animal is kept within restricted movement enclosure for 1 -1 month.
2. After 1-1month of regular care and dressing all the visible sutures are removed and wound dressing and restrict of movement Is carried out up to 3 months till complete wound closure.

Photo Feature of Digital Tendon Repair

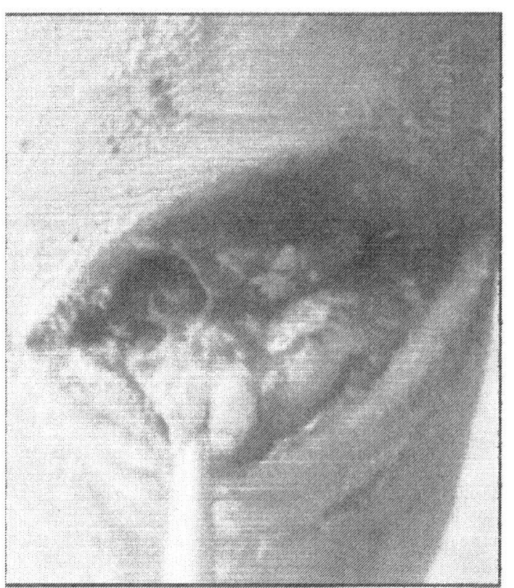

Fig. 1: Identification of individual tendons.

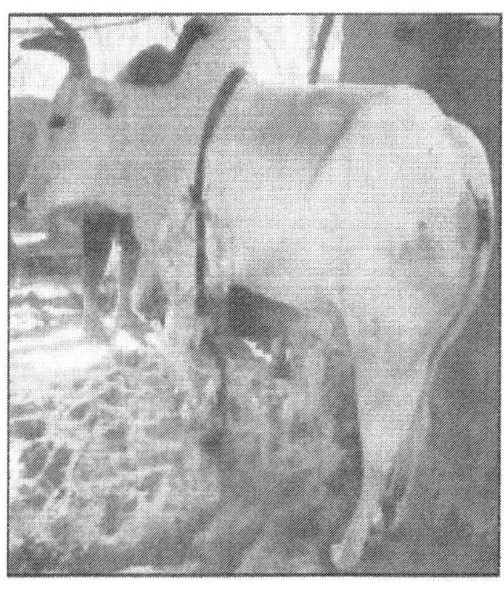

Fig. 2: Animal after Thomas splint application

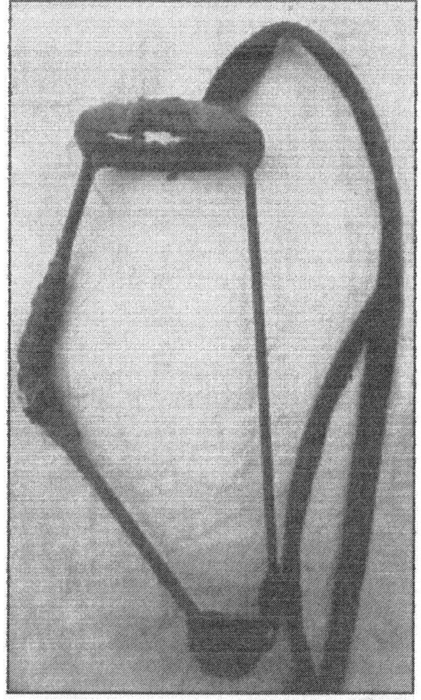

Fig. 3: Fabrication of angular frame device.

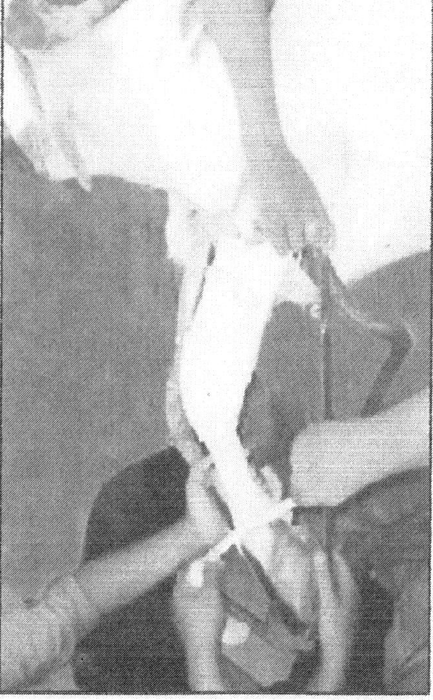

Fig. 4: Immobilization of the limb inside the splint angular frame.

93

Suturing Technique of Transected Gastrocnemious Tendon

Aim

To depict the detail method of tendon suturing of transected gastrocnemious tendon for union.

Procedure

After cleaning, debriding and flushing the transected site thoroughly local antiseptic and antibiotic is applied.

1. To expose the tendon ends clear visual as well as proper exposer the site was enlarged by two vertical incision placed at dorsal and ventral part of the transected site.(Fig.1).
2. The three different tendons and their locations is identified. The both end of tendon of a particular group are brought close together and joins end to end and retained with strong polyester suture putting to interrupted knots at 90 degree to each other.(Fig. 2).
3. Their peritendon cover are pulled over the suturing site from their either ends and are also retained in position with additional interrupted suture running at 90 degree to each other.(Flg. 3). In this way 4 interrupted suture are required for approaching one tendon.
4. In this way all the 3 tendons are joined with their respective other ends with suture. Total no of 12 interrupted suture are required for joining all the 3 structure of the gastrocnemious tendon. At the end the suture tendons are strengthened by placing to interrupted stainless steel suture. (Fig. 4).

Finally a flushing catheter was placed at higher level and the suture site is covered with a thick dry antiseptic absorbent cotton padding.

Suturing Technique of Transected Gastrocnemious Tendon

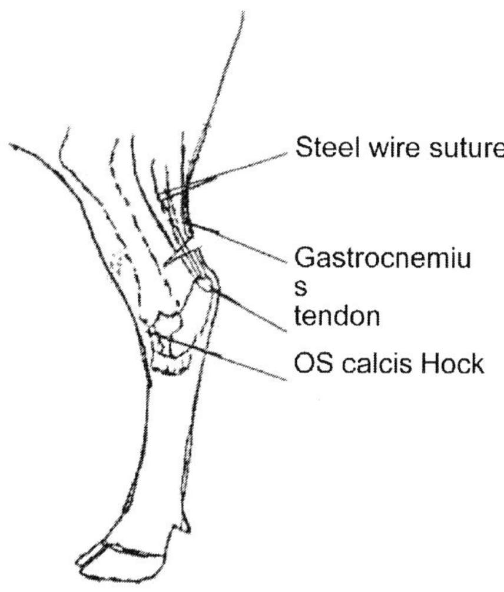

Fig. 1: Transected gastrocnemius tendon.

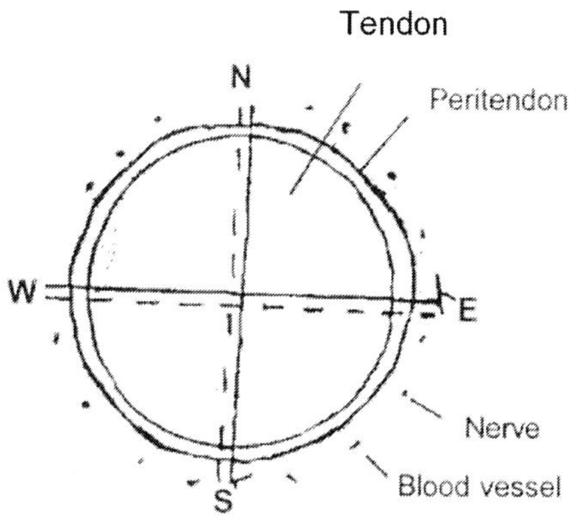

Fig. 2: Suture passing technique.

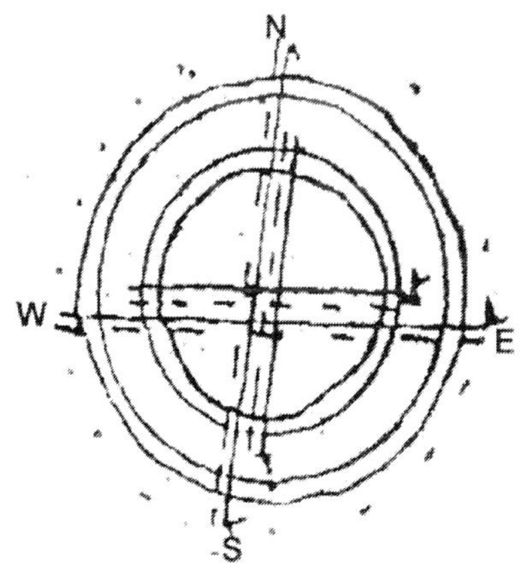

Fig. 3: Tendon & peritendon apposition suture.

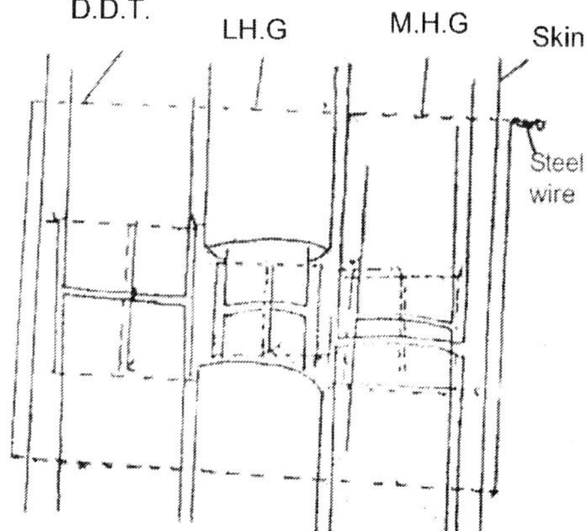

Fig. 4: Suturing technique of gastrocnemius

D.D.T. - Deep digital tendon
L. H.G. - Lateral head of gastrocnemius tendon

94

Immobilization of Hind Limb for Tendo Achiles Repair

Aim

To know the method of immobilization of the limb after repair of the transected gastrocnemius tendon (tendo achiles).

Procedure

The immobilization procedure of limb after gastrocnemius tendon repair is done in 2 stages.

1ST Stage

1. Immobilization of limb for avoiding movement at tendon suture site.
2. It is done by placing the sutured area within a pre- fabricated metal frame so as to keep the limb undisturbed at the suture site.
3. The frame is given in Figure 1.
4. The purpose of addition of the metal frame is to immobilize the limb keeping the fetlock and foot away from in a flexed manner to avoid weight bearing during healing period.
5. The limb is immobilized with netted bamboo splint (Fig. 2).
6. The immobilized limb is placed within the metal frame keeping the fetlock and foot in a flexed manner.

2nd Stage

1. After immobilization of the limb within netted bamboo splint and metal frame the limb is further kept immobilized within a Thomas splint. (Fig. 4).

Post Operative Care

1. The animal is kept with restricted movement for a period of 2-3 months.
2. Naphthalene is sprinkled.
3. Wound care is taken of as per the requirement.

Immobilization of Hind Limb for Tendo Achiles Repair

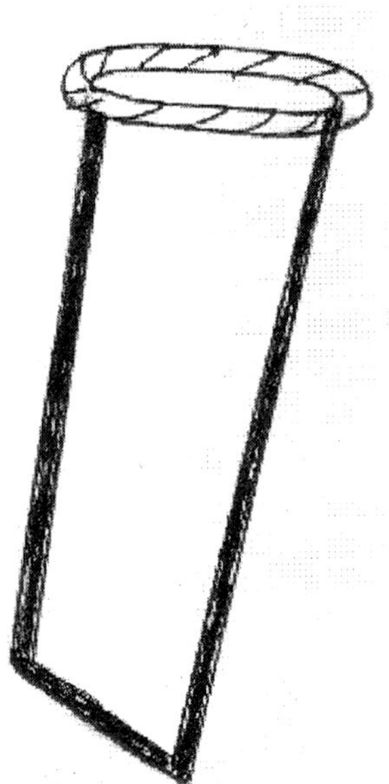

Fig. 1: Metal Frame

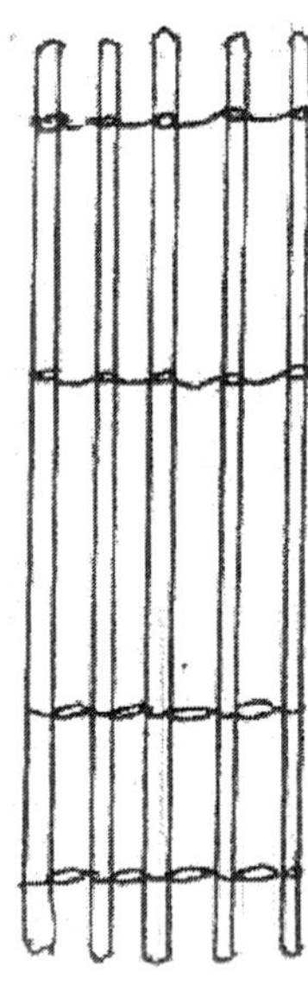

Fig. 2: Netted bamboo splint

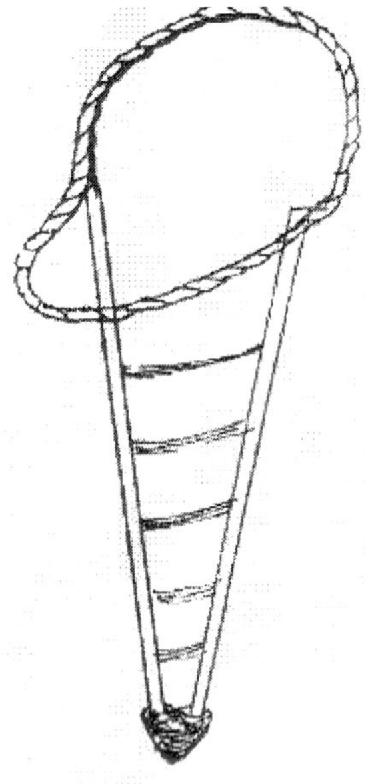

Fig. 3: Thomas splint

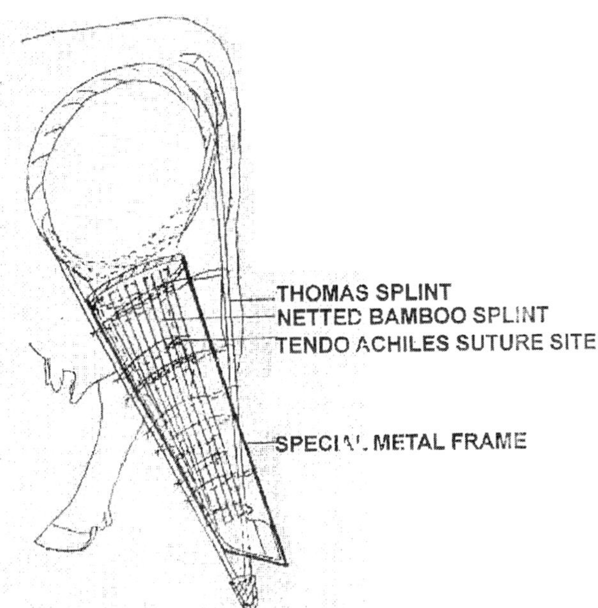

Fig. 4: Immobilization of hind limb for lendo achiles repai

Coxofemoral(Hip) Luxation

Introduction

Coxofemoral luxation is commonly seen in dairy cattle Traumatic in origin and often related to postpartum events.

Jersey cows may be predisposed to this condition.

Clinical Signs

1. The animal is unable to bear weight on this leg which is rotated so that the stifle and digits are directed outward.
2. The external pelvic landmarks are abnormal.
3. Crepitus ("bone on bone") and localised pain may be elicited on rotational manipulation of leg.
4. Radiographic facilities should be made to confirm the diagnosis and direction of luxation.

Differential Diagnosis

1. Pelvic fracture
2. Proximal femoral fracture.
3. Separation of the proximal femoral epiphysis
4. Fracture of the femoral neck
5. Sacroiliac luxation
6. Acute septic arthritis of hip or stifle joints.

Treatment

Non surgical reduction is related to the internal and using the appropriate manipulative procedures within 48 hours of occurrence.

Reference: Greenough, P.R. and Weaver, A.D.(1997). Lameness in cattle, 3'^^ Edition, W.B.Saunders Co. Philadelphia, P.P. 175-177.

Coxofemoral(Hip) Luxation

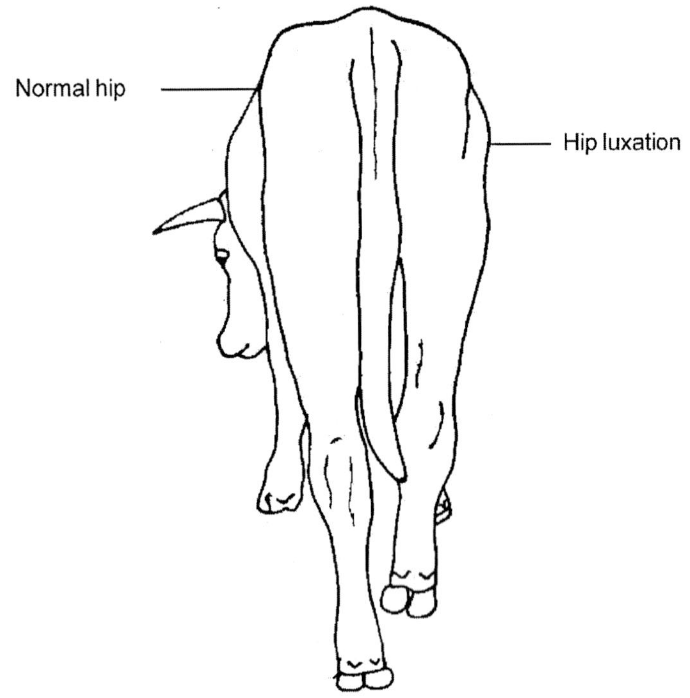

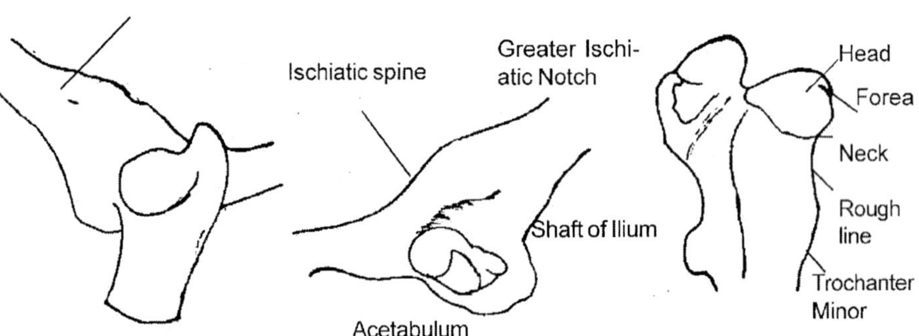

Fig. 5: a) Normal Hip joint. **b)** Pelvic bone showing Acctabulum **c)** Femur of ox.

Reference: Greenough, P.R. and Weaver, A.D. (1997). Lameness in cattle, 3rd Edition, W.B. Saunders Co. Philadelphia, P.P. 175-177.

95

Hip Dislocation and It's Correction

Hip joint is a ball and socket joint which involves cotyloid cavity of os-coxae and head of femur. Hip dislocation can be corrected by external immobilization of the area with POP cast and keeping the animal in a mobile sling for several weeks.

(1) The dislocation involves cotyloid cavity and head of femur and the affected limb deviate outward. (Fig.1)

(2) The fracture site is immobilized extending joint below and joint above level initially with plaster of Paris.(Fig.2)

(3) Cloth bandage is applied over it for support involving joint above and joint below which should not be too tight or too loose.(Fig.3)

(4) Second layer of cloth padding is provided over the first layer to provide more strength and further immobilization.(Fig.4)

(5) Final immobilization is done by application of rubber belt or suspensory bandage. (Fig.5)

(6) At the end the entire animal is kept in mobile sling for proper immobilization for some weeks and housed in limited space(Fig.6)

Hip Dislocation and It's Correction

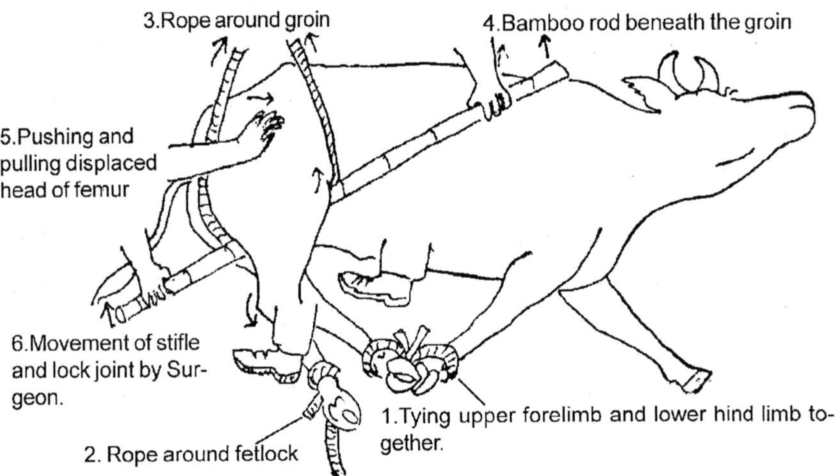

Fig. 1: Hip dislocation in cattle

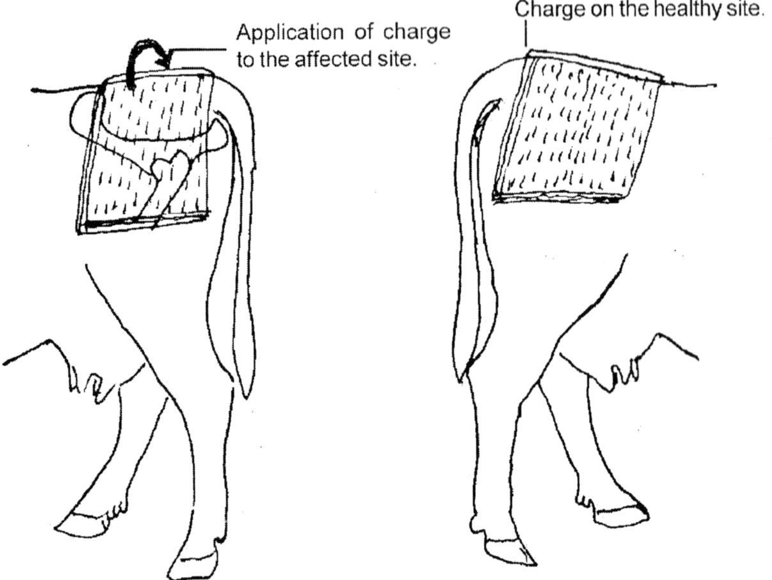

Fig. 2(a): Application of charge over the affected hip

Fig. 2(b): Extension of charge in the healthy site

Reference: O'conner, J.J. (2003) Dollar's Veterinary Surgery, 4th Edition, CBS Publishers and Distributors, New Delhi

Hip Dislocation and it's Correction

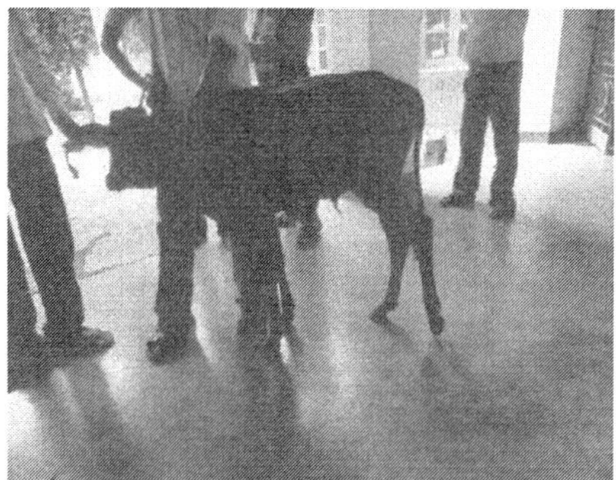

Fig. 1: Bone showing fracture site

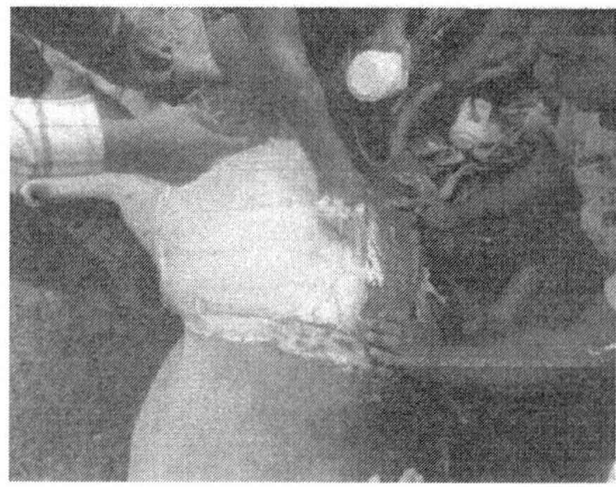

Fig. 2: Application of plaster of pahs

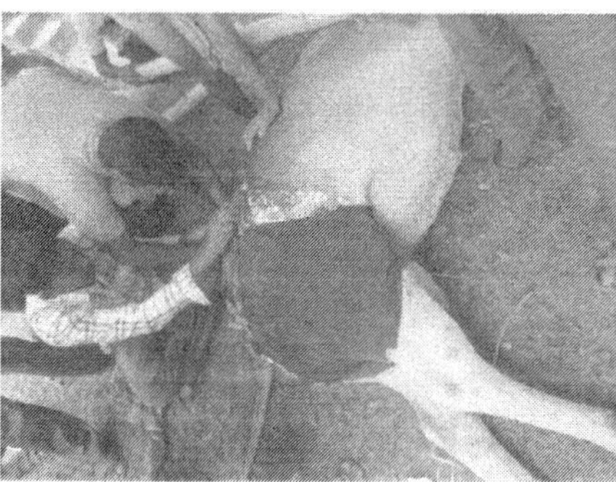

Fig. 3: Immobilisation of fracture site with cloth bandage.

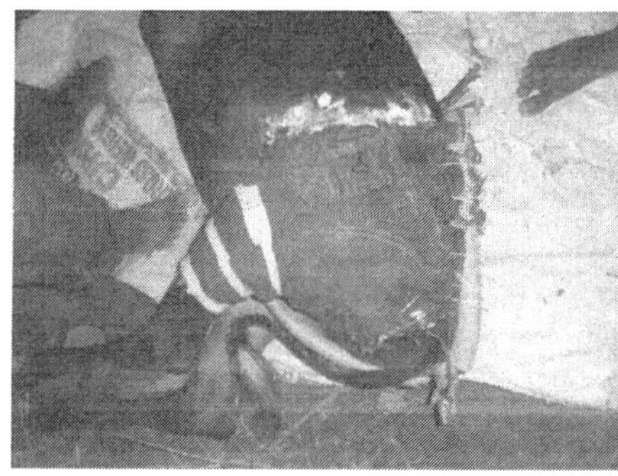

Fig. 4: Immobilisation of fracture site with second layer of cloth padding

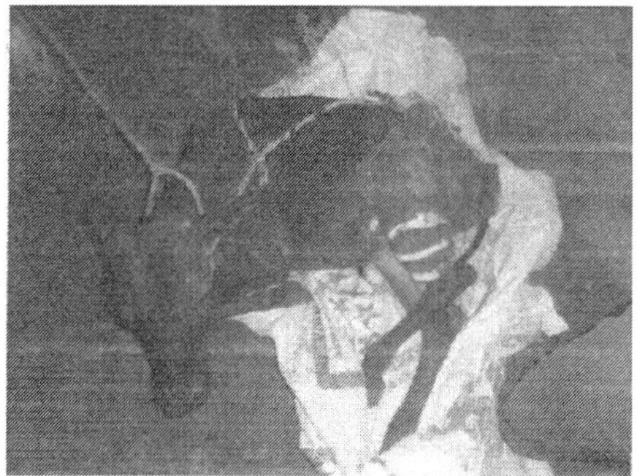

Fig. 5: Final immobilised limb with Rubber belt or suspensory bandage

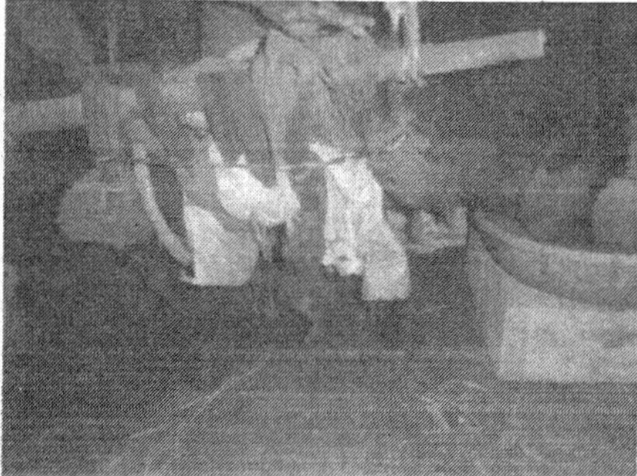

Fig. 6: Animal kept in mobile sling for proper immobilisation

96

Contracted Leg in Calves

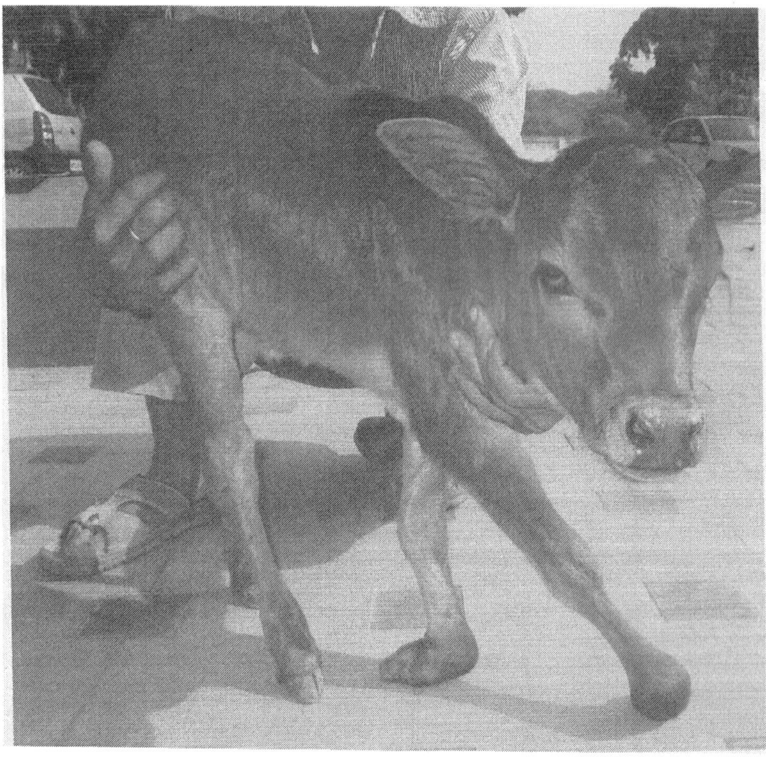

Fig. Calf showing bilateral contracted leg.

Contracted Leg in Calves

Definition

A shortening or contraction of the deep and superficial digital flexor tendons and associated muscles, sometimes also the carpal flexors, leading to abnormal flexion of the fetlock, possibly also of the pastern and carpal joint.

Signs

1. If only superficial tendon contracts there will be knuckling of fetlock.
2. When deep digital flexortendon contract the hell tends to life from the ground.
3. When severe DDF contracted that calf walks on dorsal surface of fetlock causing open joint capsule.

Treatment

1. If calf can bearweighton toe, no correction is required.
2. If fetlock and pastern are knuckled then correct by manual extension and apply plaster cast.
3. If heel of the foot remain on the ground during standing only the superficial tendon should be cut.
4. If the deformity is so severe then tenotomy of DDF and SDF is advisable.

Technique for tenotomy

1. The calf is anaesthetized and small area over lateral surface of flexortendon should be prepared for operation.
2. % inch skin incision in between two flexortendon is given.
3. If only superficial tendon is to be cut, the edge of the blade should be turned out.
4. If both tendon are to be cut blade should to be inserted under the DDF, avoiding the large vessel in that area.[Fig.2(a)j]
5. The limb should be held in extension to tighten the flexortendon and one tendon cut at higher and another at lower level.[Fig.2(b)j]
6. Skin sutured by NA suture by simple interrupted pattern and limb should cast in plaster with padding.(Fig.3)]

Contracted Leg in Calves

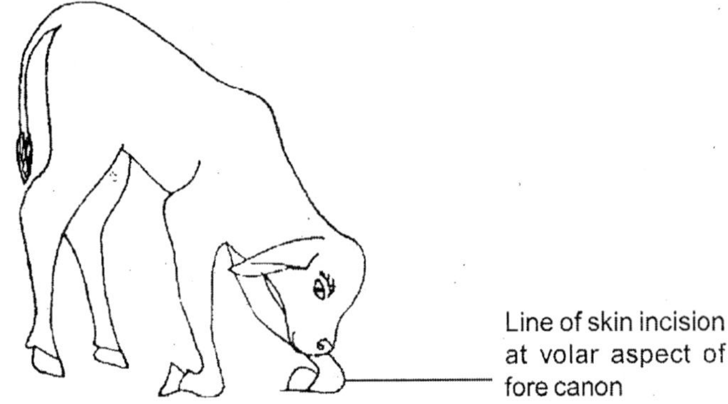

Fig. 1: Calf showing bilateral contracted leg

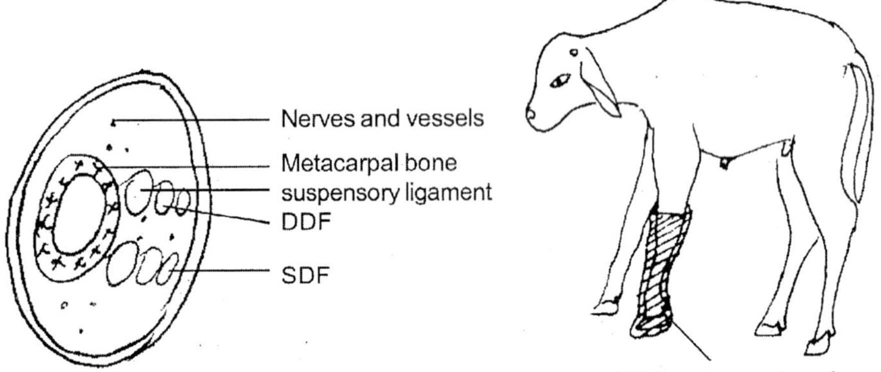

Fig. 2. (a) C.S. of fore canon at the level of operation showing structures.

Fig. 3: POP cast immobilisation of the contracted leg after operation.

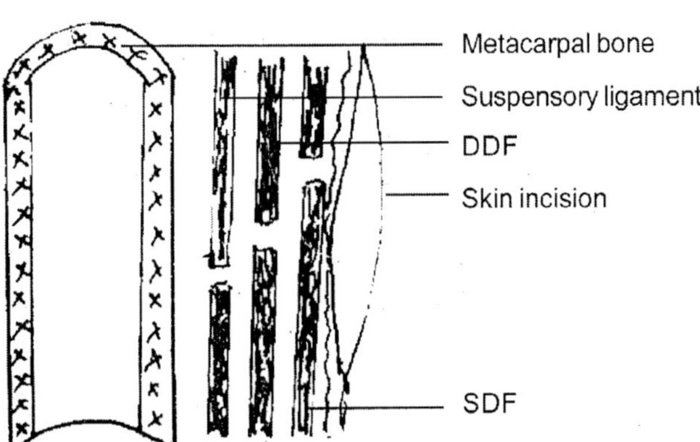

Fig. 2. (b) L.S. of fore canon showing cutting of tendon and ligament at different levels.

Pop Bandage Technique for Contracted Leg

Aim: To know the POP bandage technique for contracted legs.

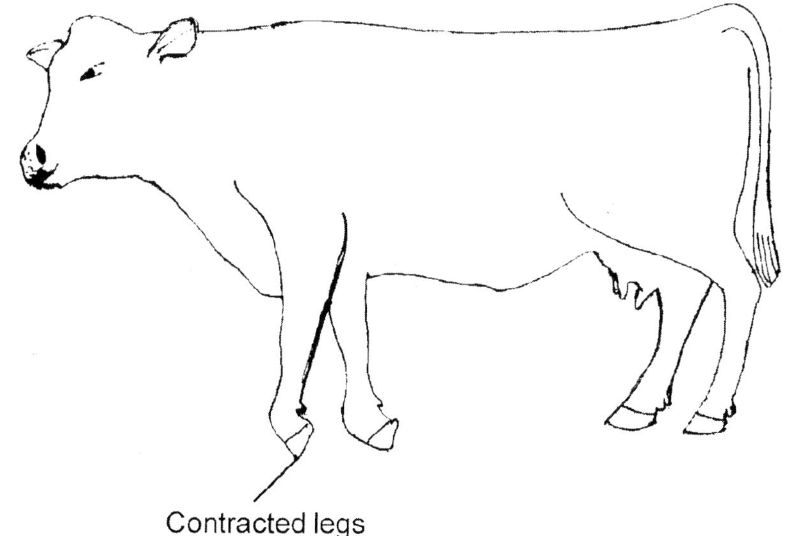

Fig. 1: Calf having contracted b: Lateral fore-limb.

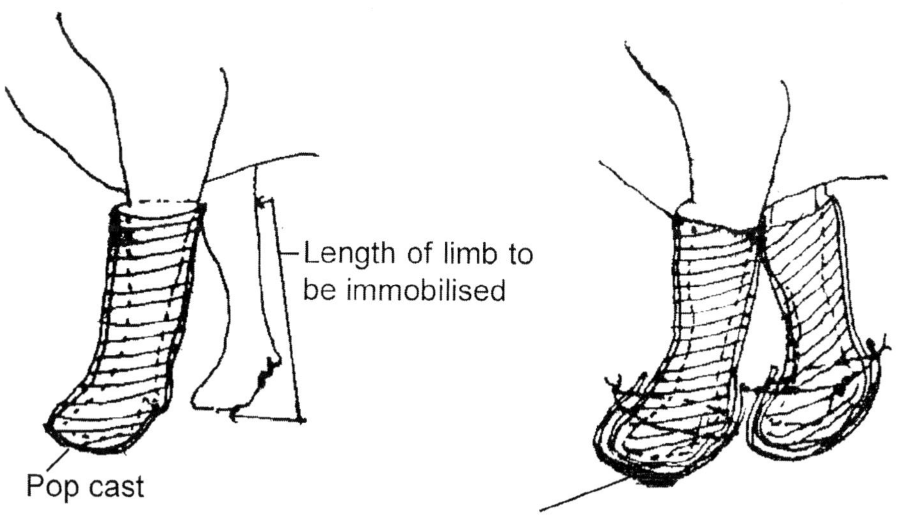

Fig. 2: Pop cast bandage.

Fig. 3: Rubber shoe protection over foot.

97

Flushing Facility of Compound Fracture

Management of Compound Fracture

An open fracture is an injury that occurs when a broken bone is exposed through the skin. This may mean that the bone is actually sticking out of the skin, or it may mean that the skin and soft-tissue is disrupted and exposes a path to the site of the fracture. Often called a compound fracture, an open fracture necessitates different treatment from the usual closed fracture.

Surgically Cleaning the Bone

Surgically cleaning the bone is one of the first steps for treating an open fracture. Most patients who sustain an open fracture undergo a surgery called "irrigation and debridement." Irrigation means washing the bone and the site of the injury. Debridement is described in the next step.

Determining the extent of injury can be difficult just by looking at an open fracture. This is especially true in high-energy injuries including automobile collisions and gunshot wounds. With these types of injuries, even small penetrations in the skin can cover very large areas of soft-tissue damage around an open fracture. Therefore, when surgically cleaning the bone, it is important to do this in the operating room (OR) under anesthesia — trying to sufficiently assess and clean the bone in the emergency room, without adequate anesthesia, may be insufficient.

Infection & Open Fractures

All open fractures are considered contaminated because of the communication between the fracture site and the environment outside of the body. While actual rates of contamination can vary, all open fractures should be considered to be contaminated. The likelihood that bacteria have entered the fracture site is dependent on a number of variables including the severity of the injury, the damage to soft-tissues, and the environment where the injury occurred.

Treatment of Open Fractures

Open fractures require urgent surgery to clean the area of the injury. Because of the break in the skin, debris and infection can travel to the fracture location, and lead to a high rate of infection in the bone. Once an infection is established, it can be a difficult problem to solve.

The timing of surgery is a subject of debate, as traditionally orthopedic surgeons have recommended surgery performed within six hours of the injury. More recently, some data has supported performing surgery with slightly less urgency, but within 24 hours of the injury.

In addition to surgical cleansing of the wound, treatment should include appropriate antibiotics and stabilization of the fracture. Patients should receive a tetanus shot if they are not up-to- date or are unaware of their vaccination status.

Recovery from an Open Fracture

Open fractures usually take longer to heal because of the extent of injury to the bone and the surrounding soft-tissues. Open fractures also have a high rate of complications including infection and non-union. Timely treatment can help avoid problems associated with open fractures. Emergency care will involve antibiotics, cleaning of the fracture site, and stabilization of the bones.

Management of Compound Fracture

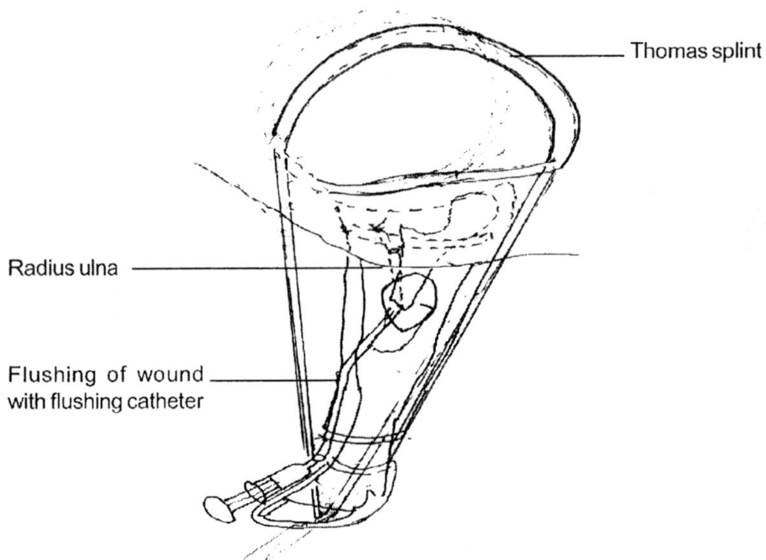

Fig. 1: Treatment of compound fracture of radius ulna.

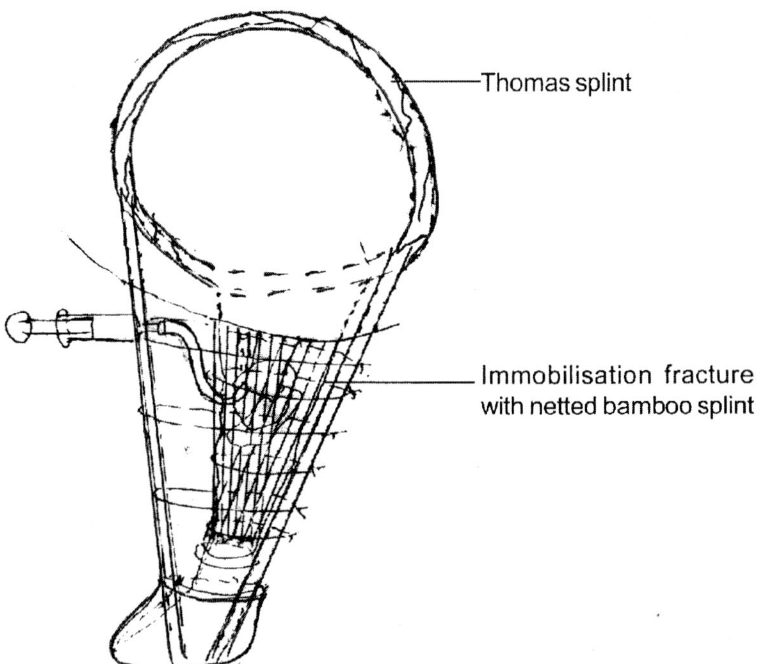

Fig. 2: Treatment of compound fracture of radius ulna.

Management of Compound Fracture

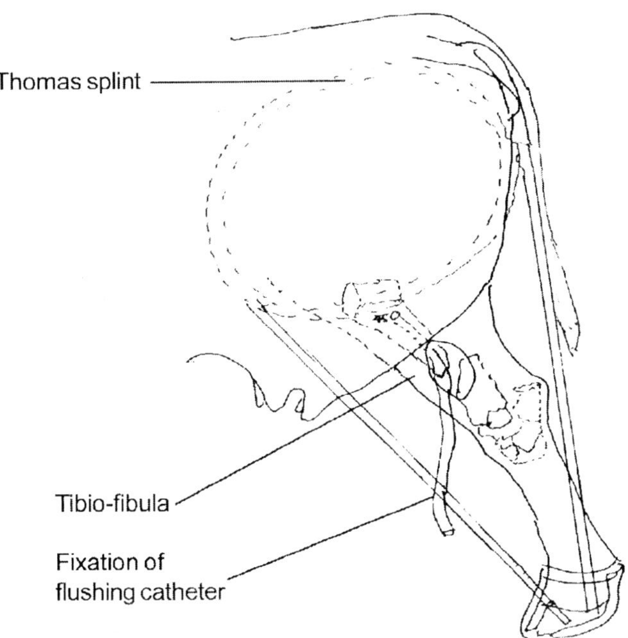

Fig. 3: Treatment of compound fracture of tibio-fibula

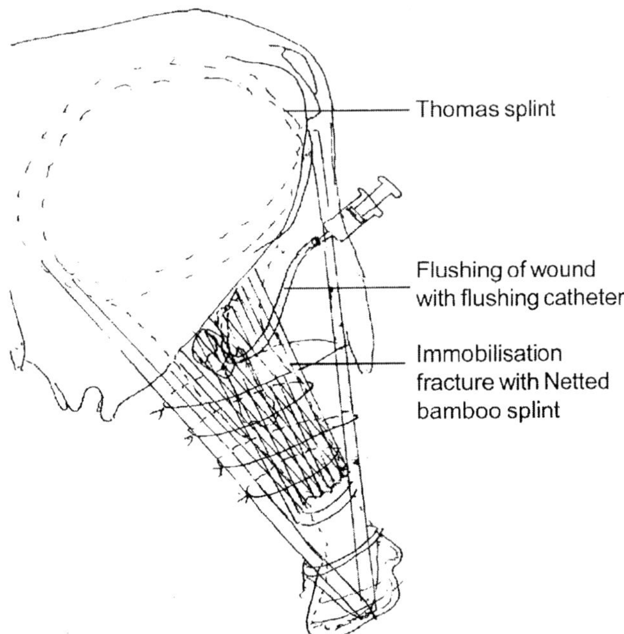

Fig. 4: Treatment of compound fracture of tibio-fibula

98

Flushing Facility of Compound Fracture

Aim: Regular flushing of compound and fracture using topical antibiotic or antiseptic required to bring the open wound and fracture either to a aseptic stage or to reduce the degree of infection and pus formation.

Procedure

1. After through cleaning the exposed bone as well as the wound of the compound fracture the wound is placed inside its part.
2. A thick walled rubber tube / plastic tube threaded with two end of a suture with a straight needle is carried to a higher site from the fracture within the wound.
3. The suture and needle is brought out, the sutures separated and again threaded and the flushing catheter is fixed with suture. Fig.1.(a) and Fig. 2. (a), (b).
4. The wound is protected with a thick absorbant sterile cotton padding, keeping the flushing catheter out through a small hole within the bandage. Fig. 1 (b) and Fig.2.(c)
5. The limb is immobilized as per the recommended procedure depending the level of fracture, outer end of the flushing catheter is kept outside, of the immobilization for carrying out regular flushing of the wound.

Post operative care

1. A course of parenteral higher antibiotic
2. Regular flushing of the wound using Lugol's iodine 0.3-0.5% solution, teramycin topical, glycerine and paraxin, mixture or povidone iodine solution.
3. The catheter is removed after either complete scar formation of the wound or after bone healing.

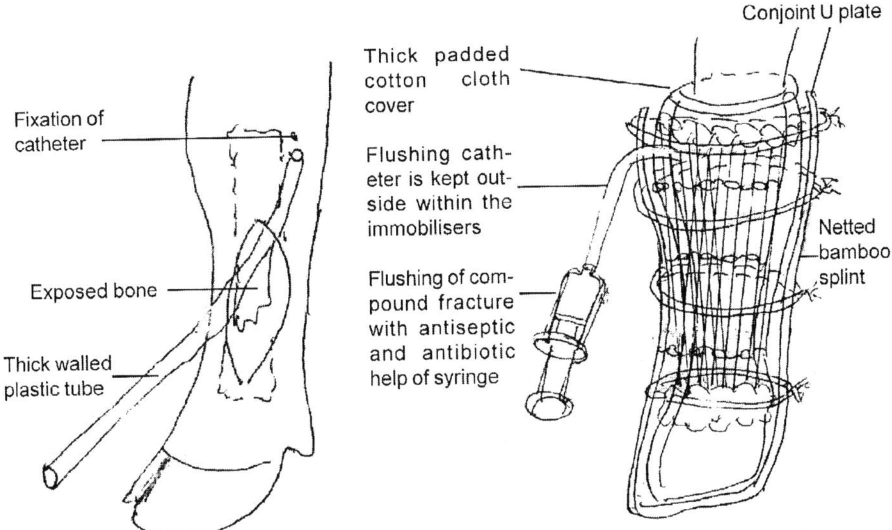

Fig. 1(a): Fixation of flushing catheter inside meta carpal compound fracture

Fig. 1(b): Immobilization of compound metacarpal fracture keeping the flushing

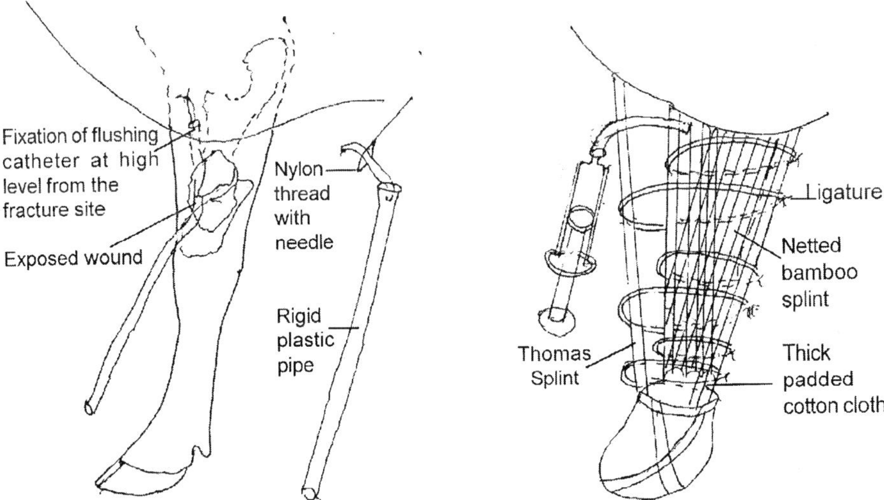

Fig. 2(a): Fixation of flushing catheter inside compound radius ulna fracture

Fig. 2(b): Preparation of flushing catheter

Fig. 2. (c): Immobilization of compound radius ulna fracture keeping the flushing catheter inside

99

Provision of Counter Opening and Flushing Catheter Fixation Within Infected Fracture

Definition

Wound with infection with 6 hours of occurrence can be brought to non infected stage by flushing.

Procedure

(1) The infected wound at fracture site is cleaned / flushed thoroughly using sufficient quantity with antiseptic solution.

(2) The site is applied with topical antiseptic / antibiotic and the size of the wound is reduced by placing interrupted stitches for skin closure.

(3) For drainage of inflammatory fluid, the counter opening is made as the distal part of the swelling of the dependent part of flushing catheter is placed inside to carry out regular flushing of the wound without removing the immobilizer.

(4) The fracture site is immobilized as per the conventional procedure using POP cast leaving two window over the opening of counter opening site.

Post operative care

(1) Along with the parenteral antibiotic regular application of local antiseptic / antibiotic inside the wound at fracture site is carried out through the flushing catheter.

(2) The immobilizer is removed after one month.

100

Classification of Tumor

Tissue of origin	Benign	Malignant
A) Tumors of mesenchymal origin		
1-Connective tissue and derivatives		
Fibrous connective tissue cell	Fibroma	Fibrosarcoma
Embryonic connective tissue cell that produces mucin	myxoma	myxosarcoma
Adipose tssue cell	lipoma	liposarcoma
chondrocyte	Chondroma	chondrosarcoma
2-Endothelial & related tissue		
Blood cells	Haemangioma	Haem angiosarcoma
Lymph vessels	Lymphangioma	Lymphangiosarcoma
Mesothelium		Mesothelioma
Meninges	Meningioma	Invasive meningioma
3-Tumors of haematopoietic cells		
Lymphoid cells	Lymphoma	Lymphoid leukemia Lymphsarcoma
Myeloid cells		Myeloid leukaemia
Plasma cells		Multiple myeloma
4-Tumors of muscle		
Smooth	Leomyoma	Leiomyosarcoma
Striated	Rhabdomyoma	Rhabdomyosarcoma
B)Tumours of Nervous tissue		
Glia	Glioma	gliosarcoma
Neuron	Neuroma	Neuroblastoma
C)Tumors of Epithelial origin	Papilloma	Squamous cell carcinoma
1. Startified squamous		
2. Basal cells of skin		Basal cells carcinoma
3. Glandular epithelium	Adenoma	Adenocarcinoma
4. Neuroectoderm(melanocytes)	Melanoma	Me I a nocarcinoma
5. Urinary tract epithelium(transitional) papilloma	Transitional cell	Transitional cell carcinoma
6. Testicular epithelium(germ cells)		Seminoma

Reference: Vegad J.L. (2007). A Textbook of Veterinary General Pathology, *2nd* Edition, PR 278-279.

101

Classification of Bone Tumours

1. ***True bone tumours.*** Neoplasms arising from cells of mesenchymal origin, derived from a common ancestry and whose function is primarily skeletal boen formation. These tumours fall into four main groups according to the predominant cell type present. By reason of the mutability of the cells metaplasia is common and intermediate stages are found.

Cell type predominating	*Simple tumour types*	*Malignant*
A. Osteoblast Tumour Cells show active ossification	Osteoma Osteoid osteoma	Osteosarcoma - Primary
B. Chondroblast Tumour cells show active cartilage formation	Benign osteoblastoma Chondroma	- Parosteal Chondrosarcoma - Primary
C. Fibroblast Tumour cells show active collagen formation	Benign chondroblastoma Chrondromyxoid fibroma	- Secondary Desmoid sarcoma Rhabdomysarcoma
D. Osteoclast Tumour cells show active bone destruction by giant cells	Fibroma Solitary bone cyst Non-osteogenic fibroma Osteoclastoma	Malignant Osteoclastoma

2. Tumours arising from tissues normally found in bone but not participating in bone formation

A. Tumours arising from fibrous tissue, forming the non-osteogenllc outer layer (fascial) of the periosteum-

periosteal fibroma

periosteal fibrosarcoma

B. Tumours arising from the elements of bone marrow -

myeloma
reticulum cell sarcoma
Hodgkin's disease of bone
lymphosoarcoma
"Ewing's sarcoma'

C. Tumours from blood vessels-

haemangioma
haemangloblastoma
aneurysmal bone cyst
angiosarcoma

D. Tumours arising from adipose tissue-

lipoma
liposarcoma

E. Tumours arising from nerves

neurilemmoma
neurofibroma

3. Tumours arising fom included tiissue

chordoma
adamantinoma

4. Metastatic tumours of bone

Exarticulation of claw in Cattle

Exarticulation of claw:- Ablation of an extremity at a level of a joint (coronate joint) inside claw.

Indications:- Suppuration of the tendon and joint.

Instruments: Sage knife, Scissors, Scalpel, Forceps, Artery Forceps, Curette or Quittor Knife, Wire or Blade Saw, Esmarch's Bandage, Bandage Material.

Anaesthesia:- Infiltration of the nerves in the region of the fetlock or high epidural anaesthesia.

Diagrams

Aim of surgery:- To perform exarticulation of claw in cattle.

Methods/procedure

- Cast the animal and tie the limb (tourniquet applied). Clean the claw with soap & water.
- Make a curved incision in an anterior and proximal direction by introducing the sage knife to the deepest part with its concavity pointing upwards.
- Make a second curve incision in a proximal and volar (plantar) direction.
- Then introduce the knife between the third phalanx and the navicular bone and make an incision at right angle to sole.
- Cut the medial wall of claw and well developed medial ligament of the interphalangeal joint through an anteroposterior direction and ligate the vessels.
- Scrap the articular surface of the sesamoid bone and second phalanx with the curette to remove the necrotic parts of tendon.
- Apply an antibiotic (Sulphonamide) under an antiseptic bandage and enclose the foot with a leather or canvas foot.
- If the infection spread to higher that is second phalanx, then amputation must be performed at the level of first phalanx.

Post Operative Care

- Administration of antibiotic parenterally or locally
- Daily change of bandage
- Rest to the animal till the problem is solved.

"Better to go for exarticulation, than to wait for unnecessary amputation"

Reference : Berge, E., and Westhues, M. (1996). Veterinary Operative Surgery, Medical Book Co. Denmark, PP. 383-384

102

Amputation of the Claw

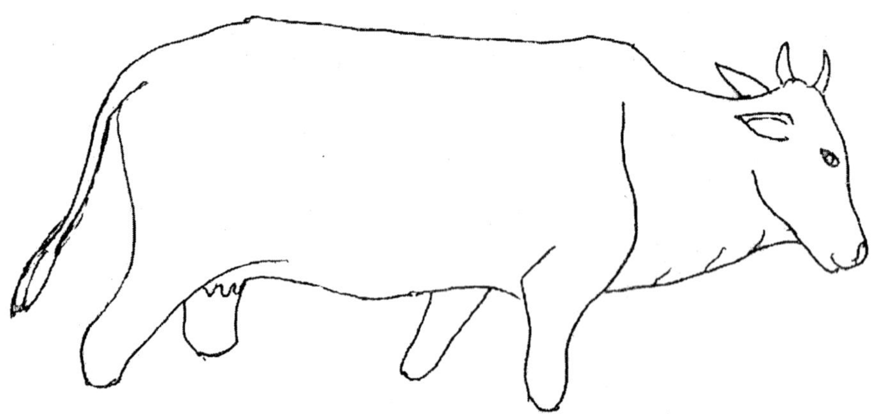

Fig. 1: An Insentire

Amputation of Claw in Cattle

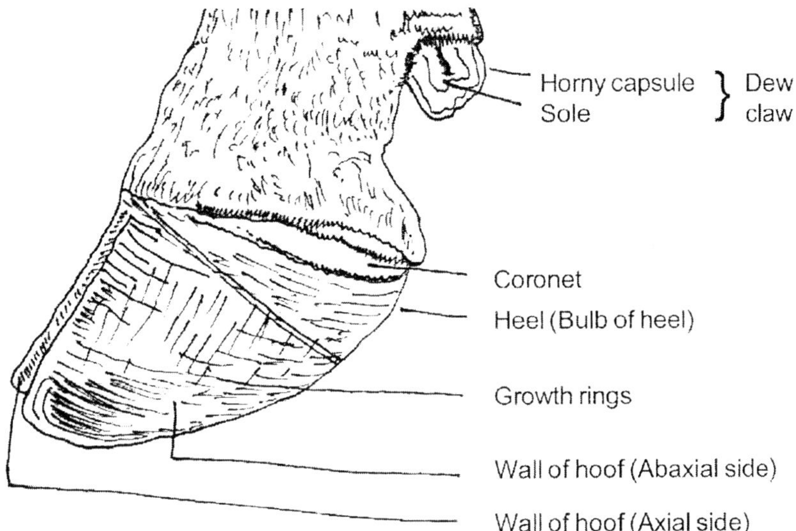

Fig. 1: Exarticulation of claw (Before exarticulation) with direction of saw cut.

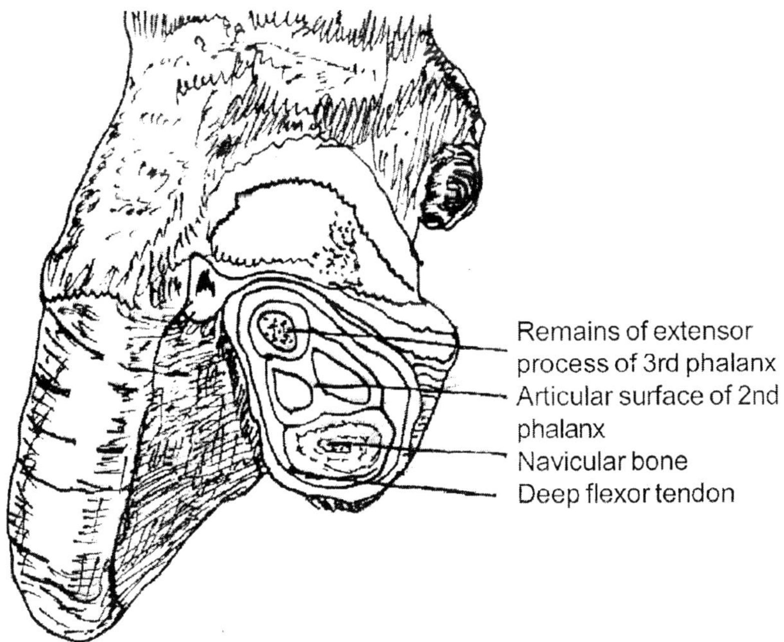

Fig. 2: Exarticulation of claw (After exarticulation).

Reference: Berge, E., and Westhues, M. (1996). Veterinary Operative Surgery, Medical Book Co. Denmark, PR 383-384.

Amputation of the Claw

Indication: Cellulitis and purulent inflammation of the pastern joint, arthritis of the 2nd interphalangeal joint and cellulitis in the phalangeal region.

Instruments: Esmarch's bandage, drawing knife, paring knife, retractor hooks, scissors, scalpel, suture material.

Anaesthesia: Infiltration of nerves above the fetlock or high epidural anaesthesia. In pig, general anaesthesia is used.

Technique

- The animal is cast and foot is tied to the diagonally opposite one so that the affected claw is uppermost.
- A tourniquet is applied proximal to the carpal (or.tarsal) joint, cleaned with paring knife, warm water and shop followed by sharing upto fetlock joint all around and disinfected.
- Amputation of the claw is best done above the 1 interphalengeal joint because, this is the upper limit of inflammatory and necrosis process.
- The operation is started with skin incison in the midline of the dorsal surface of the toe.(Fig.l)
- The skin incision goes from the proximal end of 1 palanx to the horny claw and then to interdigital space In one hand and to lateral surface on the other, so that a triangular piece of skin Is left (1/2 -1 cm high) on the dorsal surface of the coronet.
- A second similar incision is made in the midline of the posterior surface of the toe.
- From the incision In the intergital space, the ligaments and the adipose tissue are cut. Bleeding is controlled by ligatures.
- Then, with wire saw, the 1st phalanx is sawn through In an oblique direction from distantly and medially to proximal and lateral (Fig.2).The sawing must be interrupted to avoid overheating the tissues.
- Diseased tissues are now removed with scissors /knife. Sulfonamide is applied to the wound cavity and the edges of the wound are closed with Interrupted sutures (Fig.3)
- A bandage is now applied, smeared over with tar and left unchanged for 12-14 days.

Reference: Berge, M. & Westhues, H. (1966), Veterinary Operative Surgery, Medical Book Company, Copenhagen, RR-379-382.

Amputation of the Claw

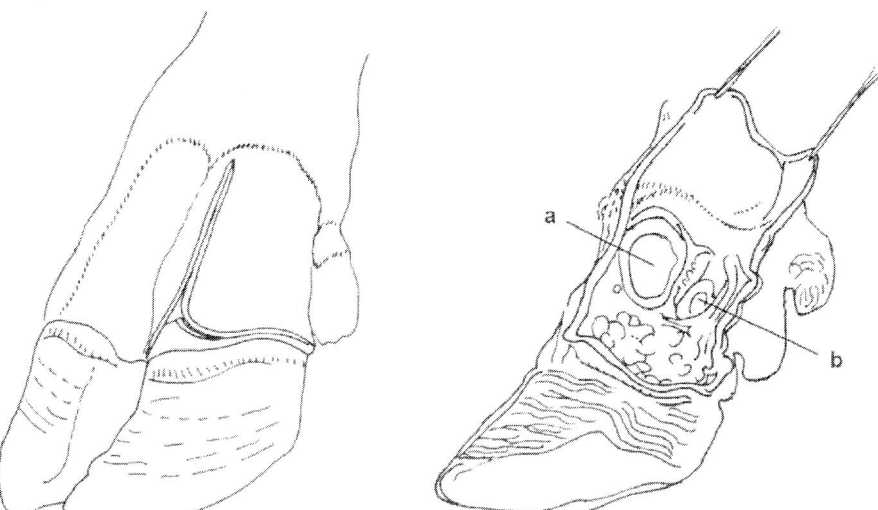

Fig. 1: Course of the skin incision on the dorsal surface of the fetlock and pastern.

Fig. 2: The skin flap is turned up. The amputation was made thorugh the first phalanx. a. Cut surface of the 1st phalanx. At surface of the flexor tendo

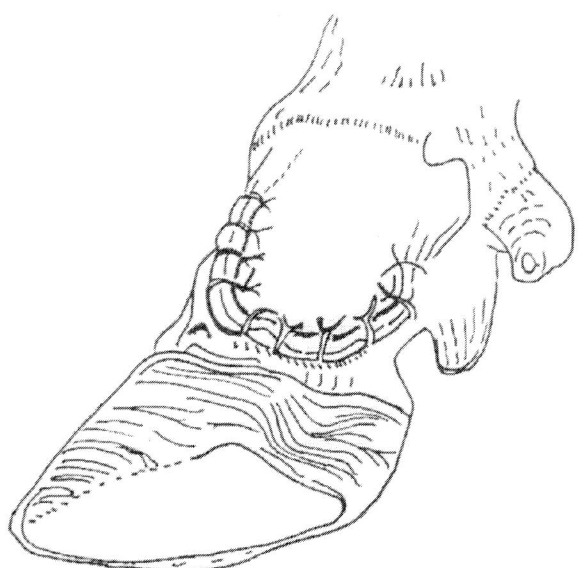

Fig. 3: Skin sutures after completion of hte operation.

Reference: Berge, M. & Westhues, H. (1966), Veterinary Operative Surgery, Medical Book Company, Copenhagen, P.P.-379-382.

103

Single Digit Amputation

Objetive

To completely exercise a cancerous hoof in presence with cauliflower like growth with regular bleeding & myosis.

Material Required

Amputation saw, thick padded with bandage roll, a mixture of powder containing resin and naphthalene ball powder, bicycle tube protection sleeper (Fig-3), local anesthesia.

Procedure

- Site is cleaned thoroughly and amputation site is saved with blade .Tincture iodine is applied around the digit over the saw line .Site is anaesthetize by local anesthesia.
- Rubbertourniquet is applied above the fetlock joint (Fig-2).
- Both the cancerous hoof are completely incise from a healthy side with help of a sharp sterile amputation saw.
- A thick layer cotton padded Is placed over the amputated stump after dusting a mixture containing resin naphthalene ball powder and termeri powder Fig. 3.
- The thick padded cloth cover over the stump and written in position with by wrapping rubbertourniquet.
- Bicycle tube rubber protection sleeper is cover over these area and written position with ligature.

Post Operative Care

- Parenteral antibiotic given 5-7 day.
- Animal keep in clean and dry place. Regularly dressing of wound 5-7 days interval up to 1 month.

Single Digit Amputation

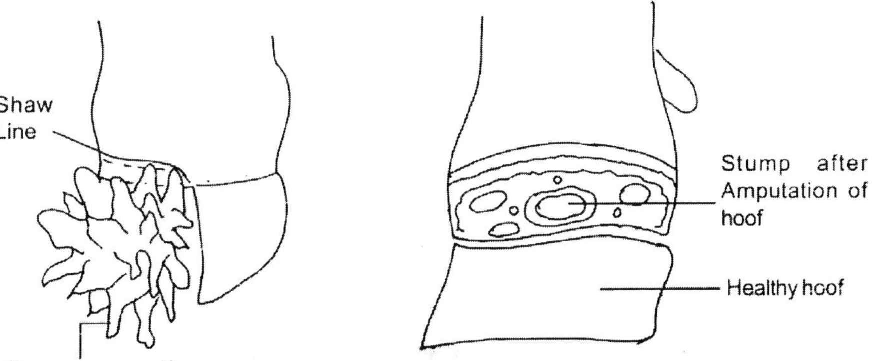

Fig. 1: Hoof growth with couliflower like growth in unilateral hoof

Fig. 2: Amputation of unilateral hoof with cancerous growth

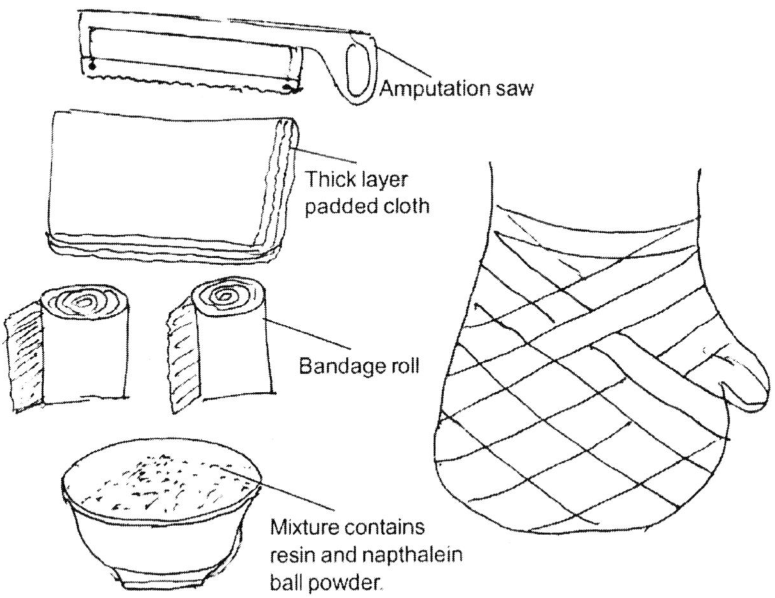

Fig. 3: Hom amputation material

Fig. 4: After bandage cover.

104

Double Digit Amputation

Indication

Bilateral digital cancerous growth cauliflower like(fig-1),cancerous growth with continuous bleeding and myasis.

Aim

To remove the cancerous growth from healthy side by surgery. (Fig. 1-2)

Material Required

Amputation saw, thick padded with bandage roll ,a mixture of powder containing resin and naphthalene ball powder, bicycle tube protection sleeper(Fig-3),local anesthesia.

Procedure

- Site is cleaned thoroughly and amputation site is saved with blade .Tincture iodine is applied around the digit over the saw line .Site is anaesthetize by local anesthesia.
- Rubber tourniquet is applied above the fetlock joint(Fig-2).
- Both the cancerous hoof are completely incise from a healthy side with help of a sharp sterile amputation saw.
- A thick layer cotton padded is placed over the amputated stump after dusting a mixture containing resin, naphthalene ball powder and termeric powder.
- The thick padded cloth cover over the stump and written in position with by wrapping rubber tourniquet.
- Bicycle tube rubber protection sleeper is cover over these area and written position with ligature.

Post Operative Care

- Parenteral antibiotic given 5-7 day.
- Animal keep In clean and dry place. Regularly dressing of wound 5-7 days interval up to 3 month.

Double Digit Amputation

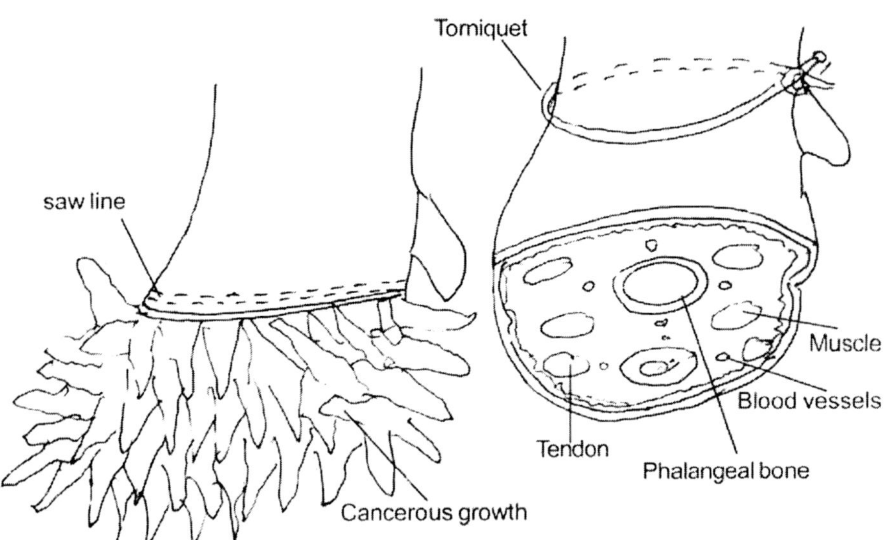

Fig. 1: Foot showing bilateral cancerous growth

Fig. 2: After amputation of bone the digit.

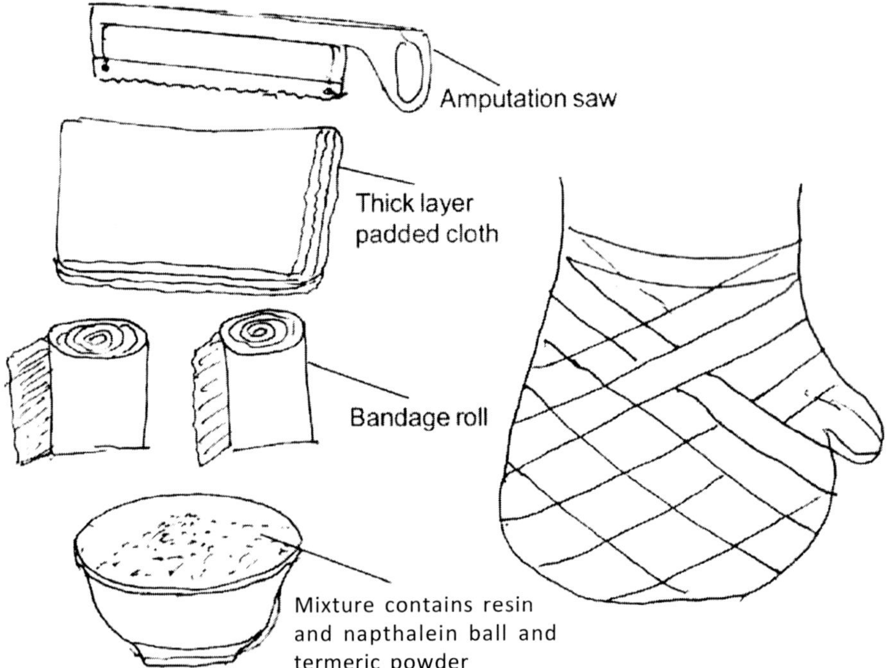

Fig. 3: Amputation material.

Fig. 4: After bandage cover.

105

Level of Amputation at Fore & Hind Limb by Bone Section Technique

Aim: Amputation of limb by bone section technique.

Indication: Irreparable injury; Gangrene; Malignant disease.

Site:

Fore-limb: Common site is junction of the lower and middle third of the radius(fore-arm).

Hind-limb: common site is the middle third of the leg region(tibia).

Anaesthesia and control: Fore-limb: general anaesthesia; Hind-limb: epidural anaesthesia. Operated in lateral recumbent position.

Procedure

1. A tourniquet is applied below the elbow or stifle as the case may be.
2. The skin flap is made by giving a bold elliptical incision running in medio-lateral direction sufficiently below from level of amputation to provide a proper cover and padding over the bone stump at indicated site as shown in Fig.1.
3. The skin and muscle flaps are reflected upward up-to the level of amputation and the bone is cut from the appropriate level from appropriate site using hand saw as indicated in Fig. 2(a) and Fig. 3(a).
4. Bleeding is controlled either by forcive pressure or by ligation of bleeding vessels. Nerve ends are crushed.
5. The site is applied with antiseptic or antibiotic solution and the stump is covered by suturing tendinous part of muscles in a systematic manner.
6. The method of covering the muscle is anterior group of muscle with posterior group and medial group with lateral group is done to bring proper stump movement: Muscle is sutured with thick catgut or prolene as indicated in Fig.2(b) and Fig.3(b).

7. Finally the skin is closed with nylon suture as indicated in fig:-2(c) and fig:-3(c).
8. The stump is covered with a thick, antiseptic, absorbent pad.

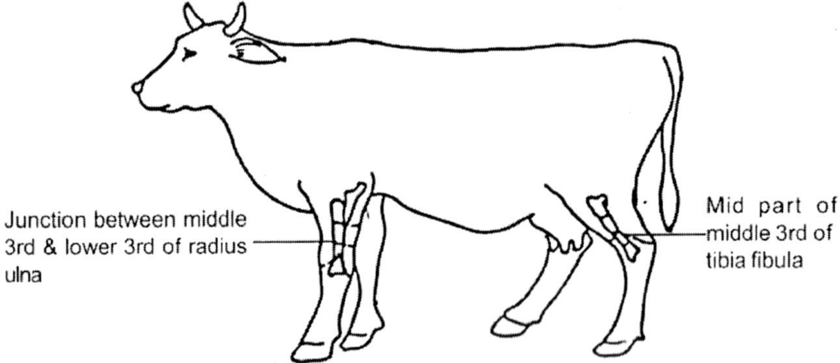

Fig. 1: Showing level of amputation at fore & hind limb.

Reference: Venugopalan. A, (2013), Essentials of Veterinary Surgery, 8th edition,Oxford & IBS Publishers, New Delhi, pp-512.

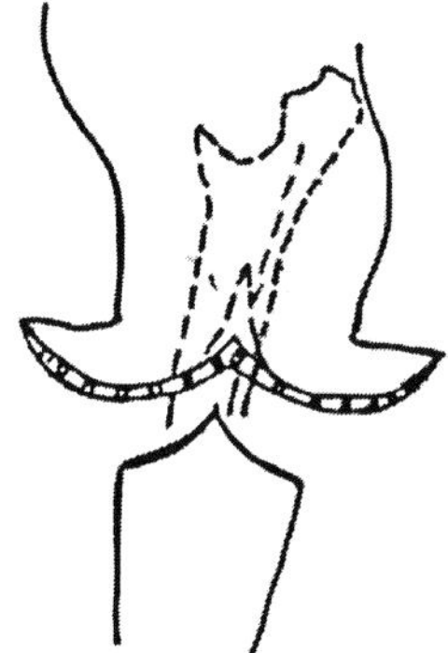

Fig. 2a: Showing skin and muscle incised and reflected upward at site of incision in radius unla

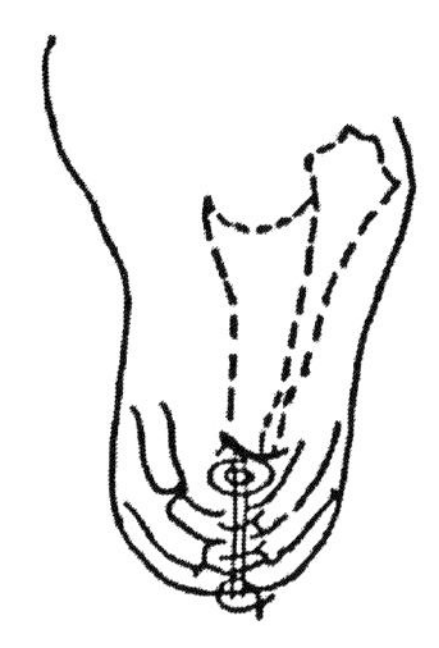

Fig. 2b: Showing cutting of bone and suturing of muscle tendons together

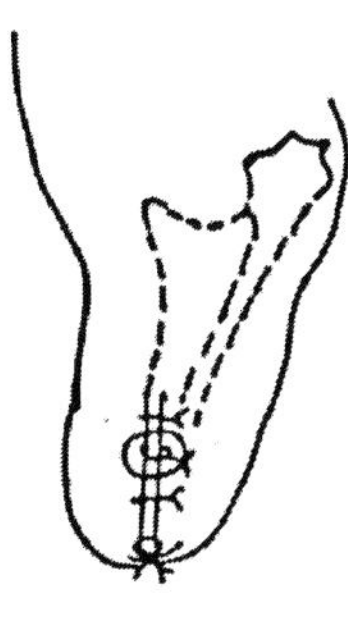

Fig. 2c: Showing skin suturing over the top

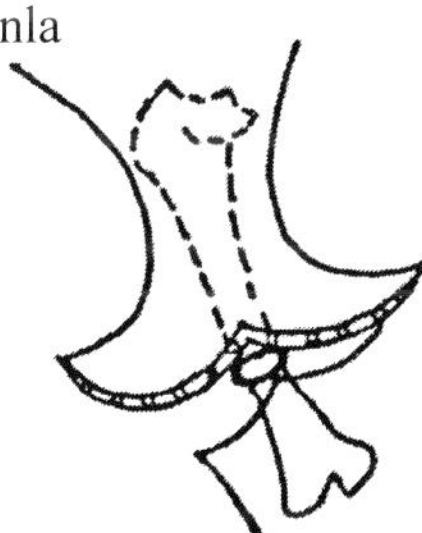

Fig. 3a: Showing skin and muscle incised and reflected upward at site of incision in tibia fibula

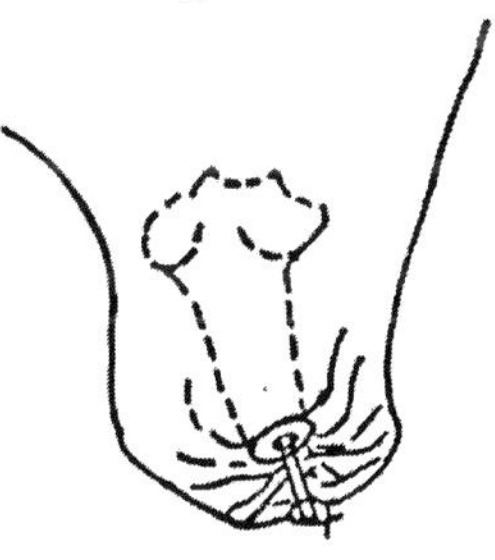

Fig. 3b: Showing cutting of bone and suturing of muscle tendons together

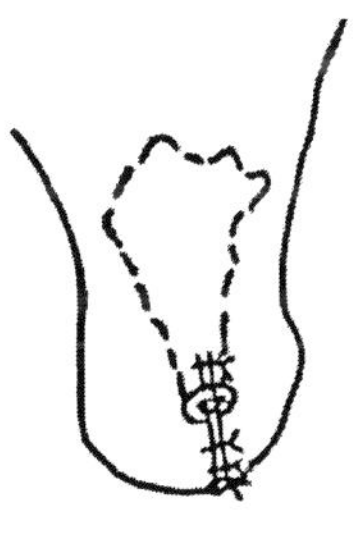

Fig. 3c: Showing skin suturing over the stump

Reference: Venugopalan. A, (2013), Essentials of Veterinary Surgery, 8th edition,Oxford & IBS Publishers, New Delhi, pp-512.

Various Level Amputation by Bone Section

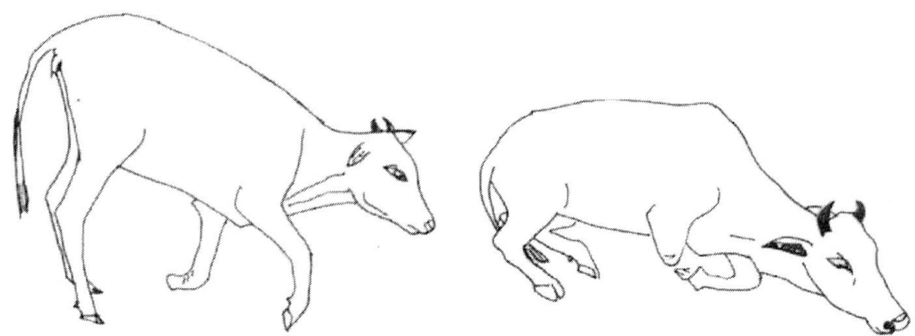

Fig. 1(a): Below knee amputation **Fig. 1(b):** Above knee amputation

Fig. 1: Forelimb amputation by bone section

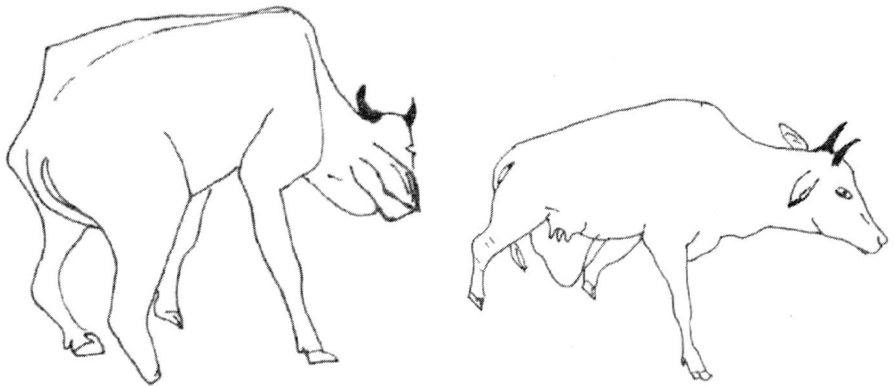

Fig. 2(a): Below hock amputation **Fig. 2(b):** Above hock amputation

Fig. 2: Hindlimb amputation by bone section

106

Method of Apposing Muscle, Fascia, Skin Over Amputed Stump

Aim

Study about method of apposing muscle, fascia, skin over amputed stump.

Indication

Proper healing of amputed stump, avoiding infections.

Description

Limb is amputed generally through diaphysis or by disarticulation method. Whatever is the amputation,the surgeon should always keep as much soft tissue as possible to cover the bone extrimities. It is difficult to achieve in large animal, when amputation is immediately below carpus or tarsus.

Surgical Techniques

1. After amputation the aiiiputed bony stump should be covered vyith surrounding muscle in such a manner that a perfect muscular pad will cover over bony stump .
2. Some articular surface are very irregular and sharp edges must be removed with a rongeur to make the surface smooth before covering it with m.uscle.
3. For apposing of muscle ,the anterior group muscle is sutured with posterior group and medial group muscle with lateral group (fig.3a) using several interrupted suture using chromic cat gut.
4. Muscular suture is covered by 2nd layer suturing of fascia. In 2nd layer covering the fascia is apposed with several interrupted suture using chromic cat gut.

5. Finally skin flap apposed with several vertical mattress interrupted suture using chromic cat gut.
6. Lastly the stump is covered by a thick bandage to prevent any trauma to suture line when animal will stand.

Precaution

1. Muscle and fascia should be kept attached to skin to improve healing and form padding between bone and skin.
2. Suture line should never be on distal aspect of stump.
3. Suture line will not be on tension surface.
4. Blood supply should be considered while apposing as it is more aboundant at distal aspect of limb than cranial.

Post Operative Care

1. NSAID are given for 3 days post operatively.
2. Parenteral antibiotics for 3-5 days.
3. Amputed cattle are generally confined to a stall to avoid premature breakdown of opposite leg.

Reference: Nayak .S, and Mohanty, J. (1999) Joint disarticulation m.ethod for limb amputation at various level in bovine practice . Indian Vet. Journal ,76 :42-44

Method of Apposing Muscle, Fascia, Skin Over Amputed Stump

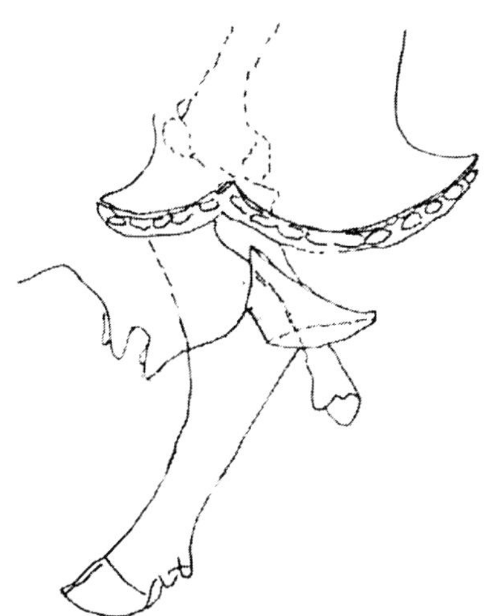

Fig. 1: Left femuro tibia amputed stump showing skin flap ratio Lateral

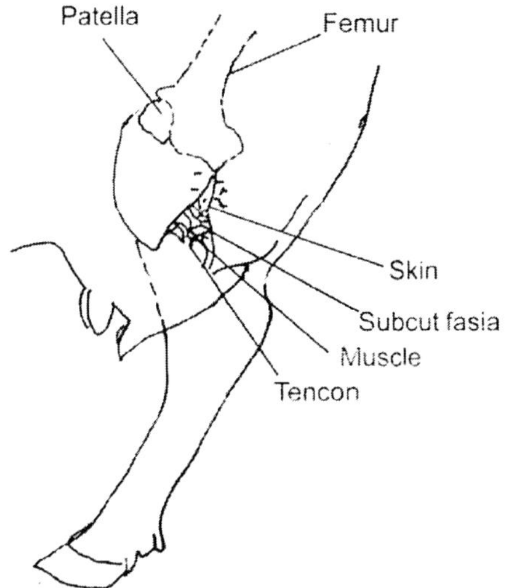

Fig. 2: Closure technique of skin facia, muscle, tendon

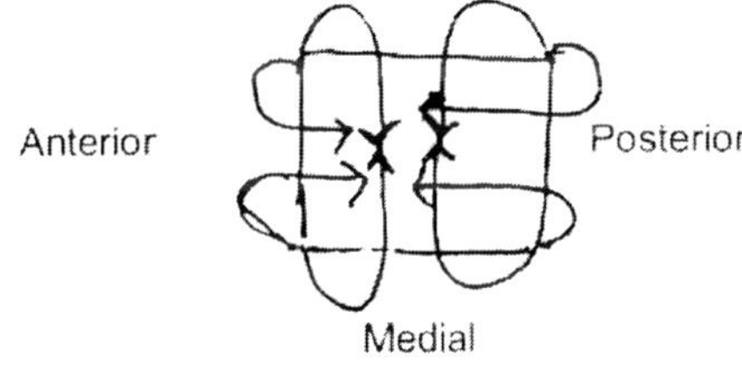

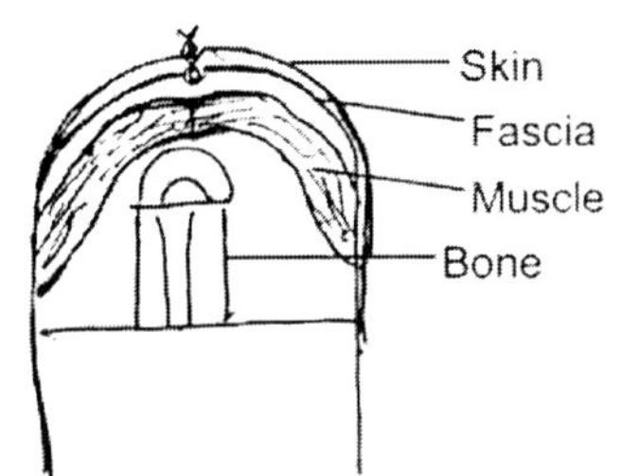

Fig. 3b: Apposition of muscle, fascia and skin over amputed stump

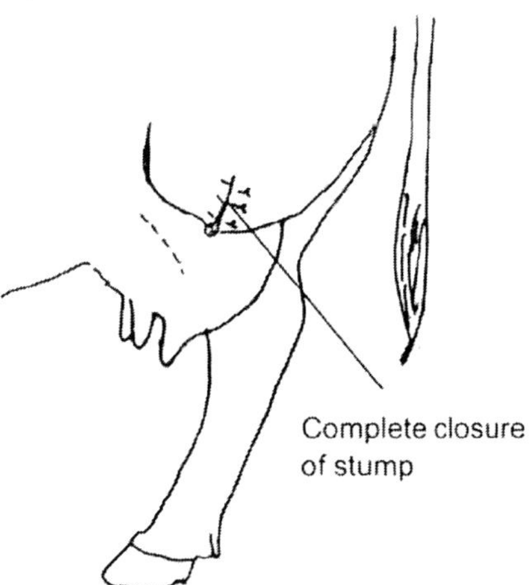

Fig. 4: Stifle amputed stump

107

Joint Disarticulation Method of Limb Amputation

Joint disarticulation: Unwanted limb is amputed by joint disarticulation method.

Site of amputation along with skin-muscle flap ratio

- Fore limb: 1. Elbow disarticulation(5:1)
  2. Carpo-metacarpal disarticulation(1:2)
  3. Fetlock disarticulation(1:4)
- Hind limb: 1. Stifle disarticulation(1:5)
  2. Tarso-metatarsal disarticulation(1:2)
  3. Fetlock disarticulation(1:4)

Anaesthesia: local infiltration anaesthesia.

Method

- After controlling the animal in lateral recumbency, skin is incised as per the recommended flap ratio (Fig.l)
- Skin, subcutaneous fascia, muscles, blood vessels, periosteum are incised by bold incision without separating the layers from each other (totoflap). Both anterior and posterior flaps are reflected from the bone up the level of the specific joint.
- The bone is separated from the joint with the help of bp blade. Bleeding vessels are controlled.
- Site is applied with topical antiseptic/antibiotic.
- The bone stump is covered with muscles of anterior flap and posterior flap by several Interrupted chromic catgut suture.

- Anterior group of muscles are anchored with posterior group of muscles. Medial group of muscles are anchored with lateral group to keep the function of the stump normal.
- Fascia of anterior flap as well as posterior flap apposition sutures is made.
- Finally skin is apposed with vertical mattress skin suture.

Post operative care

- Protection of cover bandage.
- Application of fly repellent over the affected site.
- A course of antibiotic is administered.

Various Amputation Level with Skin Flap Ratio

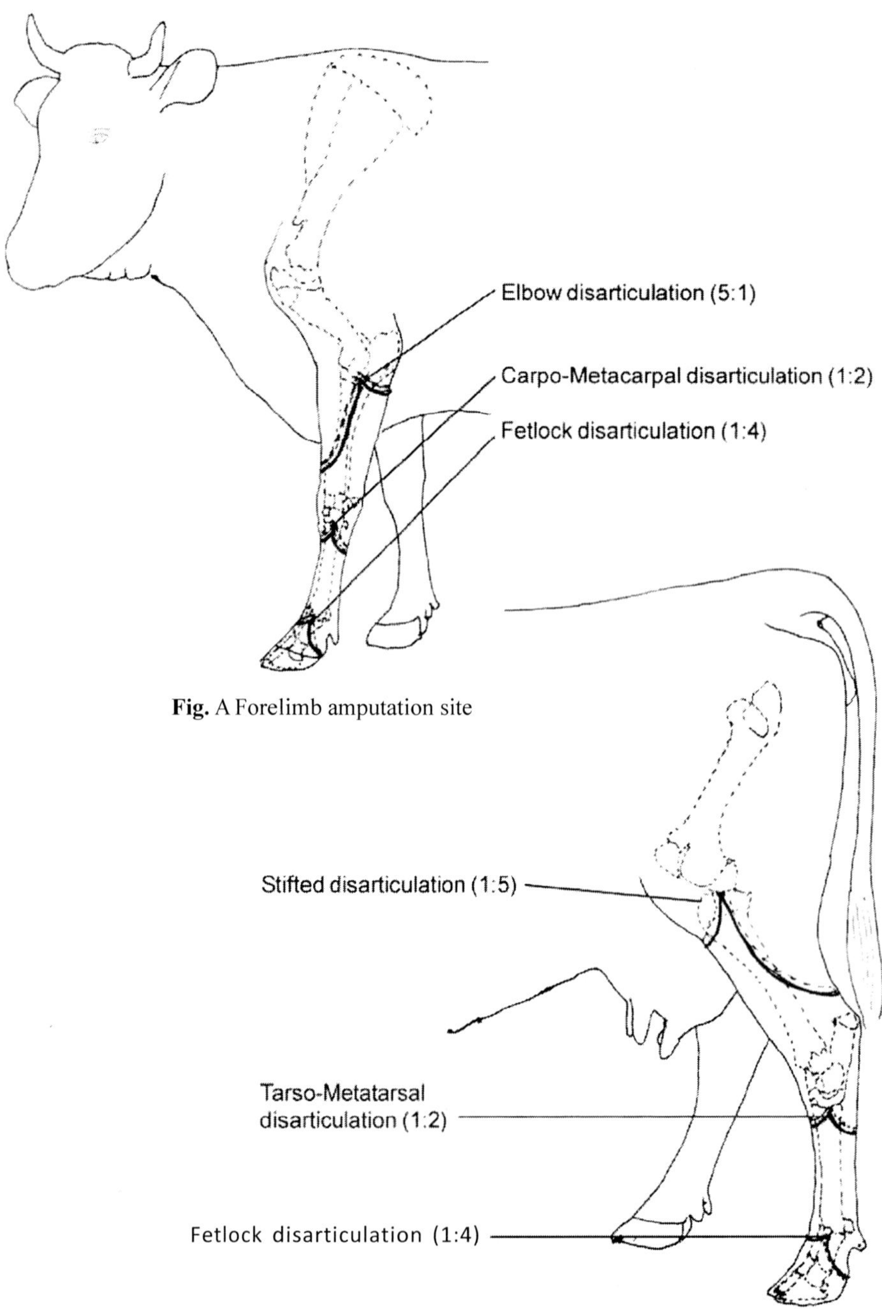

Fig. A Forelimb amputation site

Fig. 1: B Hindlimb amputation site

108

Fetlock Disarticulation

Indicaton: Irreversible damage of both the bovine digits & to provide a foot pad for comfortable walking of animal

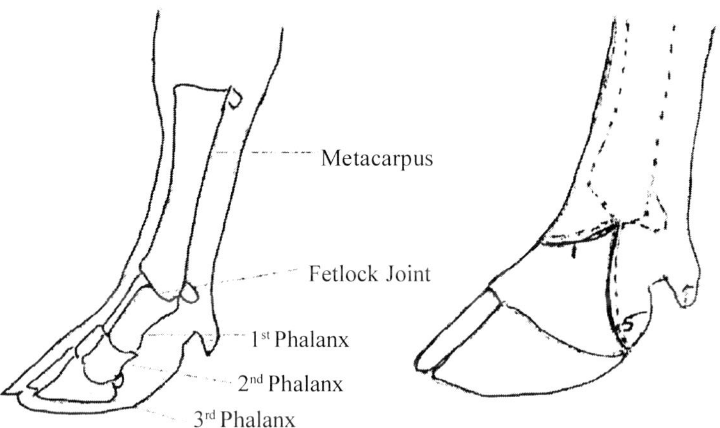

Fig. 1: Fetlock joint

Fig. 2: Skin in laceration in relation to bovine

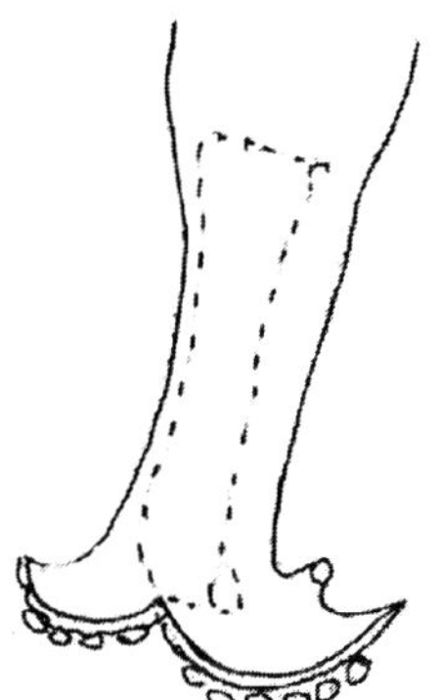

Fig. 3: After both disarticulation

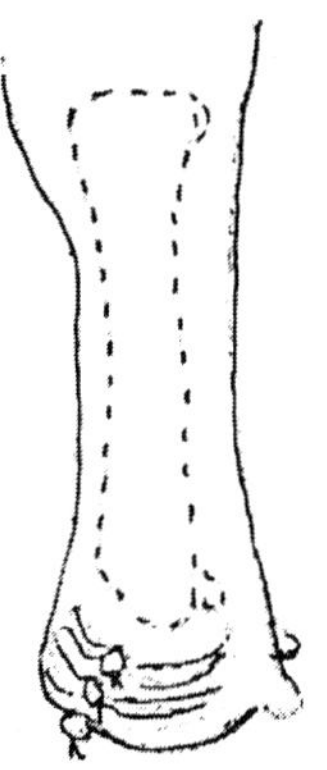

Fig. 4: Apposition of muscle and nerves

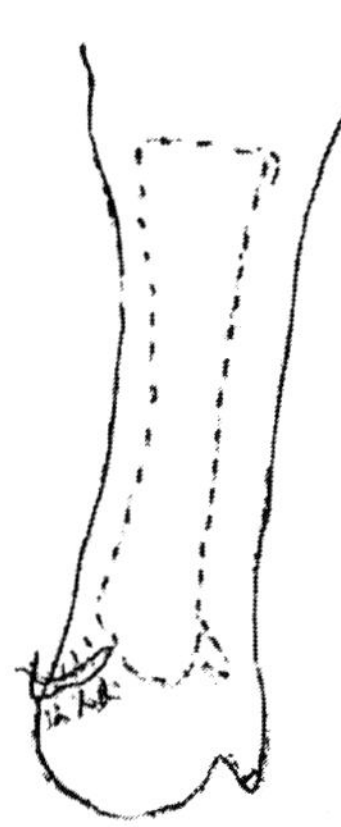

Fig. 5: Fircal skin closure with stem

109

Carpo-Metacarpal Joint Disarticulation

Indication: Irreparable damage of metacarpal bone.

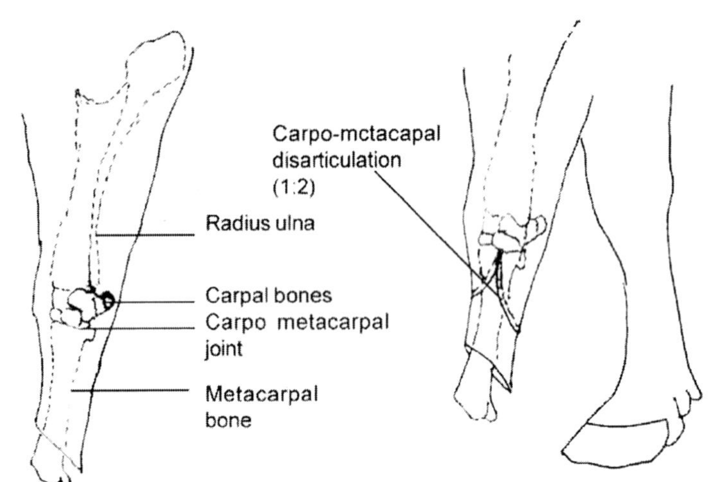

Fig. 1: Noarmla anatomy of carpo-metacapal joint

Fig. 2: Skin muscle flap ratio in relation to bone (1:2)

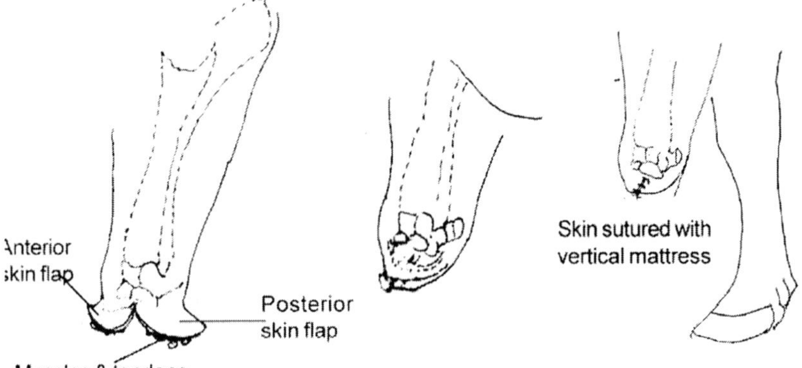

Fig. 3: Skin muscle flaps

Fig. 4: Appositional suture of muscles and tendons

Fig. 5: Skin closure

110

Elbow Disarticulation

Definition : It is a technique in which foreiirnb is amputed from elbow joint.
Indication : Incurable damage of radius ulna.

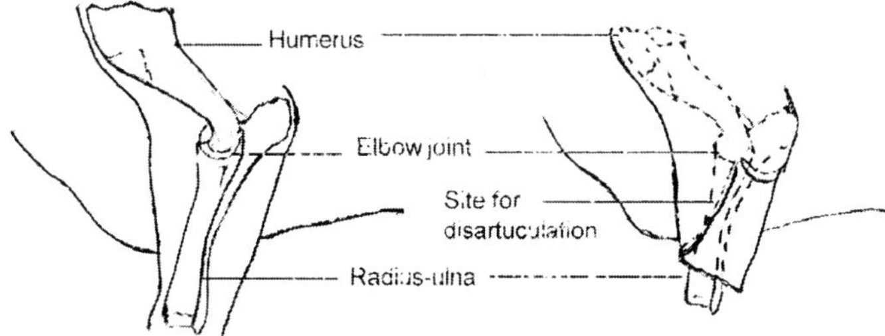

Fig. 1: Normai anatomay of elbow joint

Fig. 2: Skin muscle flap ratio in relation to bon

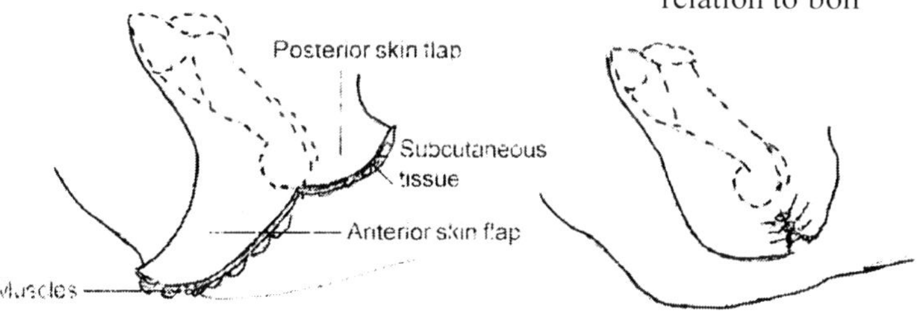

Fig. 3: Skin flaps

Fig. 4: Appositional suture of muscle and tendons

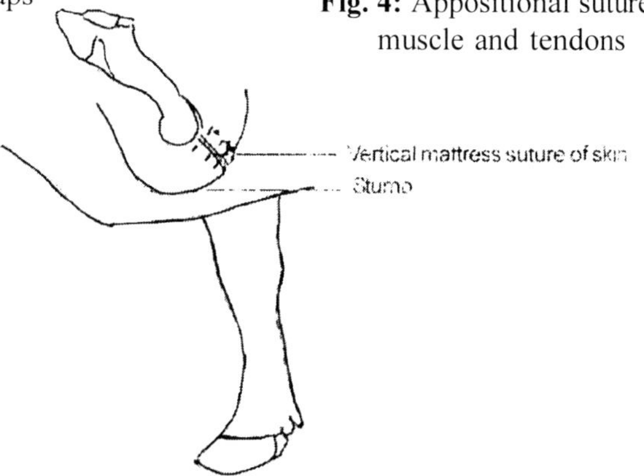

111

Shoulder Disarticulation

Indication

- Irreparable injury.
- Frost bite, burn.
- Malignant neoplasia.
- Incurable peripheral vascular disease.
- Necrosis, gangrene, extensive injury of nerve of fore limb.

Control & Anaesthesia

Lateral recumbency under regional anaesthesia.

Site

Caudal angle of axilla and above elbow joint (Fig. 1).

Surgical Technique

1. A circular incision around the elbow is given.(Fig-2)
2. Then a linear straight line incision over the humerus bone is given.(Fig-2)
3. The groove between the long head of triceps and deltoid is separated bluntly to approach the humerus bone.(Fig-3)
4. Importance is given to avoid damage to major blood vessels and nerves.
5. The humerus bone is disarticulated from the joint.(Fig-4)
6. After disarticulation the separated muscles are closed in continuous fashion.
7. Lastly the skin is closed in inverted T fashion.(Fig-5)

Post Operative Care

1. Antiseptic dressing is done till healing is complete.
2. A course of antibiotic and analgesic should be administered.
3. Suture should be removed 8-10 days after surgery or after complete healing.

Reference: Ghosh, R.K., (2012), Primary Veterinary Anatomy, Edition, Current Books International, Kolkata-13, P.126.

Shoulder Disarticulation

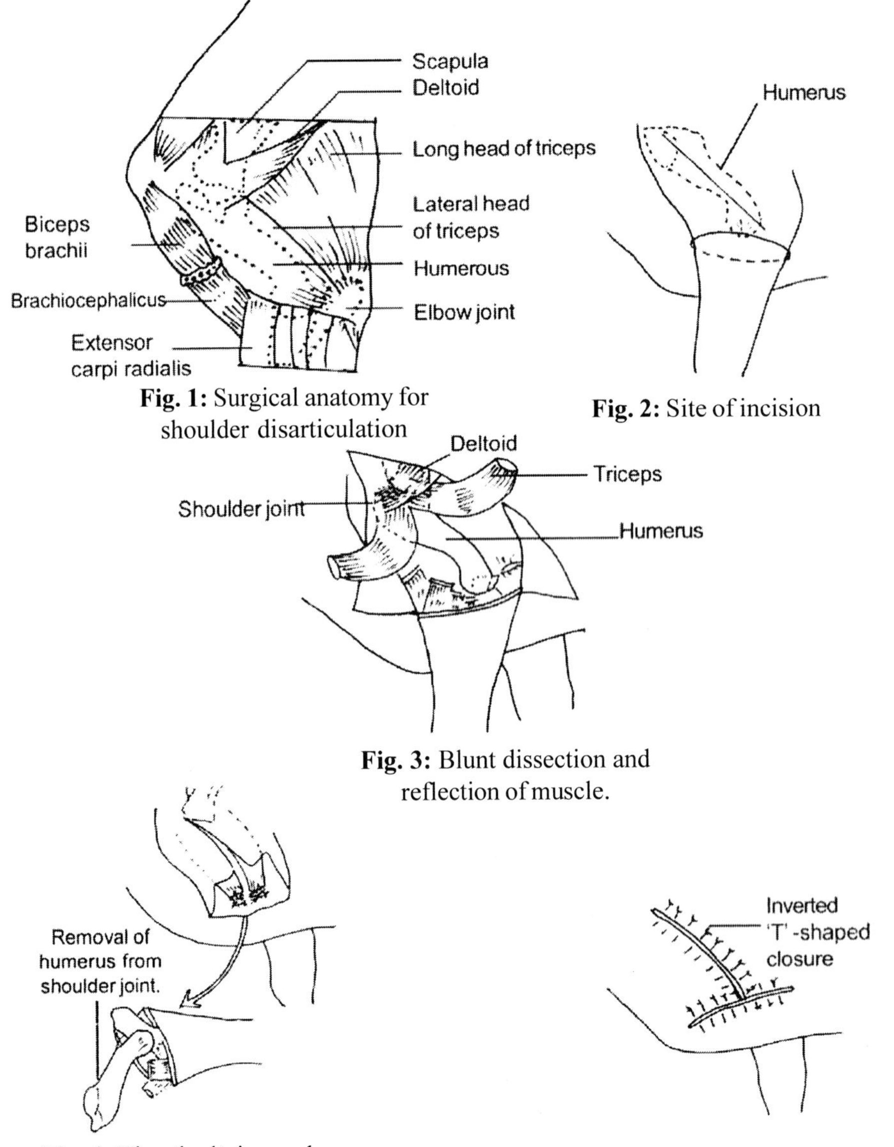

Fig. 1: Surgical anatomy for shoulder disarticulation

Fig. 2: Site of incision

Fig. 3: Blunt dissection and reflection of muscle.

Fig. 4: Disarticultuion and apposition of muscle

Fig. 5: Final colosure

Reference: Ghosh, R.K., (2012), Primary Veterinary Anatomy, Edition, Current Books International, Kolkata-13, P.126.

112

Tarso-Metatarsal Joint Disarticulation Technique in Large animal

Indication : Irreparable damage of the meta tarsal joint.

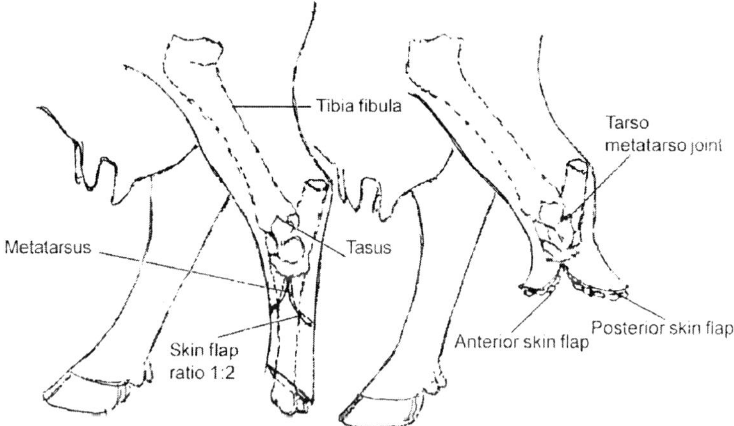

Fig. 1: Anatomy of tarso meta tarso joint

Fig. 2: Skin flap after joint disarticulation

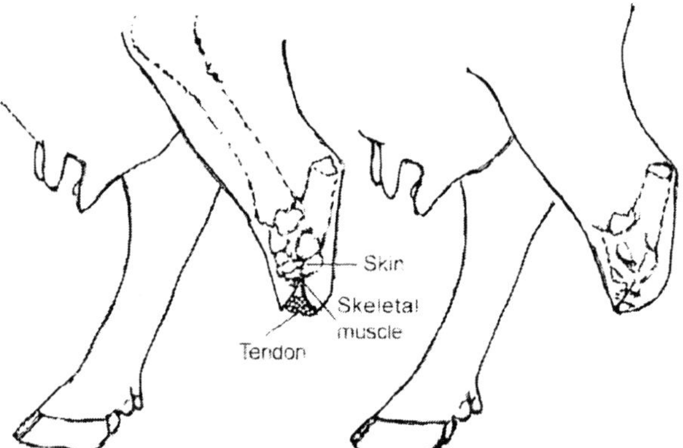

Fig. 3: Appositon of tendon & muscle (closure of skin)

Fig. 4: Complete closure of metatarsa joint

113

Stiffle Disarticulation

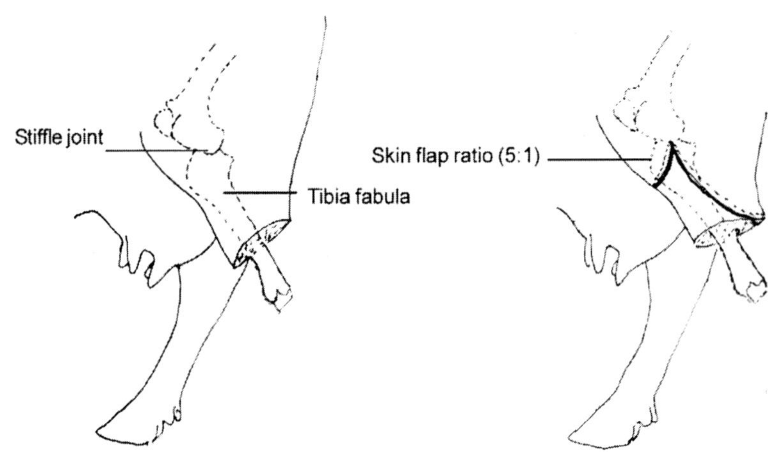

Fig. 1: Reparable fracture of leg

Fig. 2: Skin flap ratio (5:1)

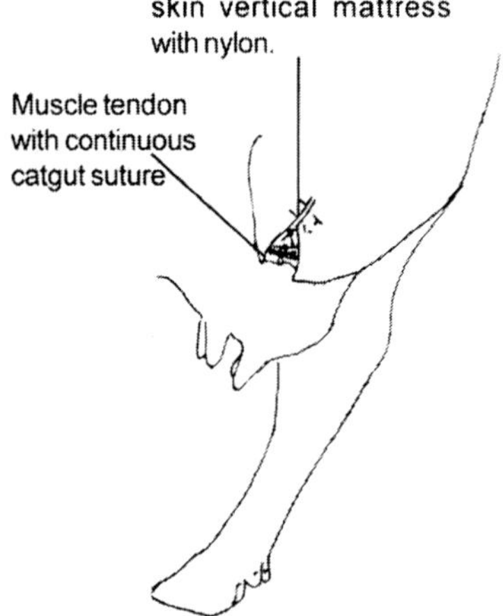

Fig. 3: Stump closure in process

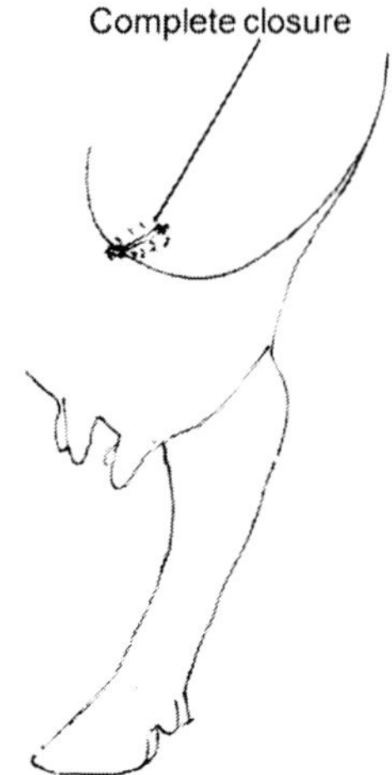

Fig. 4: Complete closure of stiffle joint

114

HIP Disarticulation

Indication

1. Necrosis, Gangrene, Extensive injury of nerve of hind limb.
2. Malignant neoplasm
3. Frost bite. Burns
4. Incurable peripheral vascular disease.

Surgical Anatomy

- Femur is surrounded by two major groups of muscle i.e. Muscles of medial and lateral groups.
- Muscles of lateral group include-Tensor fascia latae. Biceps femoris, Semitendinosus, Semi-membranosus and Adductor muscle.
- Muscles of medial group include-Sartorius, Gracillis, pectineus and part of quadriceps and biceps femoris muscle.
- Entire limb is supplied by femoral and popliteal arteries where as blood is drained by satellite veins, nerve supply by Sciatic, saphenous and external popliteal nerves.

Site of Operation

Lower third of femur, above stifle joint.

Control & Anaesthesia

Lateral recumbency under regional anaesthesia.

Surgical Technique

- A Semicircular, lateral and medial skin incision are made after proper draping of entire limb.

- After reflecting skin flap on medial aspect at the middle of femur, muscles are transected by blunt dissection.
- The femoral vessels are isolated and divided betw'een two ligatures.
- After reflecting the muscles proximally, sciatic nerve is identified where it is served.
- The femur is thus cut by bone saw and leg Is removed, haemorrhage is carefully checked.
- The stump of femur is completely covered by rest of the muscles.
- The fascia and skin flaps are brought in apposition and edges are sutured finally with interrupted or mattress suture in inverted Y-shaped / T-shaped fashion with silk suture.

Post Operative Care

- Antiseptic dressing is done till healing is complete.
- A course of antibiotic and analgesic should be administered.
- Sutures should be removed 8-10 days after surgery or after complete healing.

Reference: Ghosh, R.K., (2012), Primary Veterinary Anatomy, Edition, Current Books International, Kolkata-13, P.133.

HIP Disarticulation

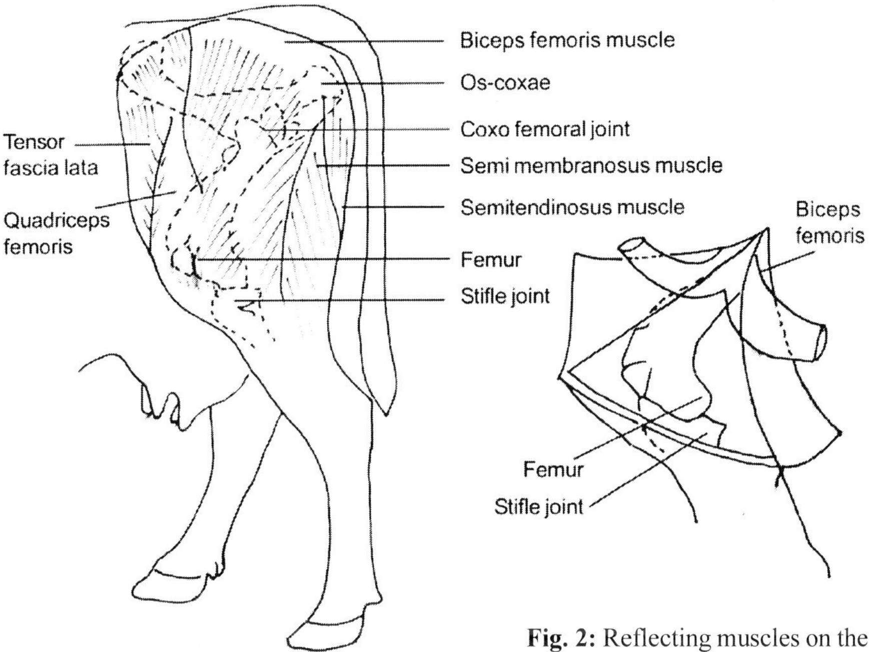

Fig. 1: Surgical anatomy of hip

Fig. 2: Reflecting muscles on the temur and their blunt dissection.

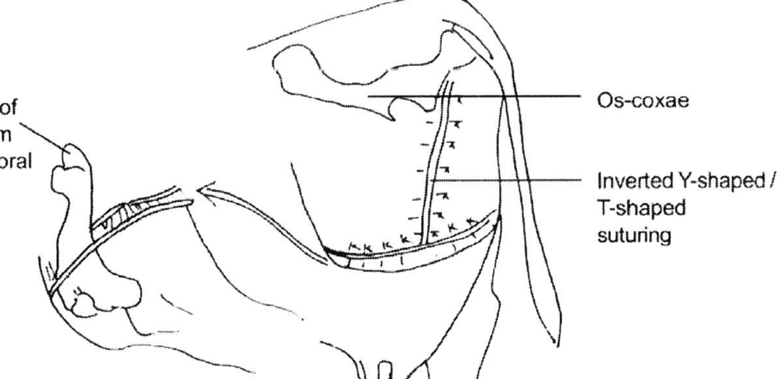

Fig. 3: Excision of femur and sturing

Reference : Ghosh, R.K., (2012), Primary Veterniary Anatomy, 5th Edition, Current Books International, Kolkata-13, P.133.

115

Figures of Various Amputees by Joint Disarticulation Method

Forelimb Amputees

Hindlimb Amputees

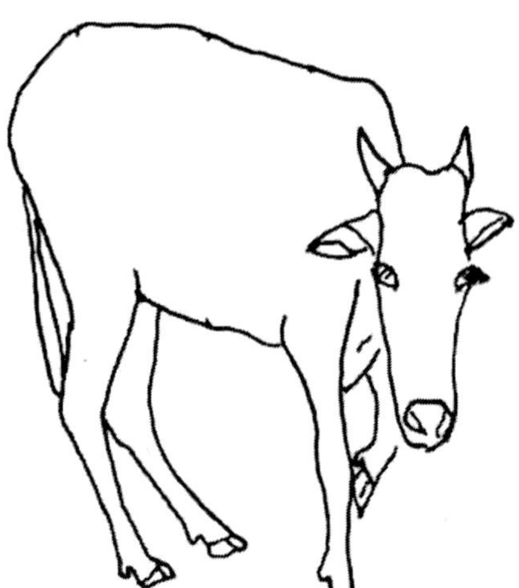

Fig. 1: Fetlock disarticulation.

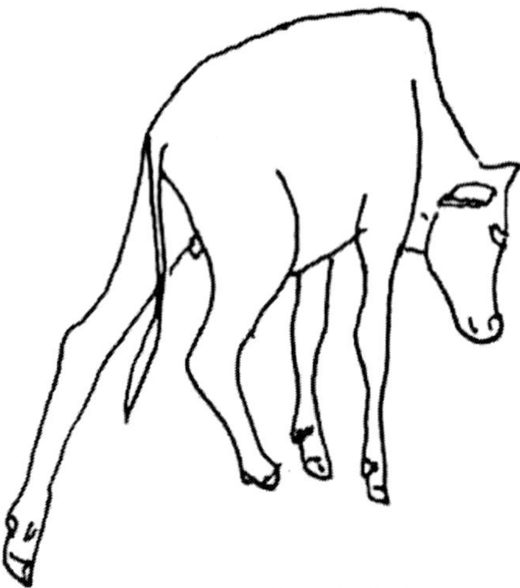

Fig. 2: Fetlock disarticulation.

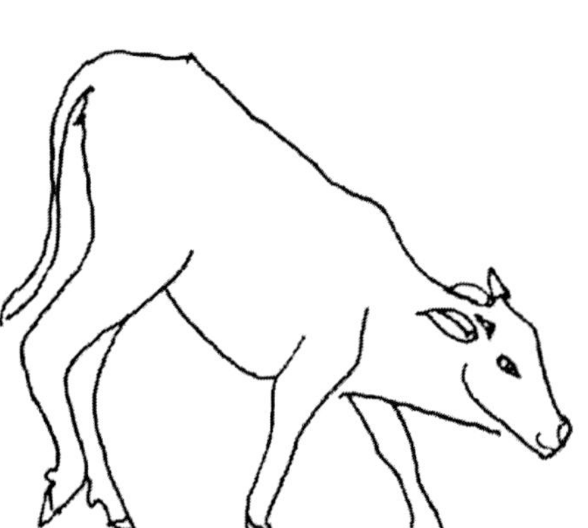

Fig. 3: Knee disarticulation.

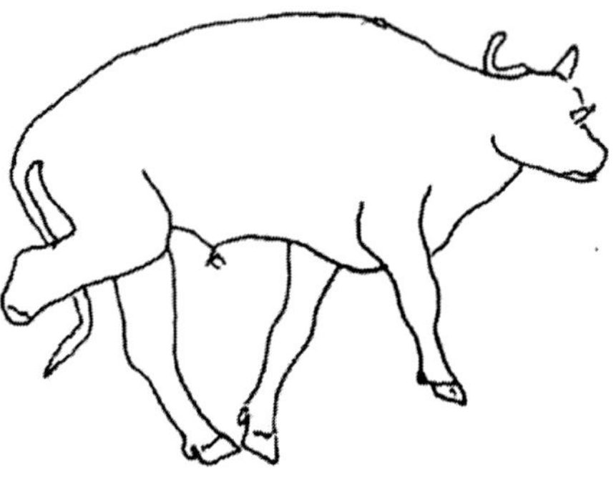

Fig. 4: Hock disarticulation.

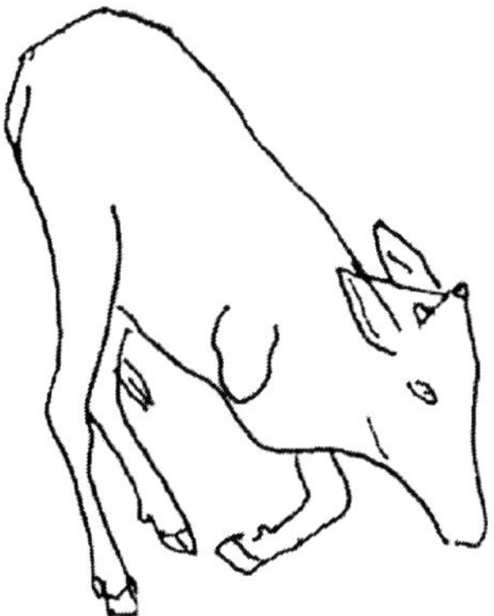

Fig. 5: Elbow disarticulation.

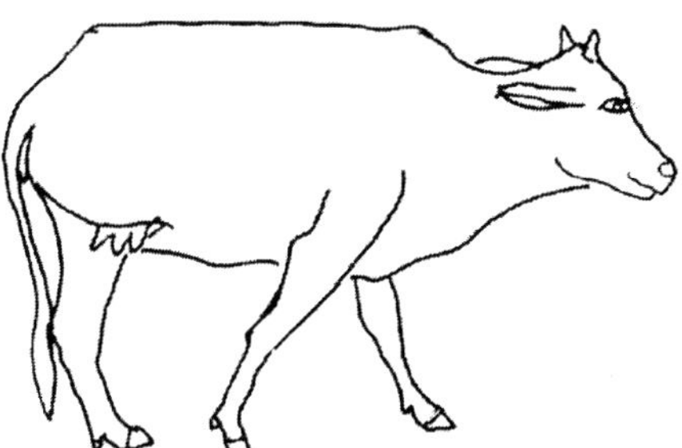

Fig. 6: Stifle disarticulation.

116

Comparison Between Bone Section and Joint Disarticulation Method of Limb Amputation

Bone section method

Advantage

1. Recommended for artificial limb fitting.
2. Non-weight bearing of stump is marked. Fig- 2a.

Disadvantage

1. Bone saw is used for amputation.
2. Bone marrow is exposed.
3. Animal cannot walk without artificial limb.
4. Walk become unbalanced.
5. Body symmetry disturbed. Fig-2a, 3a, 4a, 5a.
6. Chances of osteomyelitis is there.
7. Joint function cannot be retained.

Joint disarticulation method

Advantage

1. Artificial limb not recommended.
2. No chance of osteomyelitis is there.
3. Joint function is retained.
4. Walk is balanced.

5. Normal body symmetry. Fig-6b, 5b.
6. Bone saw not used.
7. Bone marrow is not exposed.

Disadvantage

1. Weight bearing of stump is noted. Fig-1 c, 2b, 4b.

Forelimb Amputees

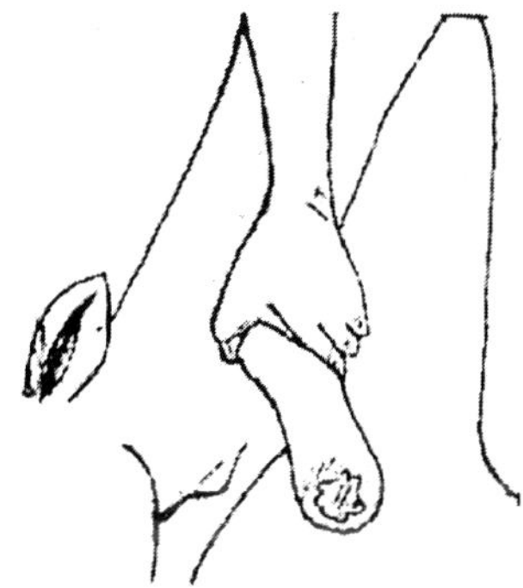

Fig. 1a: Fetlock disarticulation.

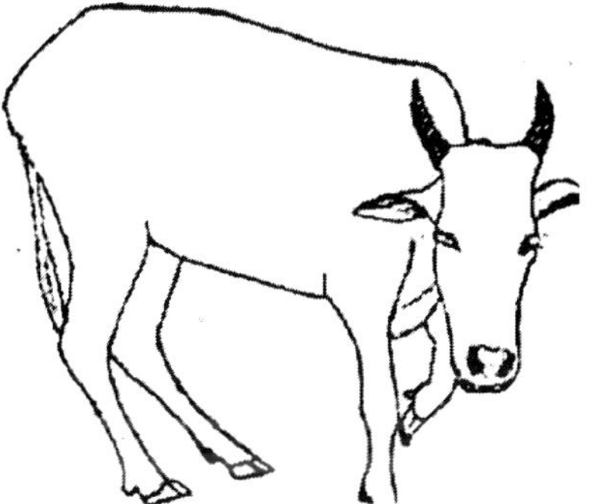

Fig. 1b: Fetlock disarticulation.

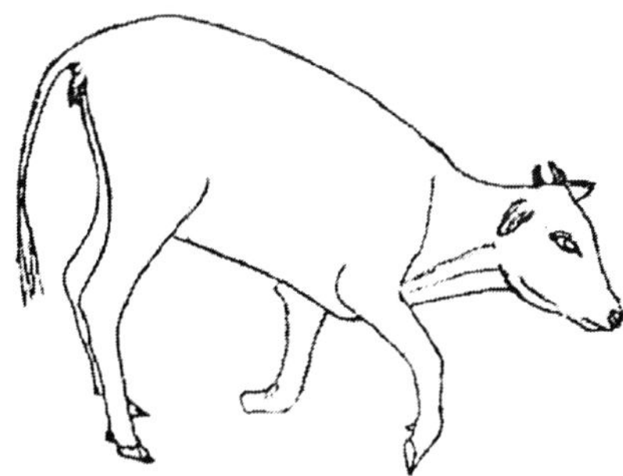

Fig. 2a: Below - knee amputation

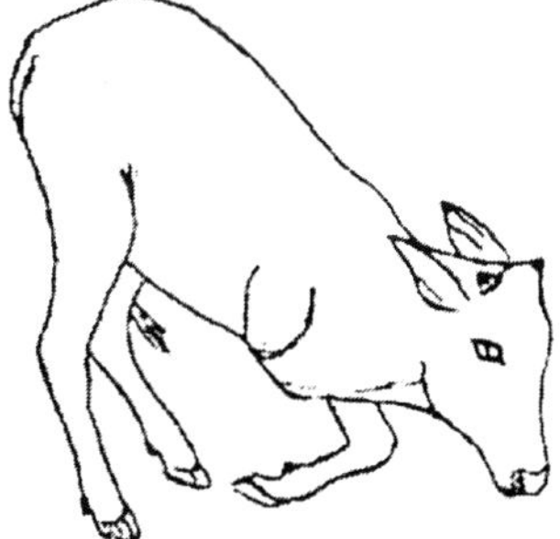

Fig. 2b: Below - knee amputation

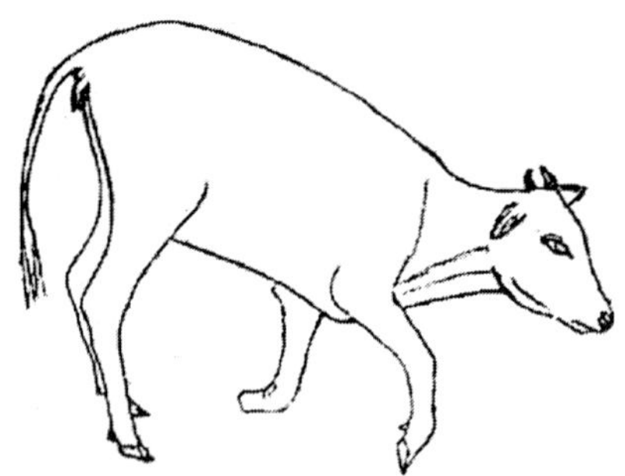

Fig. 3a: Above - knee amputation

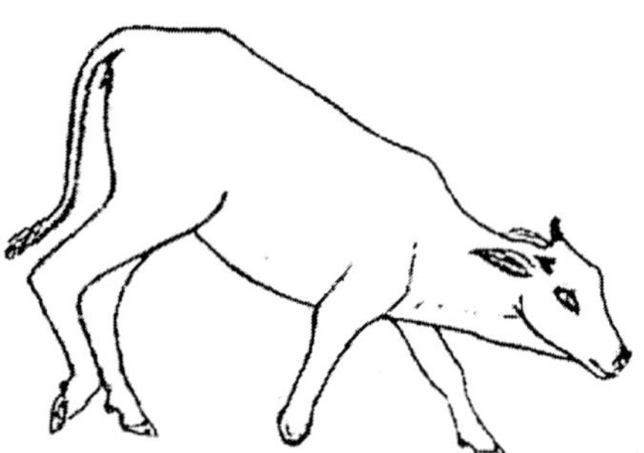

Fig. 3b: Above - knee amputation

Hind Limb Amputees

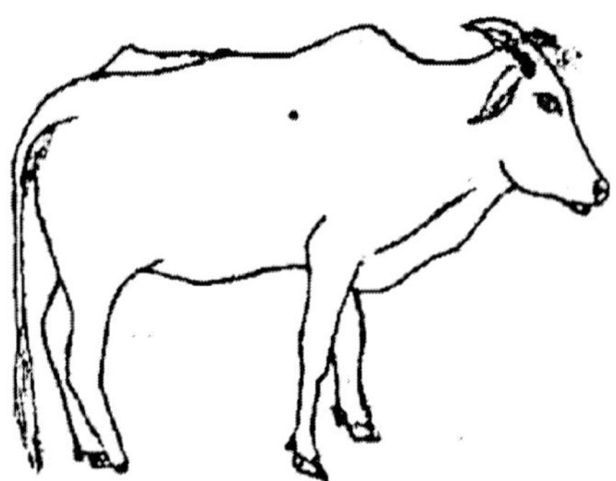

Fig. 4a: Fetlock disarticulation

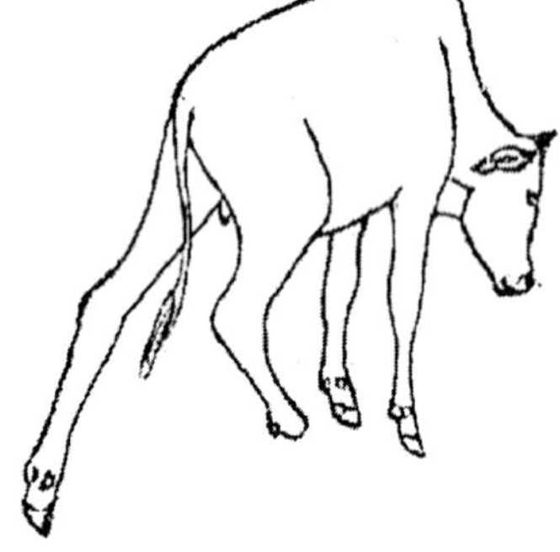

Fig. 4b: Fetlock disarticulation

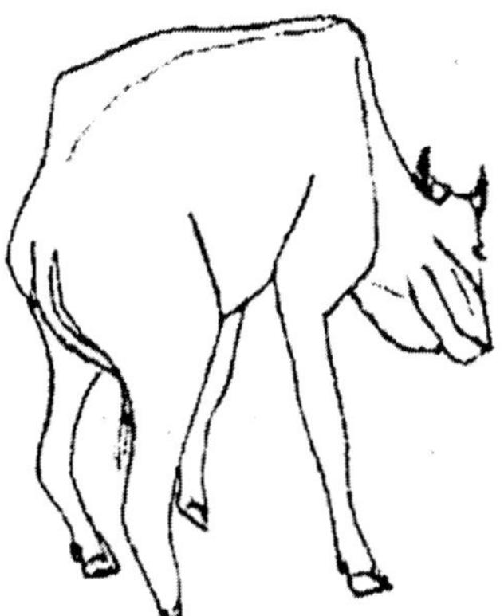

Fig. 5a: Below - hock amputation.

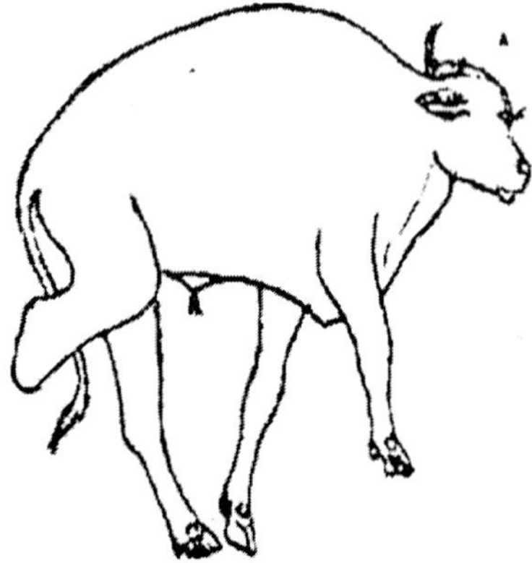

Fig. 5b: Below - hock amputation;

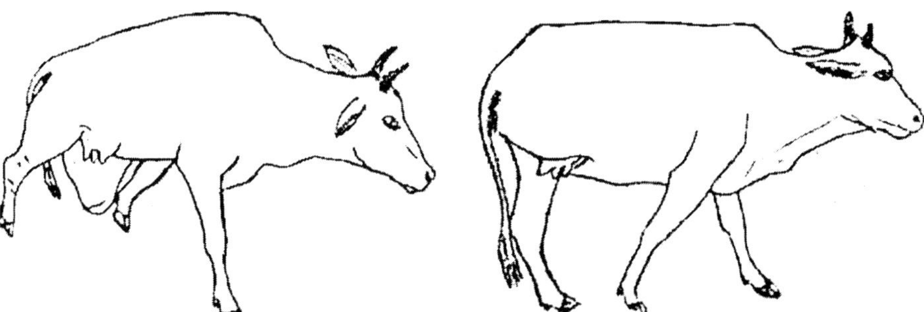

Fig. 6a: Above - hock amputation.

Fig. 6b: Above - hock amputation.

117

Different Steps in Preparation of Permanent Prothesis

1. The plaster-bandage wrap cast :(Negative cast)

- The amputee was restrained on lateral recumbency keeping the amputed leg upwards.
- A thin, moistened stockinet was pulled over the stump and it was maintained snugly in place by tying with a string at the top.
- The moistened cast stockinet was marked with indeliable pencil indicating prominences with a cross and other sensitive areas with a circle (Fig.1).
- Plaster bandages were then wrapped as pen requirement unit I the shell has a thickness of approximately 3mm in proximal third.
- After plaster hardened, it was removed either by pulling out or longitudinal splitting with a cutter (Fig.2).

2. Preparation of positive cast

- The splitted part of the cost was brought to exact apposition and was covered with thin strip of wet plaster bandage.
- The warp cast was filled with plaster of pairs.
- A 450mm, long 13mm iron pipe was inserted to a depth of 150mm.
- After plaster has set, the wrap was stripped off by cutting lengthwise down the posterior surface.
- Model was checked again using the measurements taken previously in respect of the diameter & circumferences of the stump at various heights & sides.
- Smoothening of the model was done.

3. Fabrication of the plastic shell

- 2 tapered P.V.C. (Poly vinyl chloride) sleeves of desirable size suiting the model were fabricated.
- One of the P.V.C. sleeve was stretched over the model & insert. P.V.C. adhesive tape was painted around the cut edge.
- The mandrel was tied off all around & all loose material wire trimmed off.
- Fiber glass cloth was wrapped around the model & was held in place by overlapping 5-6 layers of cotton cast stockinet.
- The resin was poured in to the small tapered extension of the P.V.C. sleeve (Fig.4). The resin was pressed to move through & thoroughly into the fabric layers.
- Plastic was allowed to cure.
- The trim line was cut with a sharp knife before the plastic cooled.
- Shell was removed from model.
- Anterior brim of the socket was kept as high as possible where as the posterior brim at a lower level for easy flexion of the limb.
- Holes were perforated on the socket for ventilation.

Different Steps in Preparation of Permanent Prosthesis

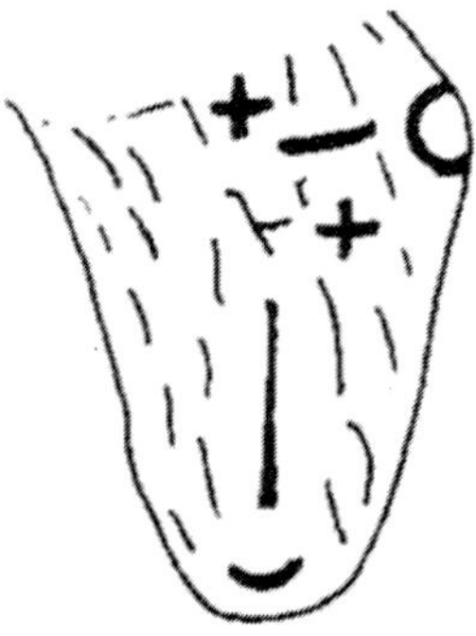

Fig. 1: Marking on the moistened cast stokinet.
0 - Outline of sensitive area, " - Oepression
+ - Prominences
1 - Border of bone
U - Distal end of bone

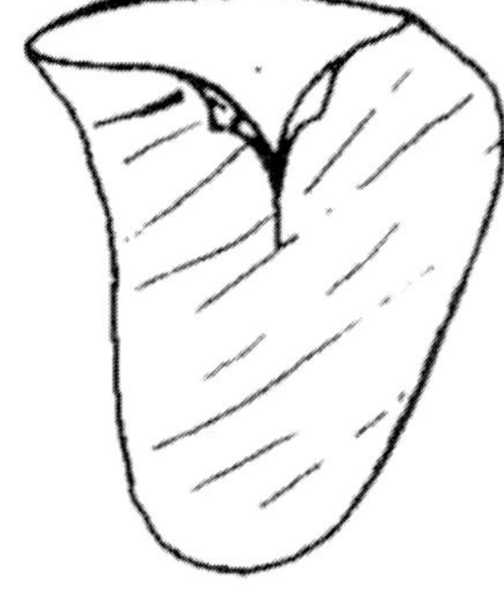

Fig. 2: Negative plaster cast.

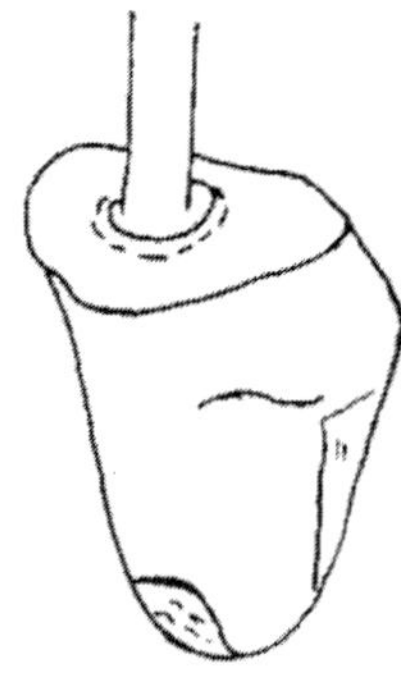

Fig. 3: Plaster mold or positive cast.

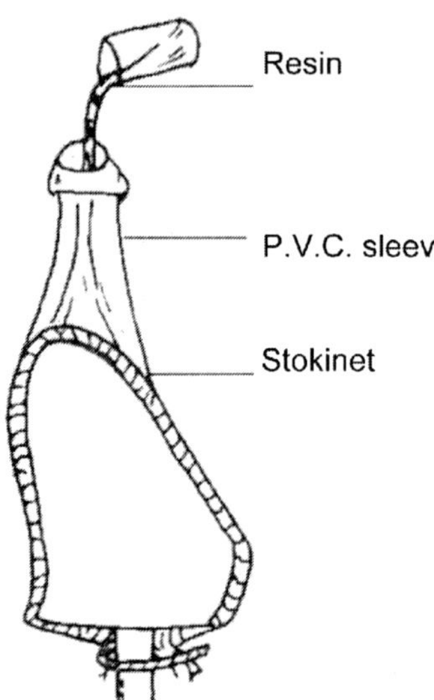

Fig. 4: Fabrication of the plastic shell.

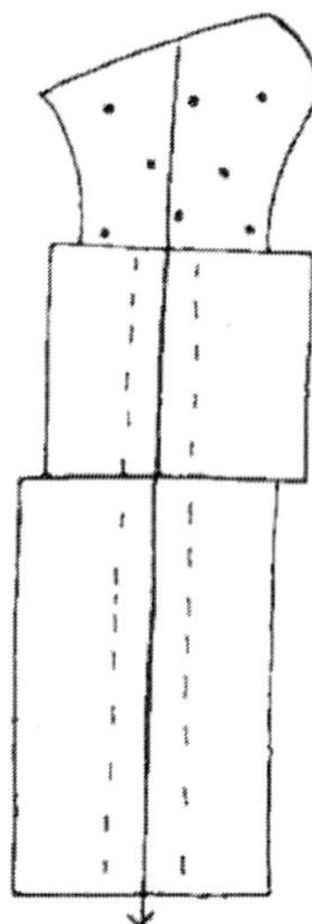

Fig. 5: Alignment of duplication

118*

Different Steps in Preparation of Fore Limb Prothesis

*Table starts from next page

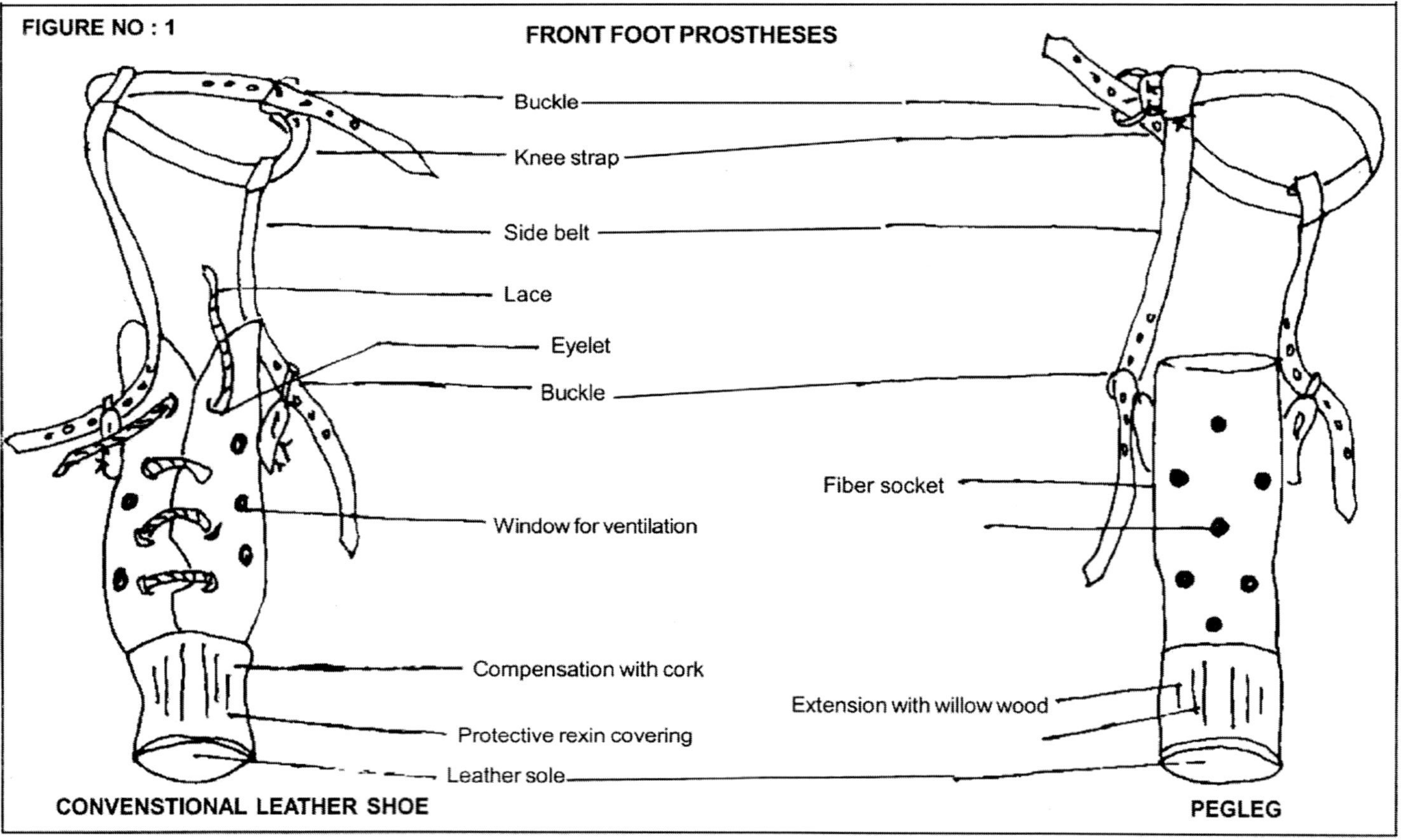

Fig. 1: Front Foot prostheses

119

Below knee (B.K) Prosthesis

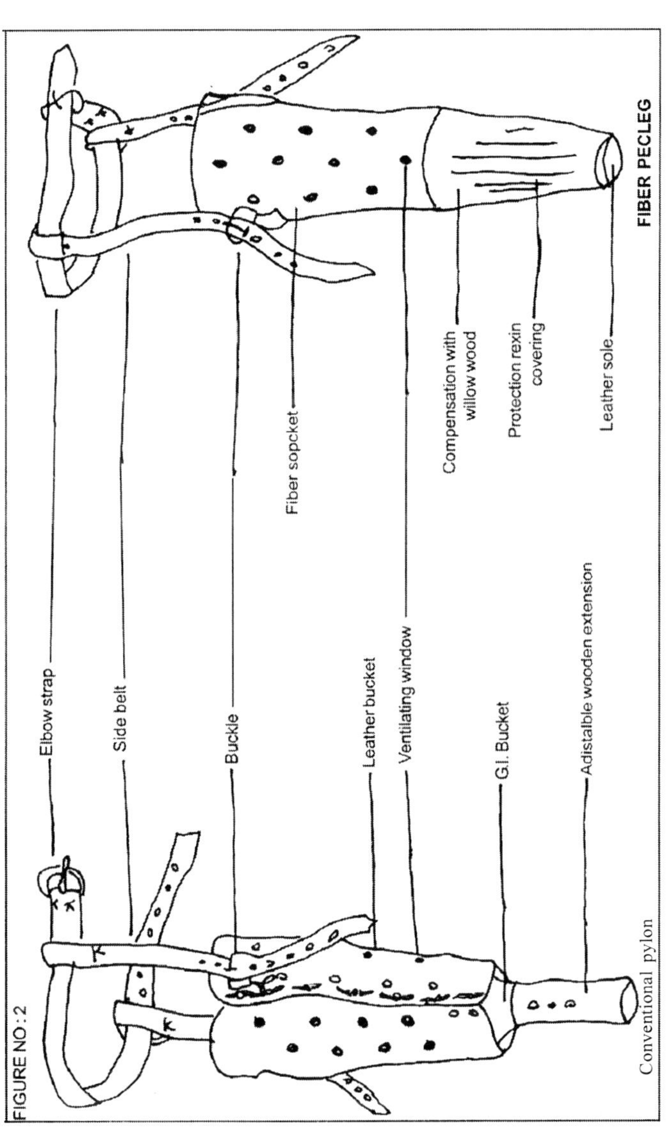

FIGURE NO : 2

120

Above Knee (A.K.) Prothesis

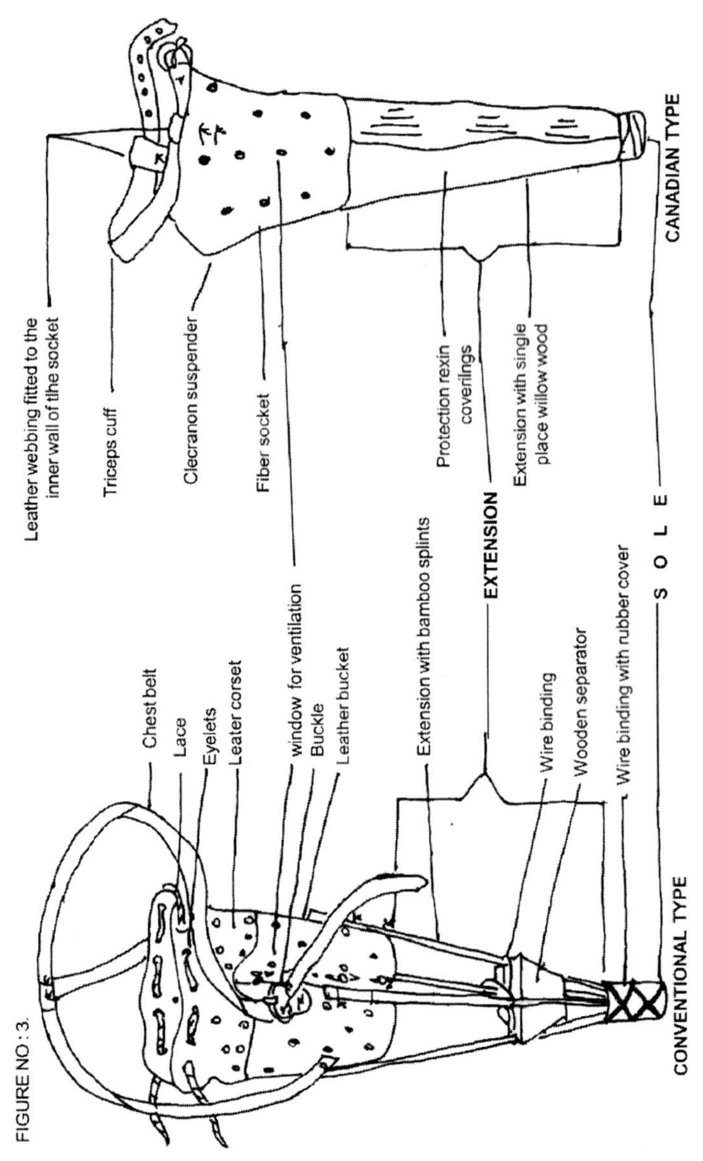

FIGURE NO : 3.

121

Hind Foot Prosthesis-I

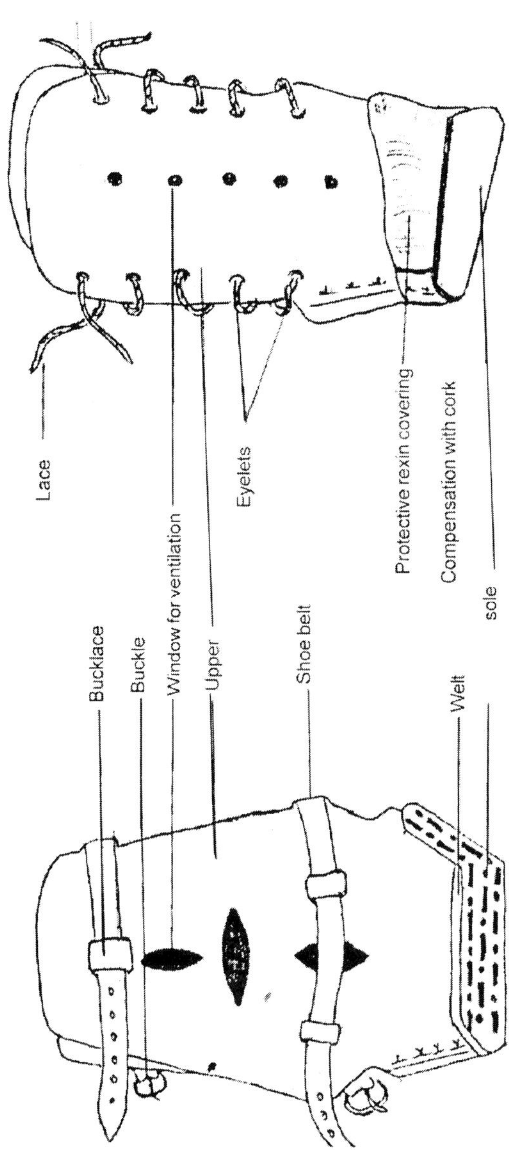

Fig. a: Conventional Lattershoe

Fig. b: Heel Flare

122

Below hock (B.H.) Prosthesis -II

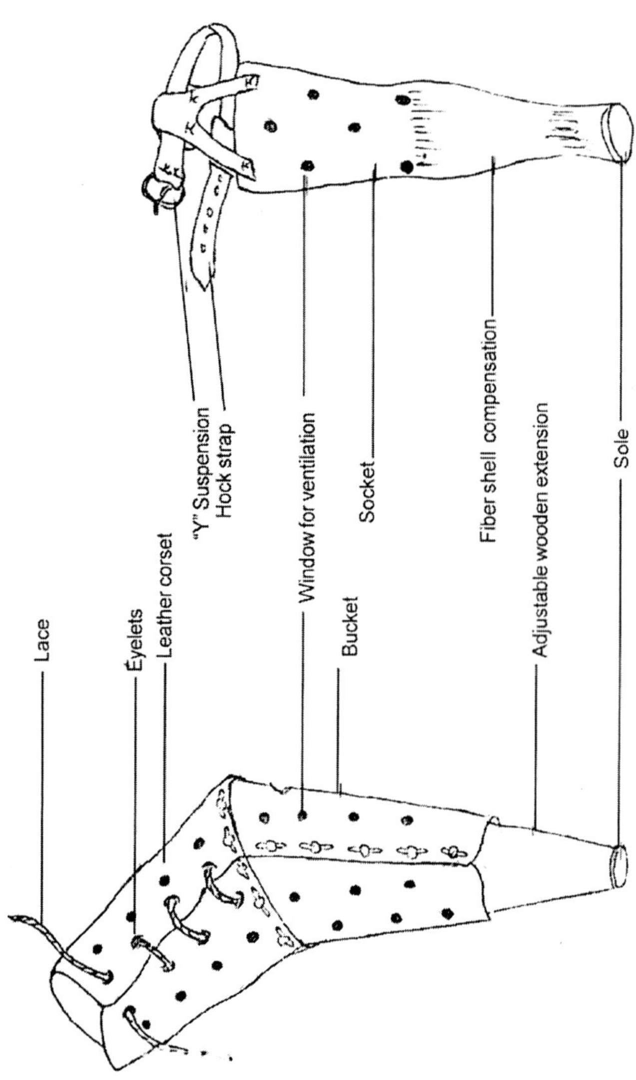

Fig. a. CONVENTIONAL TYPE PYLON.

Fig. b. CANADIAN TYPE PEGLEG.

123

Above Hock (A.H.) Prosthesis– III

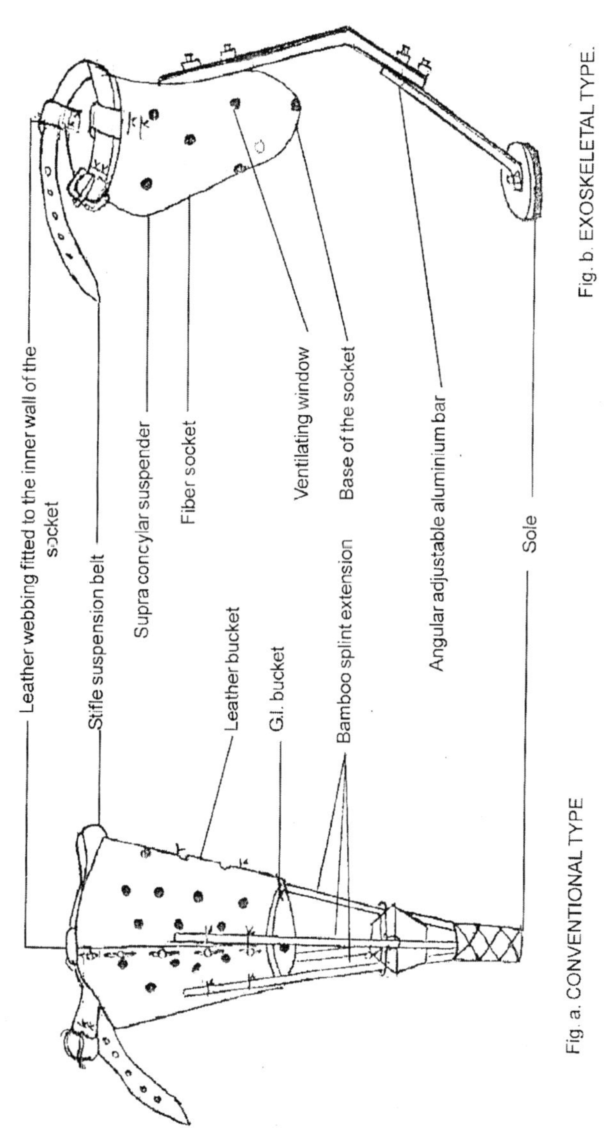

Fig. a. CONVENTIONAL TYPE

Fig. b. EXOSKELETAL TYPE.

124

Amputation and Prosthetic Limb Below Carpus in Cattle

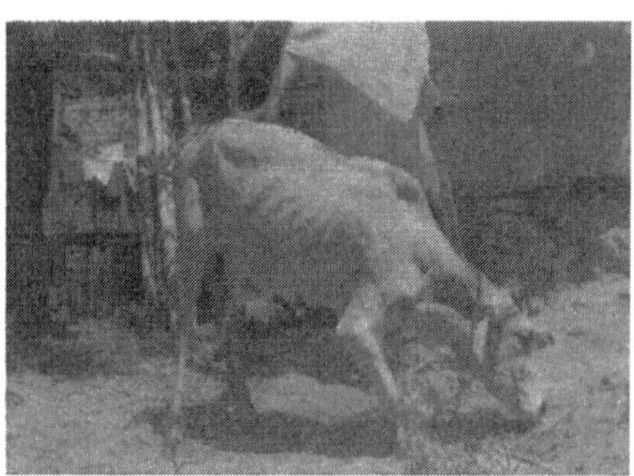

Fig. 1: The below knee stump showing free mobility of radio-carpal joint.

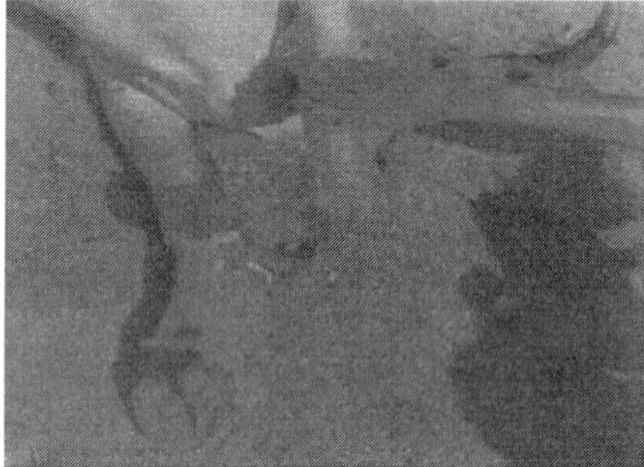

Fig. 2: The below knee stump showing semi-flexed position.

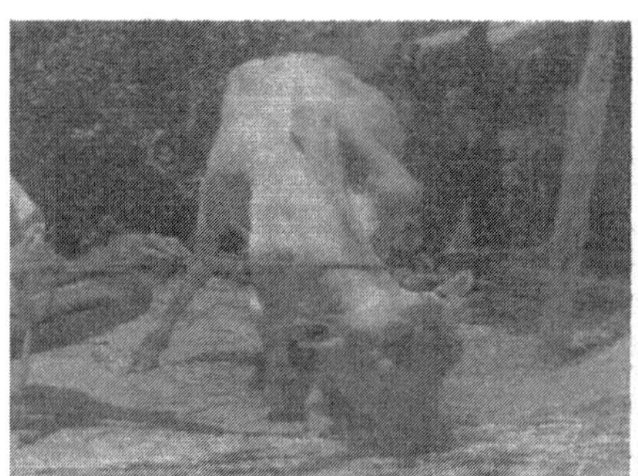

Fig. 3: Stance of the below knee amputee.

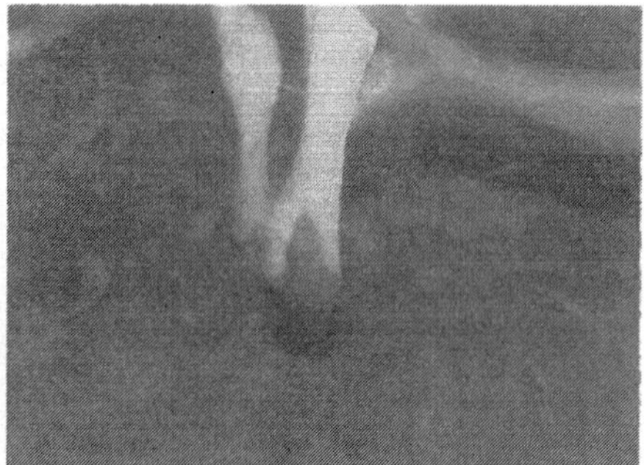

Fig. 4: Stump of the below knee amputee showing well covered and thickly padded distal end.

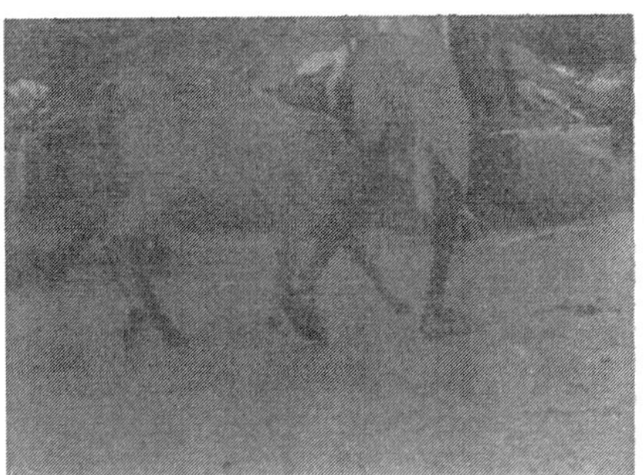

Fig. 5: Below knee amputated heifer using the stump in each step of walk.

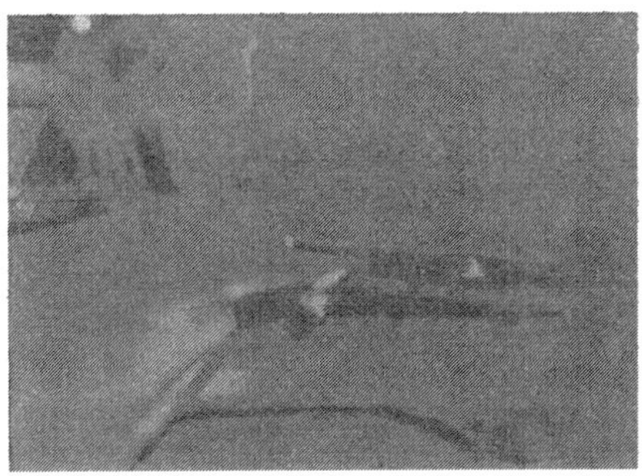

Fig. 6: Application of bamboo splint bandage In case of below knee amputee during training.

Amputation and Prosthetic Limb Below Elbow in Cattle

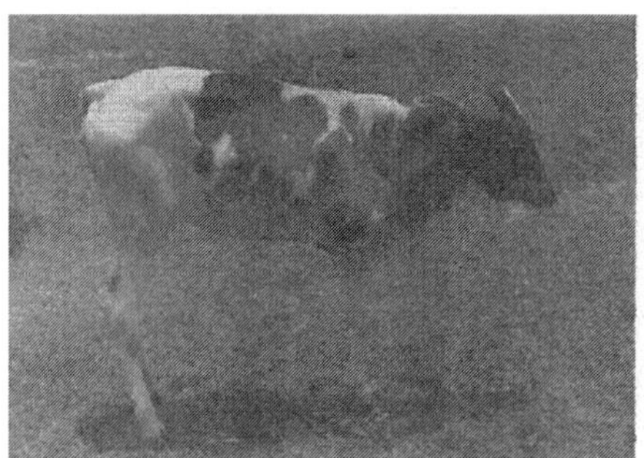

Fig. 7: Stance of elbow disarticulated amputee showing undisturbed symmetry.

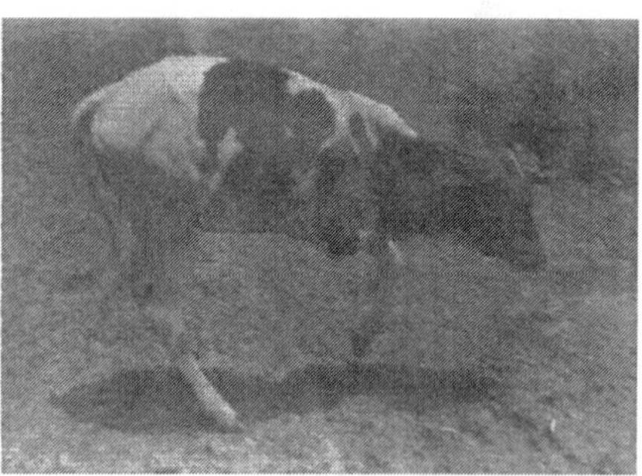

Fig. 8: Propulsion of the intact forelimb with a hopping movement, lifting the head upward.

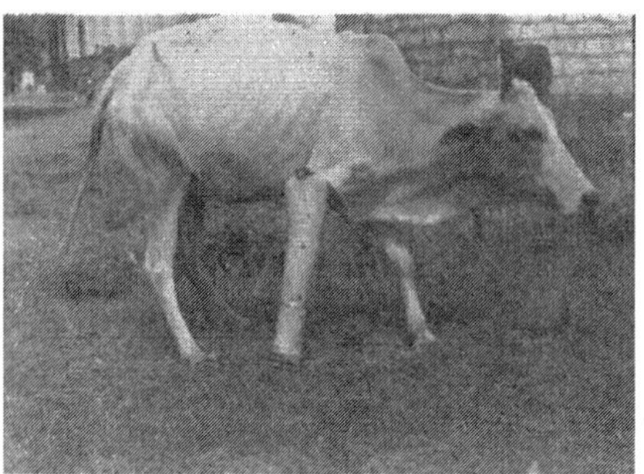

Fig. 9: At walk, below elbow amputee showing propulsion of the prosthetic limb.

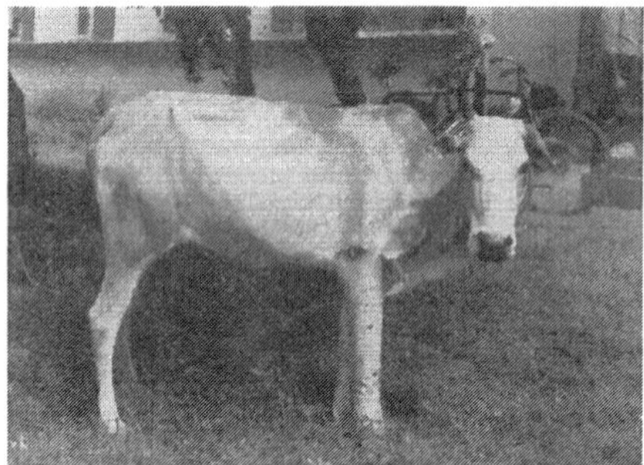

Fig. 10: At stance, below elbow amputee showing weight bearing of the prosthetic limb with canadian type

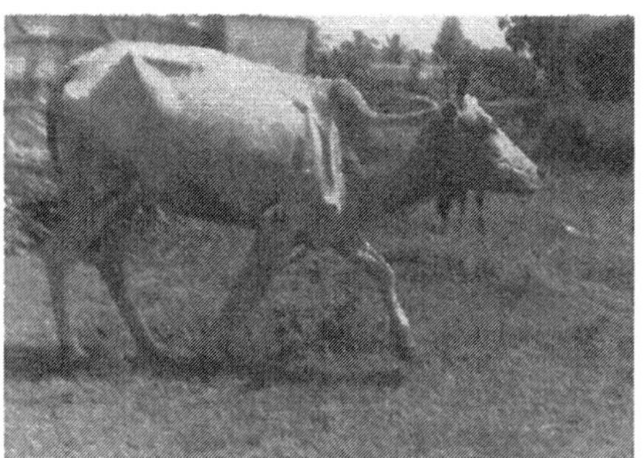

Fig. 11: At walk, below elbow amputee showing propulsion of the intact forelimb.

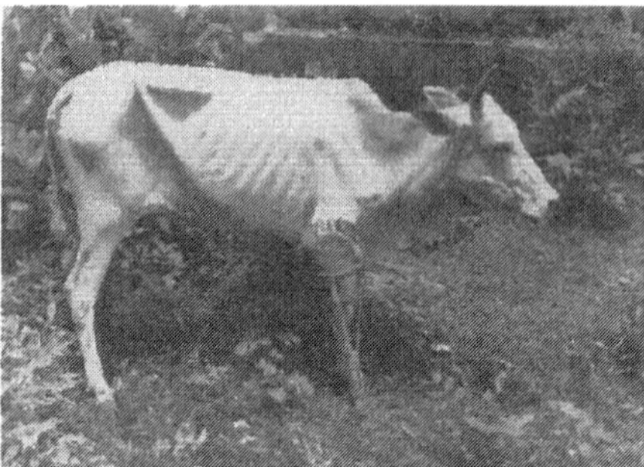

Fig. 12: At stance, below elbow amputee showing weight bearing of the prosthetic limb with conventional type

Amputation and Prosthetic Limb Below Tarsus in Cattle

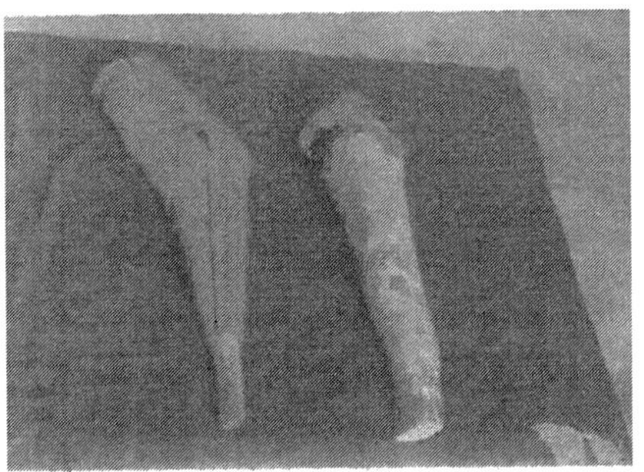

Fig. 13: Below hock prostheses (Conventional type pylon and canalian type pegleg).

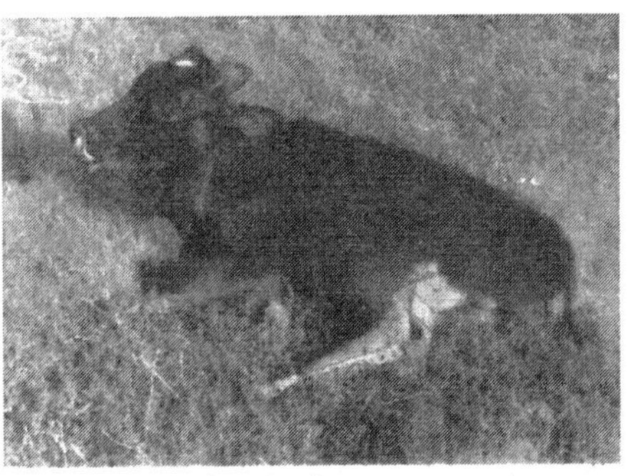

Fig. 14: Below hock amputee at sleep,

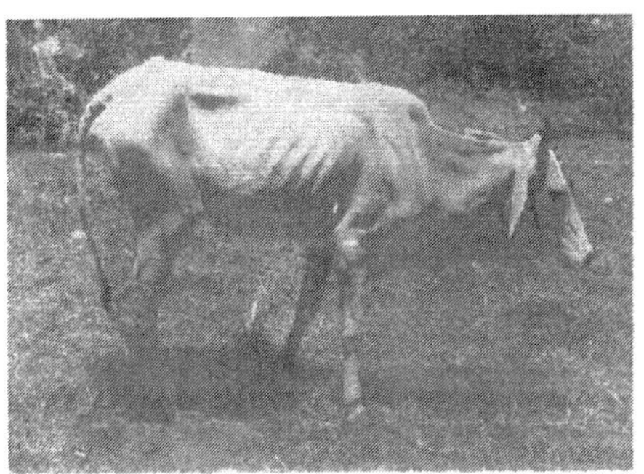

Fig. 15: At stance below hock amputee having the prosthetic limb.

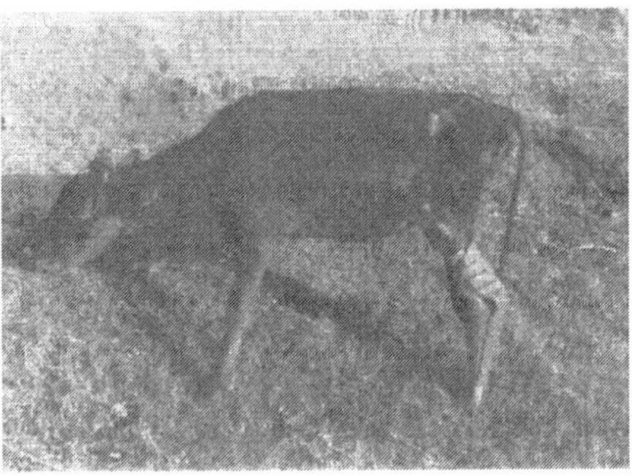

Fig. 16: At stance below hock amputee having the prosthetic limb.

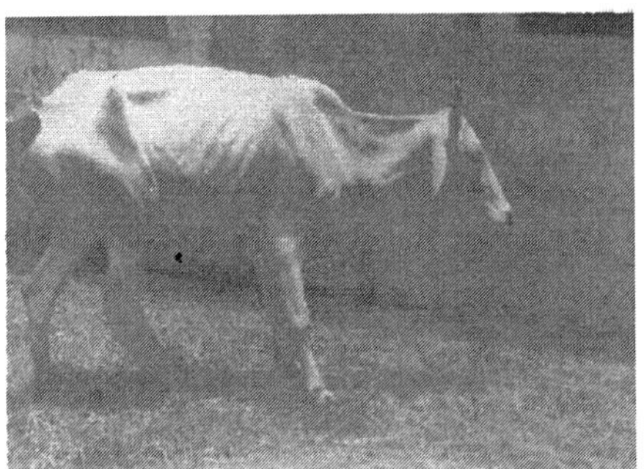

Fig. 17: Below hock amputee attempting to walk

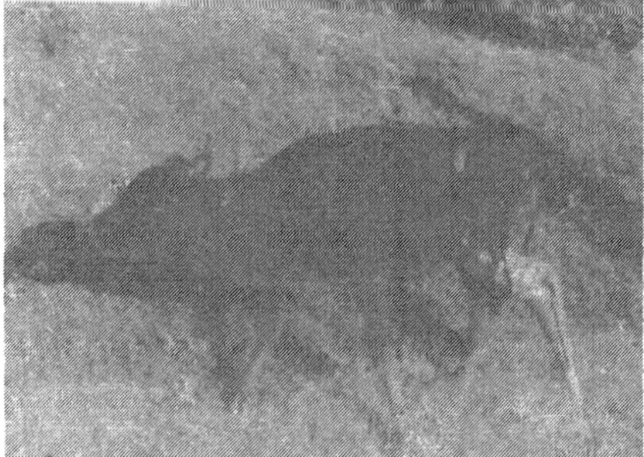

Fig. 18: Below hock amputee at walk.

Amputation and Prosthetic Limb Below Stifle in Cattle

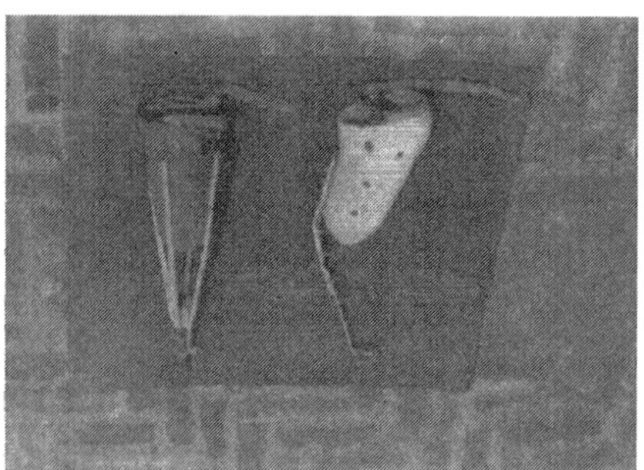

Fig. 19: Above hock prostheses conventional showing type and exoskelital type.

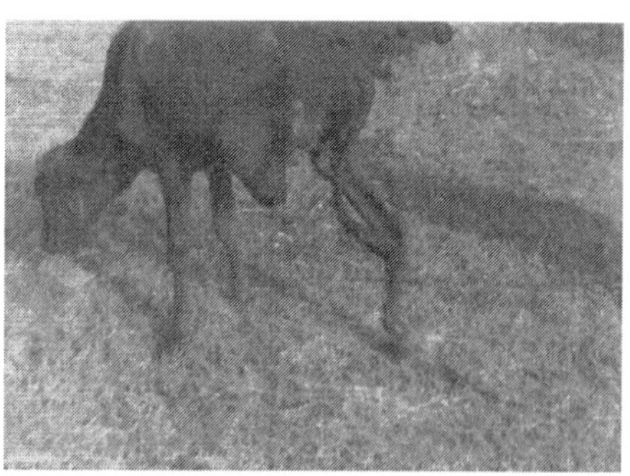

Fig. 20: Walk of above hock amputee propulsion of hind leg.

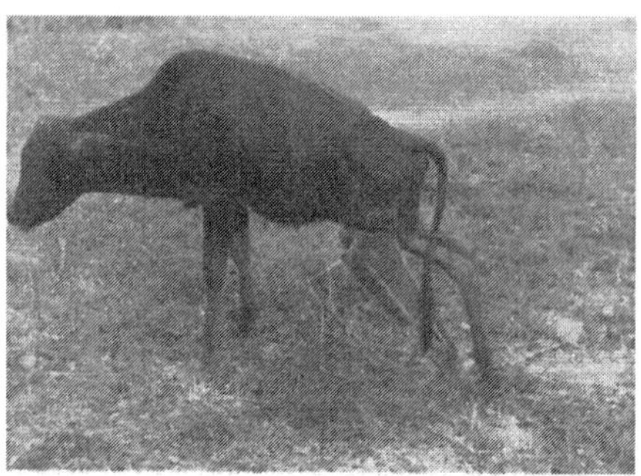

Fig. 21: Walk of above hock amputee with conventional type prosthesis showing production of prosthetic limb.

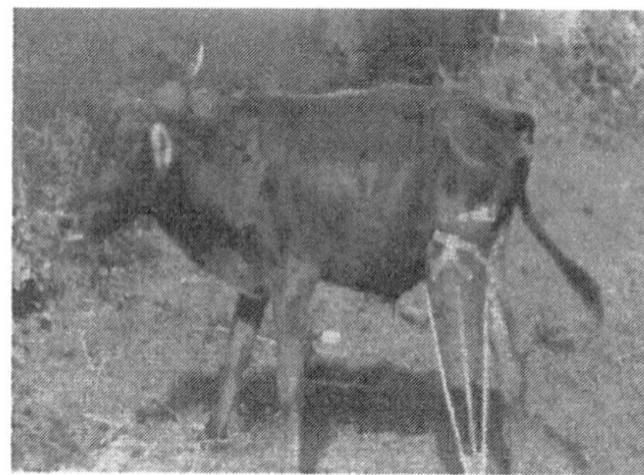

Fig. 22: Stance of above hock amputee with conventional type prostheses.

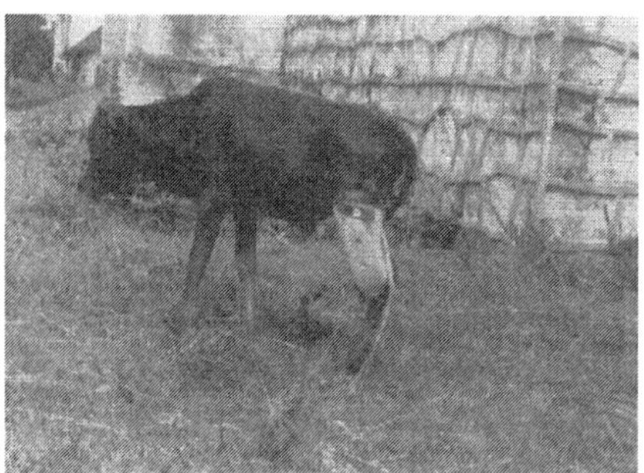

Fig. 23: Walk of above hock amputee with exoskelital type prosthesis showing propulsion of prosthetic limb.

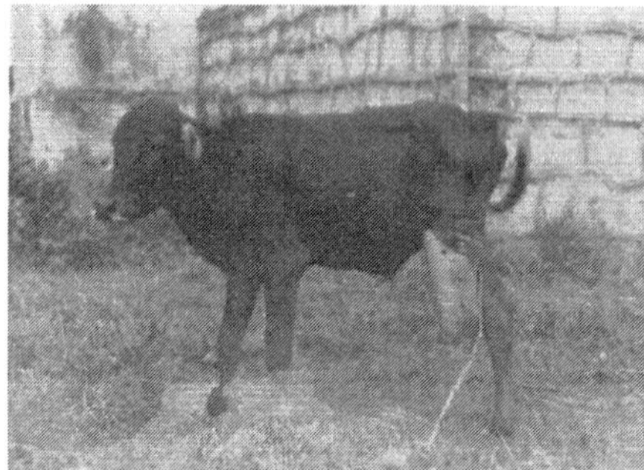

Fig. 24: Stance of above hock amputee with exoskelital type prosthesis.

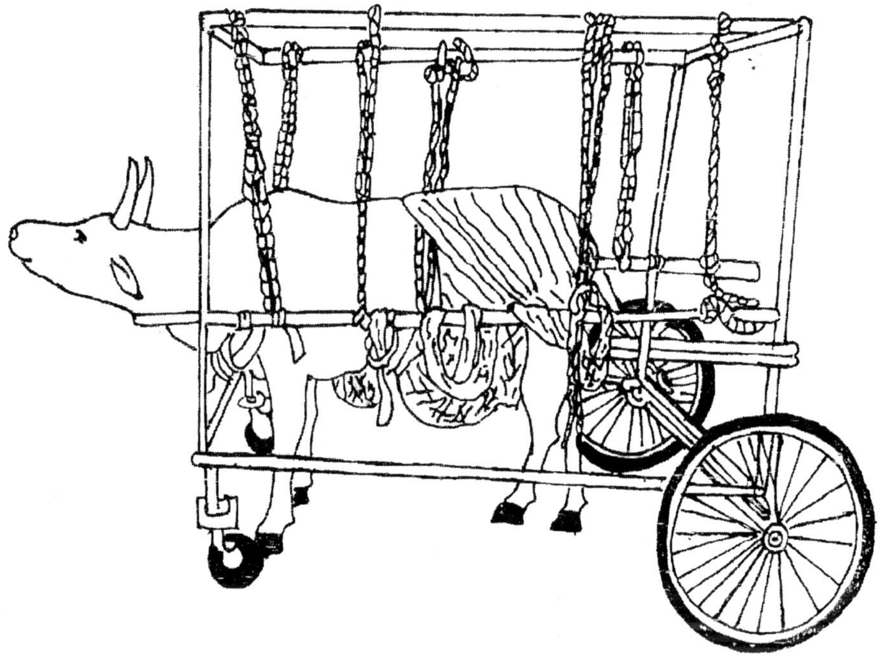

Fig. 25: Rehabilitation

125

Indications for Rehabiltation of Downer's Cow Using Mobile Sling

Introduction

A downer cow is an animal In sternal recumbency and isn't showing obvious clinical sign of hypocalcemia,hypomagnesmia or any limb or spinal Injury. Most causes are related to parturition, occurring in few days before or upto a week after calving.

Causes for Making an Animal Downer

Animals Inability to stand may be caused by illness or injury. Following may be the reasons

1. Acute mastitis
2. Metritis
3. Hypocalcemia and hypophosphatemia
4. Hypomagnesemia
5. Ketosis
6. Long bone fracture, dislocation and joint disease
7. Dystokia and neurological disorder.

- Acute mastitis- results In paresis of a milch cow for which the animal is unable to stand.
- Metritis- It causes recumbency in some cows.
- Hypocalcemia, hypophosphatemia and hypomagnesmia- This occurs due to nutritional deficiency. Milch animals also suffer from calcium deficiency due to this animals are debilitated and get downed.
- Ketosis- It produces chronic debility results in downer syndrome.
- Long bone fracture dislocation and joint diseases- Hip dislocation is

common in advanced pregnancy so that animal Is not able to get up.

- Dystokia and neurological disorder- cows getting downed due to obturator nerve paralysed.

Indications for using of Mobile Sling

- To make the animal stand.
- To make the animal walk without dragging the hind limb.
- Inside the sling comfortable bedding is available.
- Floor of the sling is non-slippery so that further injury to the animal can be avoided. Unnecessary walking of the animal can be avoided so that the healing process can be faster.
- Procedure of treatment can be easier

126

Requisite for Preparation of Large Animal Mobile Sling

Purpose

To make a list on the requisites on materials required for preparation of rehabilitation mobile sling for large animals.

Materials required

1. Bicycle/Motor cycle chain-4 nos. (Fig. 1)
2. 8 ft. long strong bamboo 12 pieces (Fig. 2)
3. Gunny Bags 8-12 nos. (as per the size of the animal) (Fig. 3)
4. Bicycle Tyre (Large size) 8-10 nos. (as per the size of the animal (Fig. 4)
5. Jute string - 300-400 gm (Fig. 5)
6. G.I. wire (6mm) 1/2 kg -1 kg (Fig. 6)
7. One saw with blade (Fig. 7)
8. Axe-1 No. (Fig. 8)
9. Coconut string 1-2 kg
10. Pliers -1 No.
11. 12-15 man power.

Requisite for Preparation of Large Animal Mobile Sling

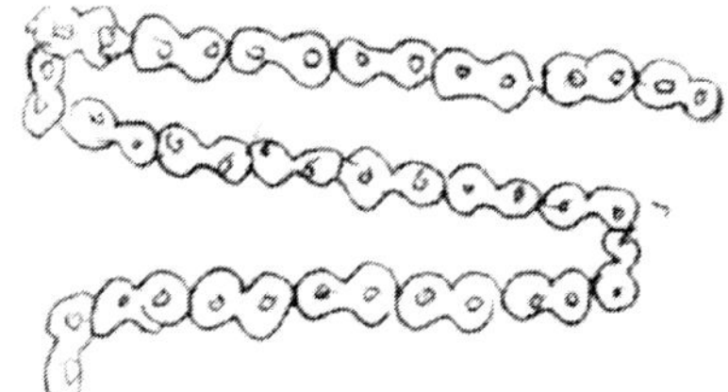

Fig. 1: Bicycle Motor cycle chain

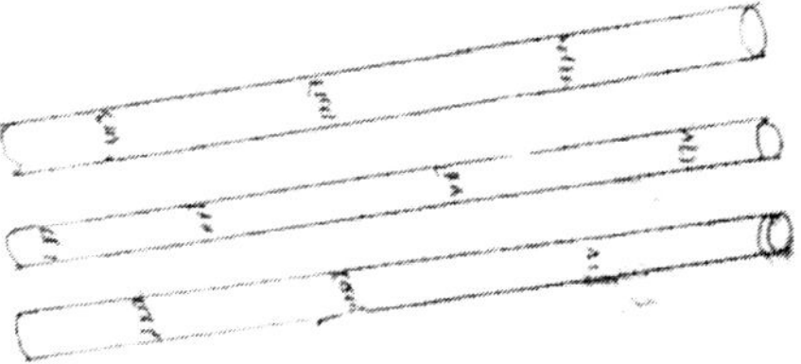

Fig. 2: to ft. long strong bamboo

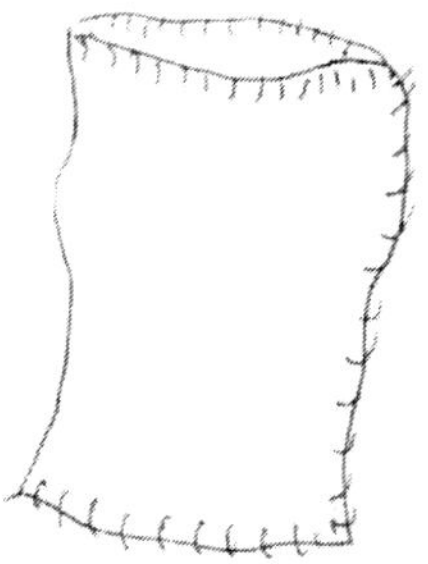

Fig. 3: Gunny bags

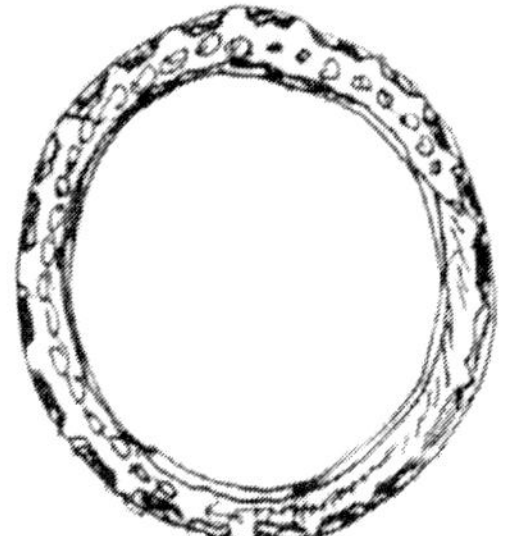

Fig. 4: Bicycle Tyre

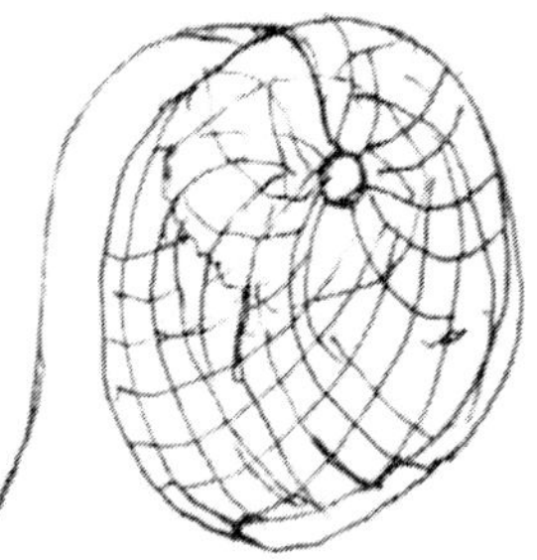

Fig. 5: Jute string

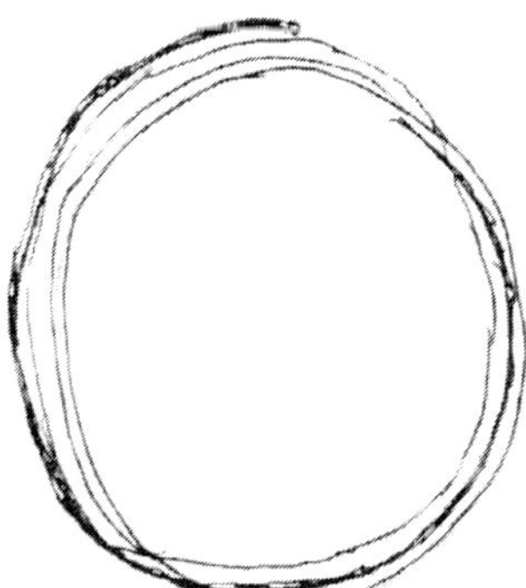

Fig. 6: G.I. wire (6mm)

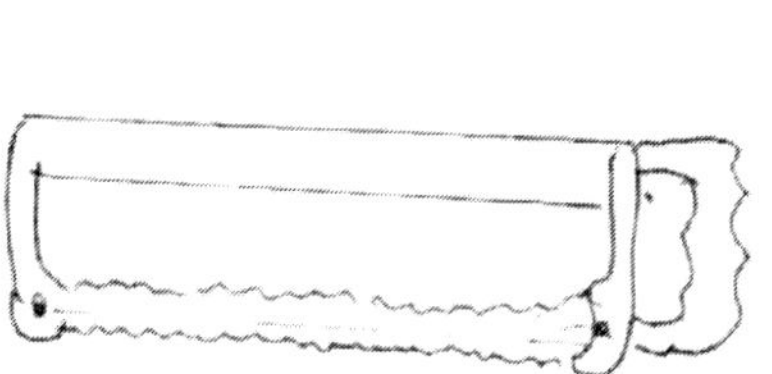

Fig. 7: Saw with blade

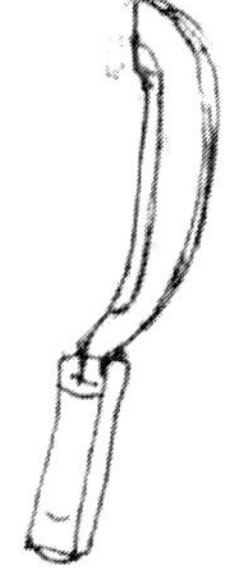

Fig. 8: Axe

127

Fabrication of Mobile Sling

It consists of 2 parts-A) fabrication of fixed supporting frame B) fabrication of animal swing frame.

A) Fabrication of fixed supporting frame -

Materials required - Bamboo pole and rope

Fabrication Technique - Size a frame 3m for large animals, 2.5m for medium sized and 2 ml for small sized animals.

B) Fabrication of animal swing frame-

Materials required - Strong fixed rectangular iron frame

Fabrication technique - The required no. of bicycle tyres are fastened upon the frame. All individual tyres are tied with jute threads at 3-4 places.

Requirement of manpower for slinging - 4 to 8 persons are required.

Procedure: Keeping the downed animal in lateral recumbency. The frame should be pushed underneath the animals's body. Then the paitent to be brought to sternal recumbency and legs should be positioned within spaces provided in frame for purpose of final positioning.

Advantages: Requirement of less man power.

It distributes body weight of animal so that there is no compression effect on chest. Animal are able to stand comfortably and there is no chance of stepping.

The patient has a free movement.

Care during slinging

1. All medicines and supporting therapies should be given before slinging.
2. The suspensory ropes should be examined so as to change damaged ones.
3. Incase of nervous patients, tranquilizers can be administered.
4. Adequate padding should be provided wherever more pressure is exerted.

5. Temperature, pulse, respiration should be checked regularly.

Duration of slinging : The number of days in sling depends upon ability of animal to adjust and for complete recovery.

Care after removing the animal from sling

Animals should be placed on lateral recumbency or in soft bedding.

Prognosis

1. Response from cases neurological disorders and older animals is usually very slow.
2. The side of animal should be changed.

128

Preparation of Padded Tyres for Sling Preparation

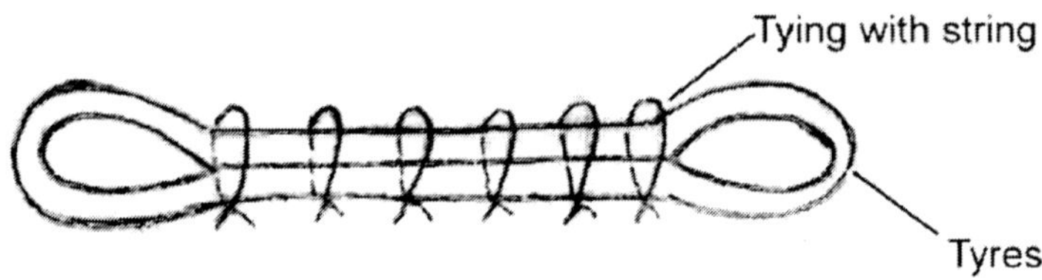

Fig. 1: Rope tying of tyres

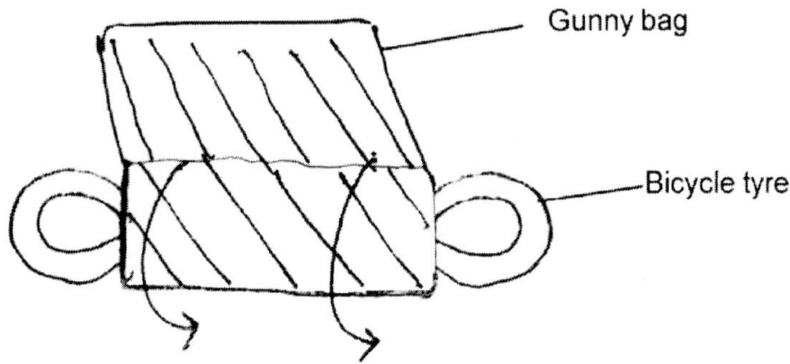

Fig. 2: Wrapping of gunny bag over tyers

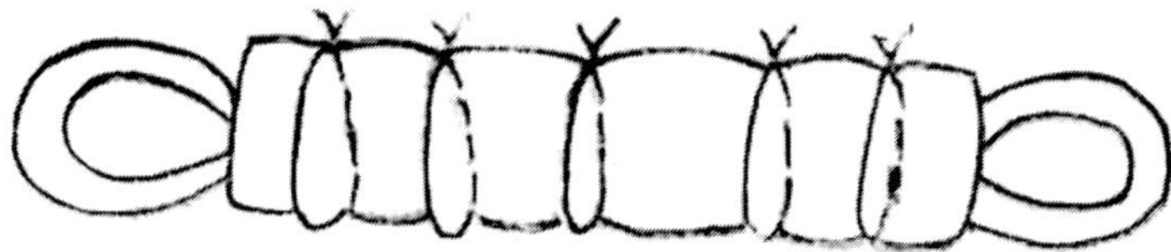

Fig. 3: Padded tyres for sling

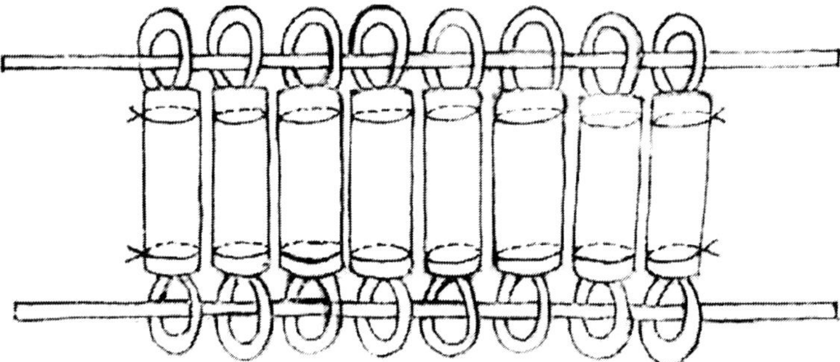

Fig. 4: Arrangement of wrap tyres within two rods

129

Supportive Sling

Indication: Rehabilitation of downer animal

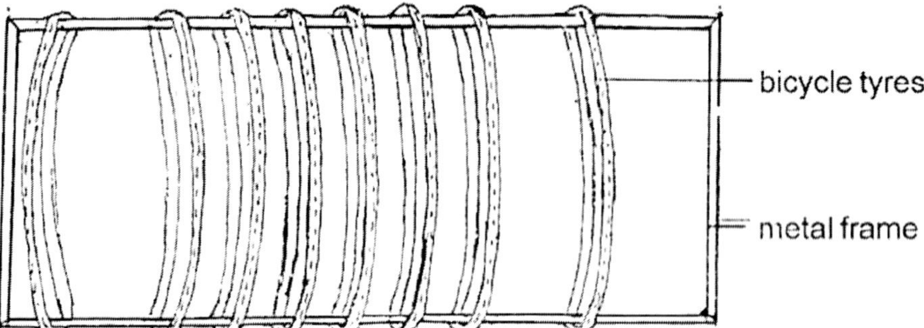

Fig. 1: Pacement of bicycle tyres over the metal frame by sliding

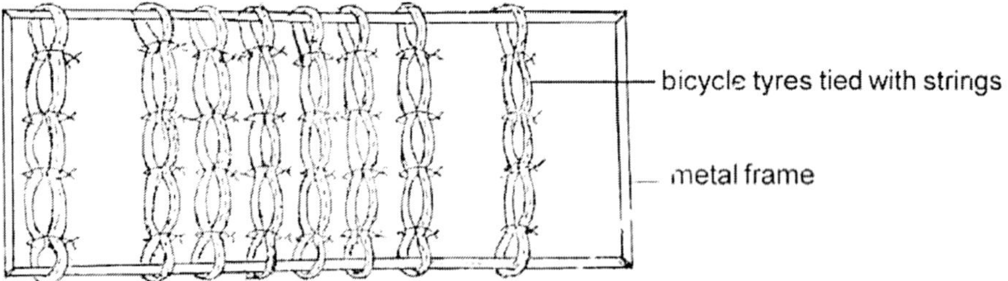

Fig. 2: Securing of bicycle tyres with strings

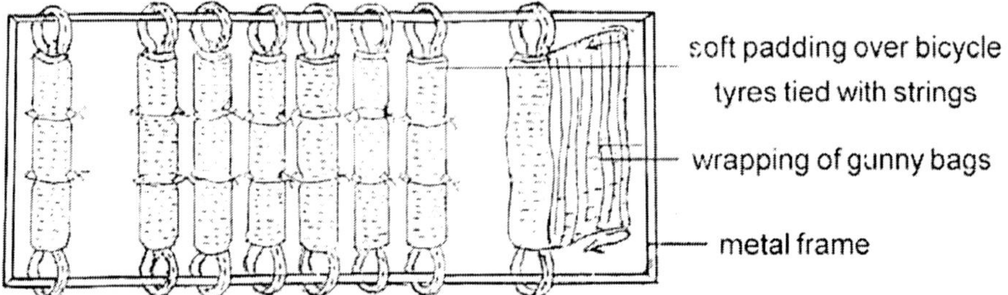

Fig. 3: Wrapping of individual bicycle tyres with gunny bags and securing in position with ropes to provide light and soft bedding

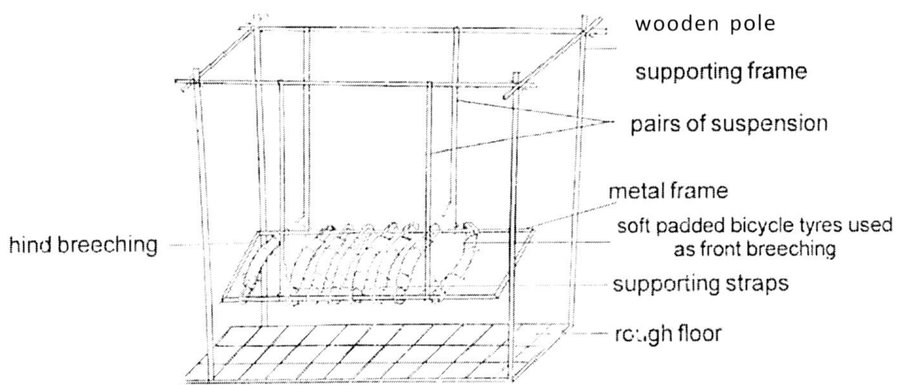

Fig. 4: Complete sling without animal

130

Fabrication of Mobile Sling

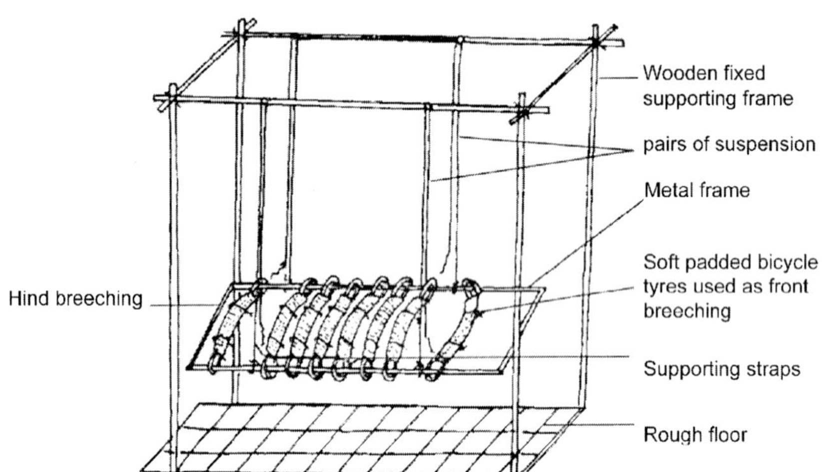

Fig. 1: Complete sling without animal.

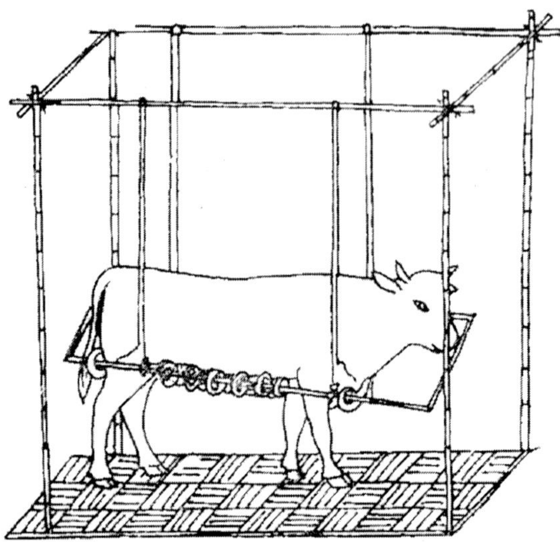

Fig. 2: Downed animal inside the mobile sling

131

Method of Placing Downer Animal Within The Sling

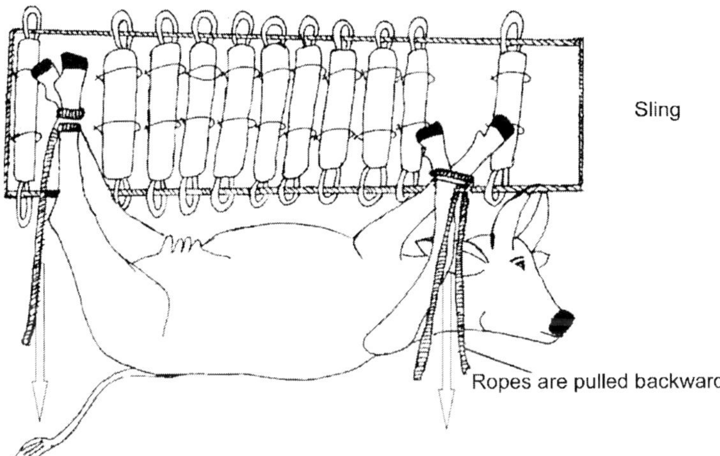

Fig. 1: All the four limbs are highly lifted from ground to put the sling under the body of animal.

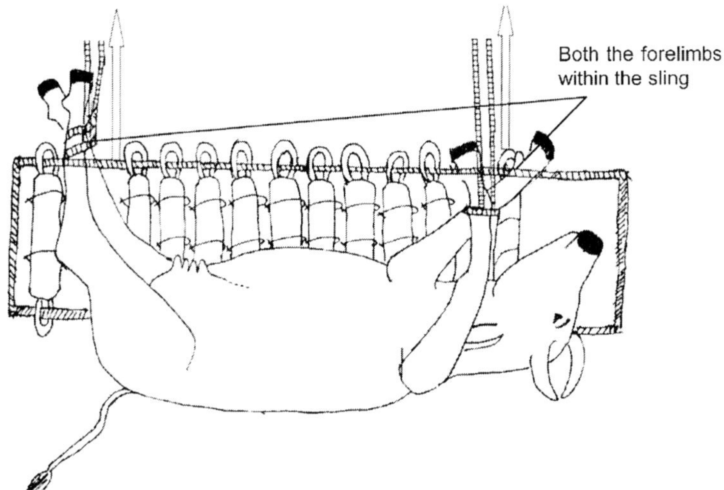

Fig. 2: Placing the animal upon the sling keeping all the four legs within the sling.

132

Method of Slinging

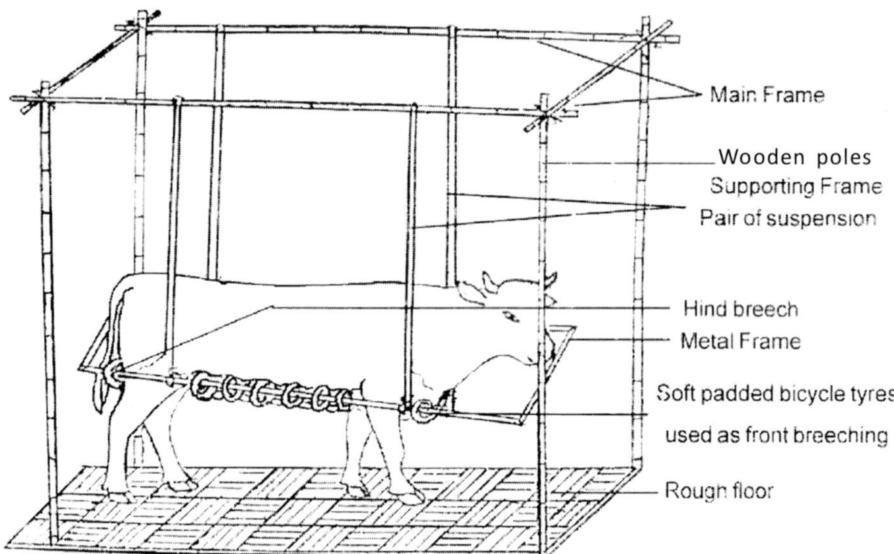

Indication- Downer cow, Sternal recumbency, hypocalcemia, hypomagnesemia, limb or spinal injury, cases related to parturition

Fig. 1: Method of slinging in large animal

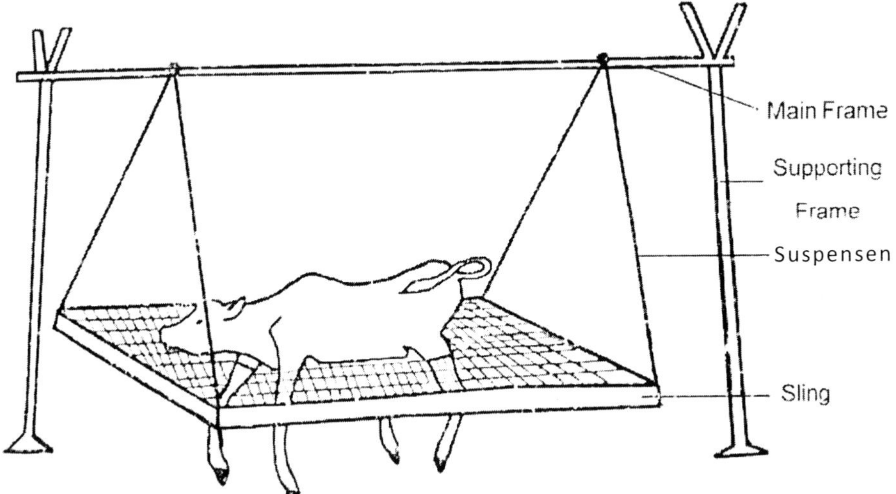

Indication- Fracture of limb, hip dislocation cr displasia, collapse of new born calf, hypothermia in hypocalcemia, hyperthermia in febrile disease

Fig. 2: Method of slinging in small animal

133

Recommended Duration for Slinging Large Animal

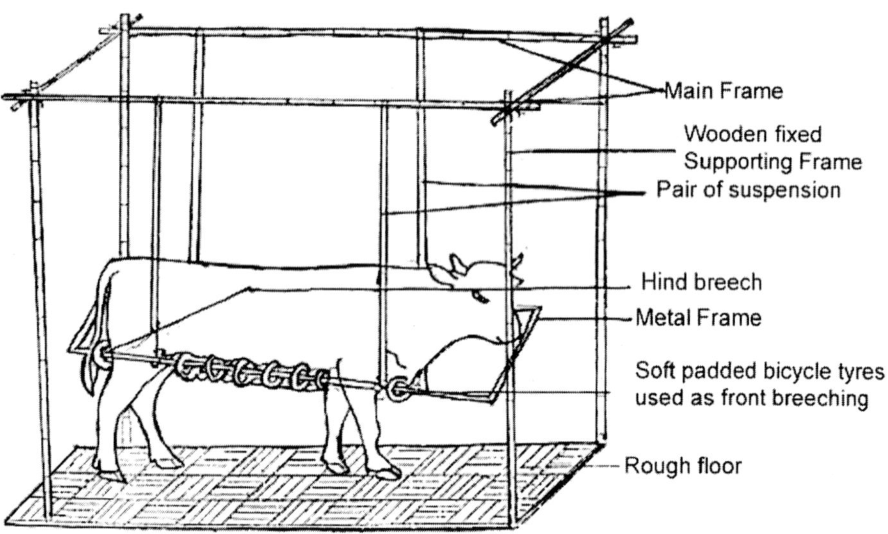

Fig. 1: Downed animal inside the mobile sling

Recommended Duration for Slinging Large Animal

Aim: To know slinging duration for large animal.

Indication: Downer cow, sternal redumbency, hypocalcemia, hypomagnesemia, limb or spinal injury, cases,related to parturition.

Duration of Slinging in the Different Condition

Duration of suffering in recumbency	Heavy Animal		Light Animal	
	Sling-rest-Sling (9pm-7am)	Totai time on Siing in a day	Sling-rest-sling-rest-sling-rest. (9pm-7am)	Total time on sling in a day
0 to 3days	6hrs-2hrs-6hrs-night rest	14hrs	3hrs-2.5hrs-3hrs-2.5hrs 3hrs-ight rest	14hrs
3 to 6 days	5hrs-2hrs-5hrs night rest	14hrs	3hrs-2.5hrs-hrs-2.5hrs night rest	14hrs
Beyond 6 days	4hrs6hrs-4hrs night rest	14 hrs	3hrs-2.5hrs-3hrs -2.5hrs 3hrs night rest	14hrs

Care After Removing The Animal From The Sling

1. Animal should be placed on lateral recumbency or sitting position comfortably on soft bedding.
2. The side of the animal should be changed at intervals of 3-4hrs
3. Animal should be provided with cold body sponging specially during summer.

Prognosis

Response from cases of neurological disorders & older animals is usually very slow. However patients which are alert and have strength can be benefitted most from slinging.

134

Sling Rehabilitation of Calf

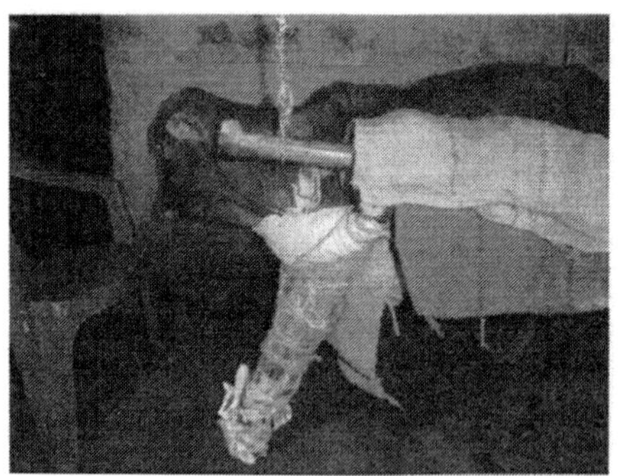

Fig. 1: Cow with fractured tibia fibula radius ulna is rehabilitated in sling.

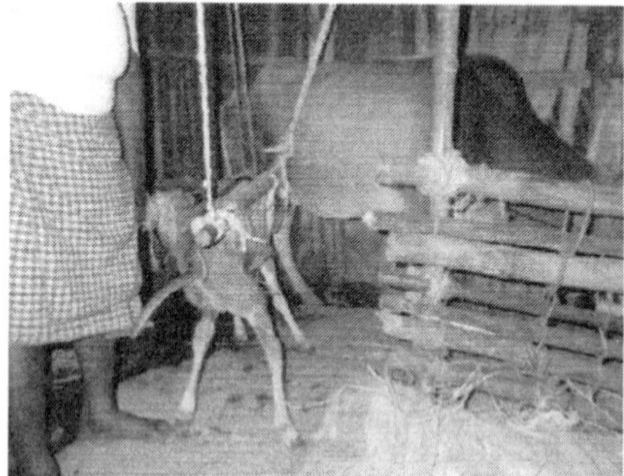

Fig. 2: A sling rehabilitated cow suckling from mother.

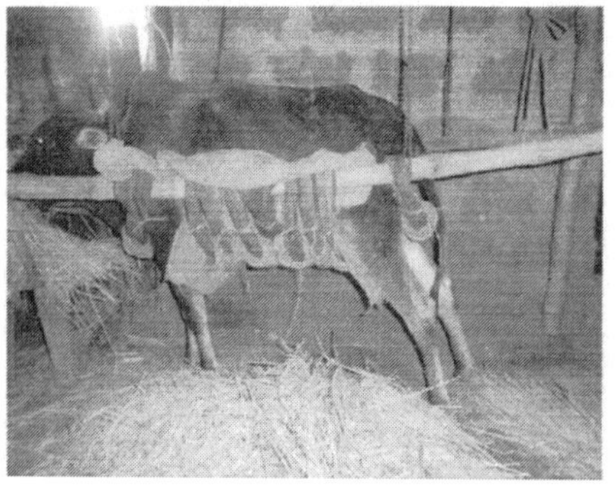

Fig. 3: A rehabilitation of a cow due to upward fixation of patella.

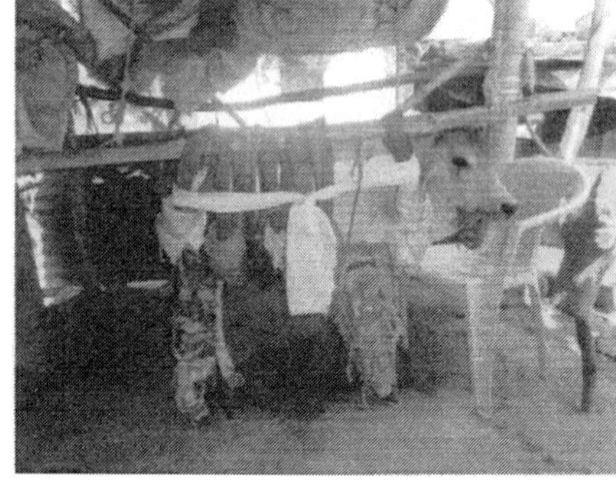

Fig. 4: Rehabilation of bilateral limb fracture of calf after immobilisation.

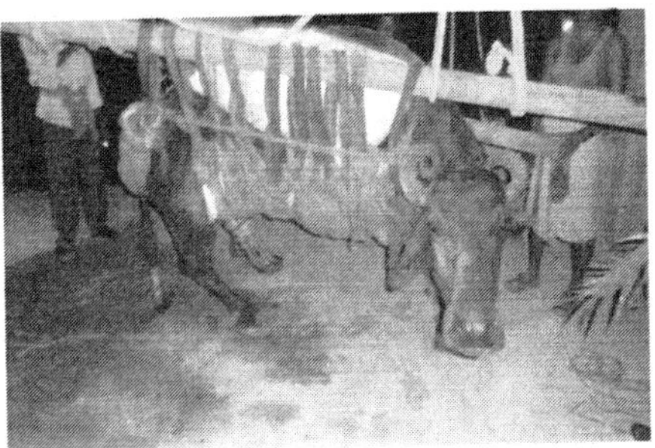

Fig. 5: Rehabilitation of metacarpal fractured buffalo under sling.

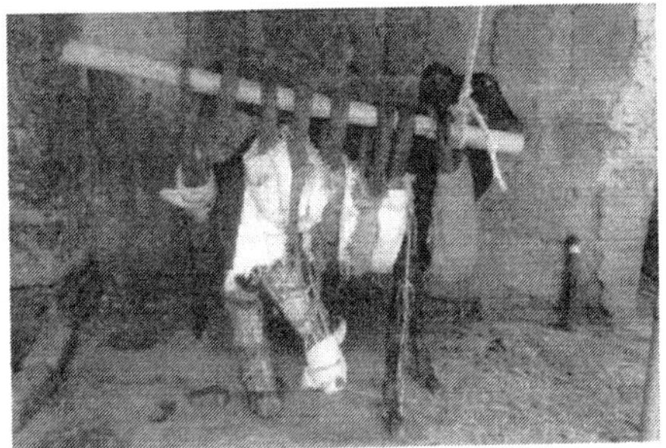

Fig. 6: Rehabilation of animal with both **hindlimb fracture.**

135

Importance of Rehabilitation of More Than one Limb Fractured Animal Within Mobile Sling

Aim of Rehabilitation

1. To assist the animal to stand.
2. To facilitate normal respiration in animal.
3. To ensure normal feed and water Intake.
4. To ensure that rumination,defaecation and urination are normal.

Management

1. Provision of soft and comfortable bedding.
2. Provision of non-slippery floor.
3. Muscle massage to restore normal muscle activity.
4. Treatment of wound and decubitus ulcer.
5. Administration of fluid therapy in case of dehydration.
6. Parental administration of calcium,phosphorus,magnesium and potassium preparations.

Reference: Greenough,P.R and Weaver, A.D.(1997), Lameness In Cattle,3rd Edition,WB Saunders Co. Philadelphia, PP: 215.

136

Rehabilitation of Large Animal in Exercise Cart

Aim

To know the method of rehabilitation of downed animal within exercise wheel cart.

Indication

Irreparable trauma to vertebral column,permanent paralysis, downed animal.

Procedure

1. A model of exercise cart has been illustrated. (Fig)
2. The downed animal Is raised to standard position transferred to exercise cart.
3. The animal is positioned in the exercise cart.
4. The affected limb is properly retained.
5. All the limbs of the animal should be placed squarely on the ground.
6. The mobile sling is moved slowly & in controlled manner to give an impetus to the animal.
7. Animal should be removed from exercise cart after its gait becomes normal.
8. Exercise is practiced dally and regularly till the working ability of animal returns to normal.

Precaution

1. Animal should not kept inside cart for prolong period because it may cause hypostatic congestlon,pressure wound.

2. Precaution may be taken against the hanging of animal inside sling.
3. Exercise should be given at regular interval

Rehabilitation of Large Animal in Exercise Cart

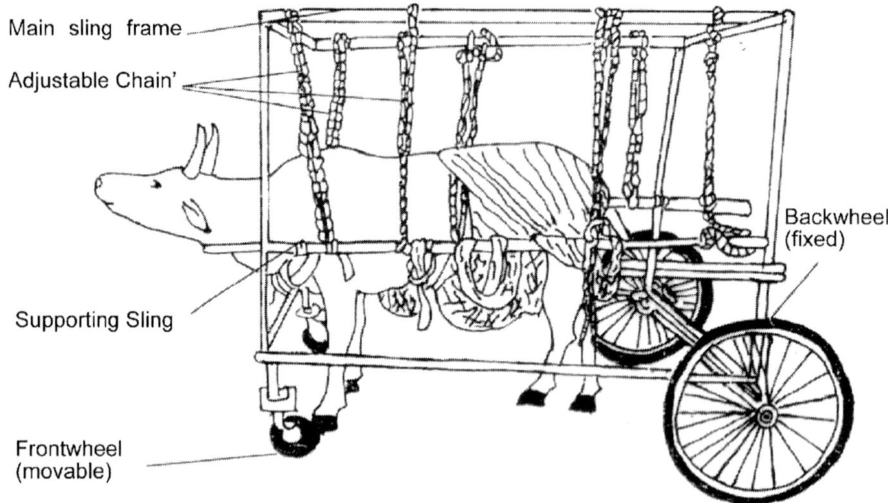

Fig. Exercise cart with supporting sling for large animal rehabilitation.

Rehabilitation of Large Animal in Exercise Cart

AIM

To know the method of rehabilitation of downed animal within exercise wheel cart.

Procedure

1. A model of exercise cart has been illustrated in figure 1 to 7.
2. The downed animal is kept upon the fixed limb and animal is transferred to exercise cart.
3. The animal is brought to standing position.
4. The fixed limb is fixed with mobile sling.
5. All the limbs of the animal should be placed strongly upon the ground.
6. The mobile sling is moved slowly & controlled manner to move the animal.
7. Animal should be removed from exercise cart after it become normal.
8. Exercise is practised daily and regularly till the working ability of animal returns to normal.

Rehabilitation of Large Animal in Exercise Cart

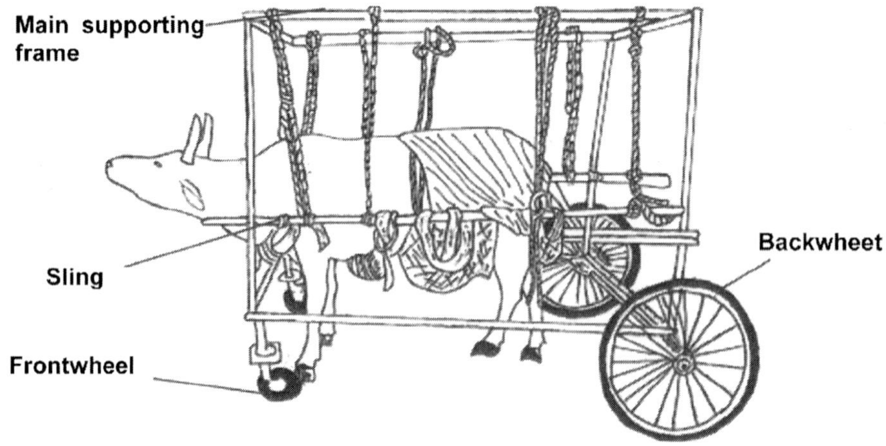

Fig. 1: Exercise cart with supporting sling for large animal with labelled path

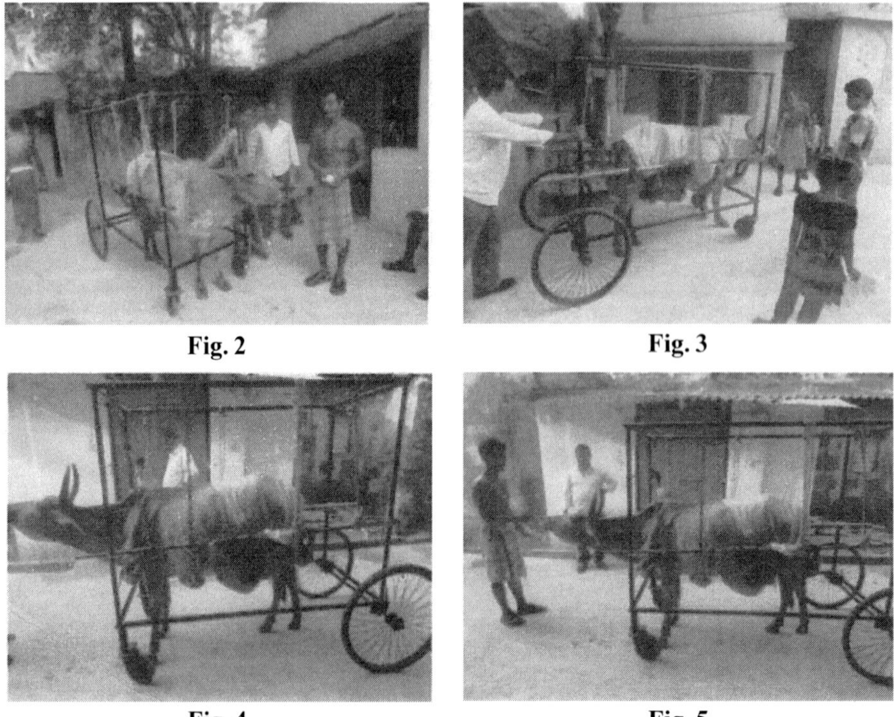

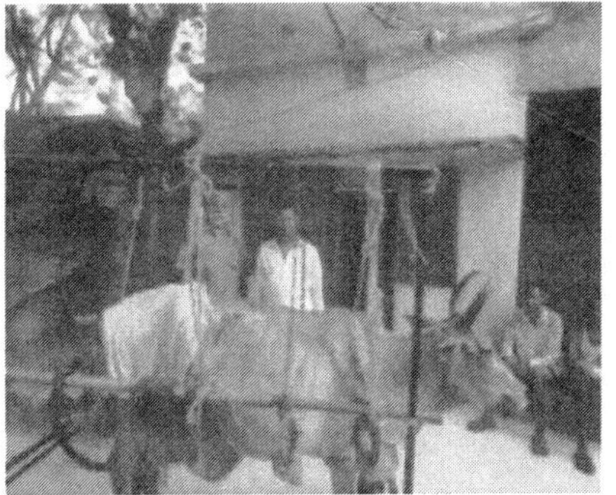

Fig. 6

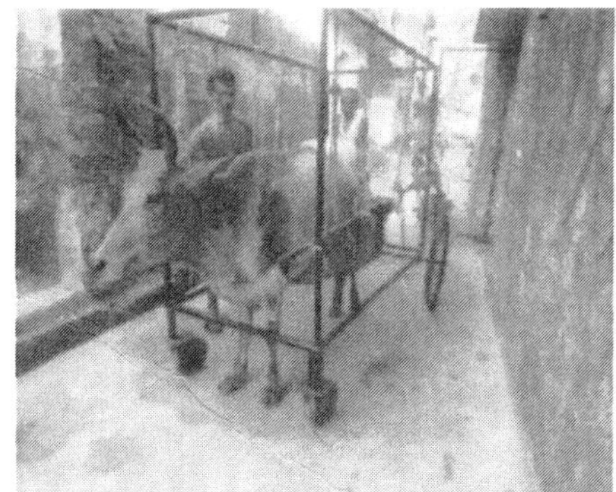

Fig. 7

137

Rehabilitation of Two Limb Fractured Animal Within Mobile Sling

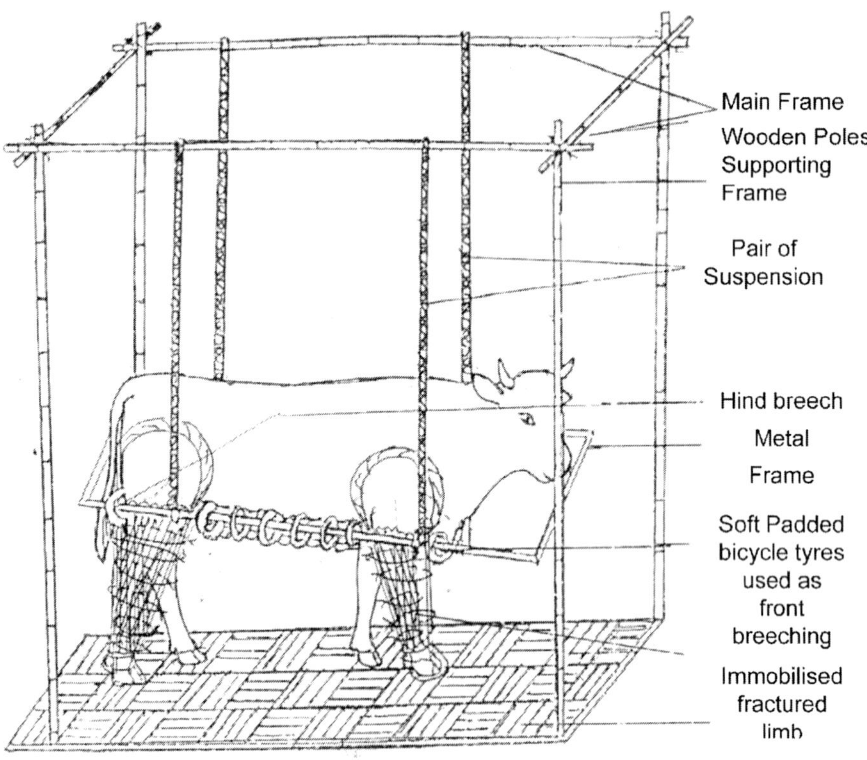

Fig. 1: Method of Slinging in Large Animal

138

Osteology

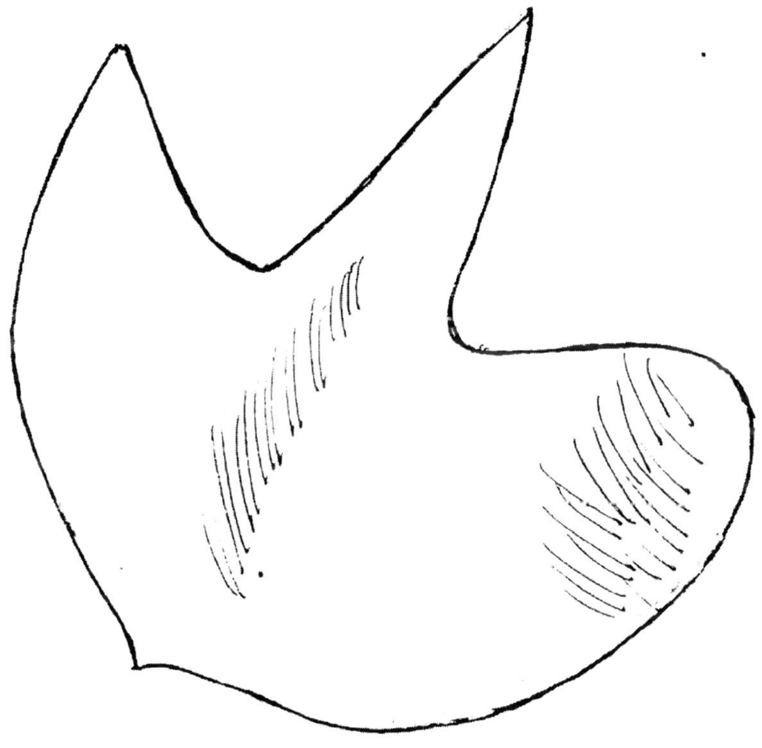

Fig. 1: Lateral maleols

GAIT of a Normal Animal, Fractured Patient and Animal with Thomas Splint

GAIT: It is the pattern of movement of the limbs of animal during locomotion over a solid substrate.

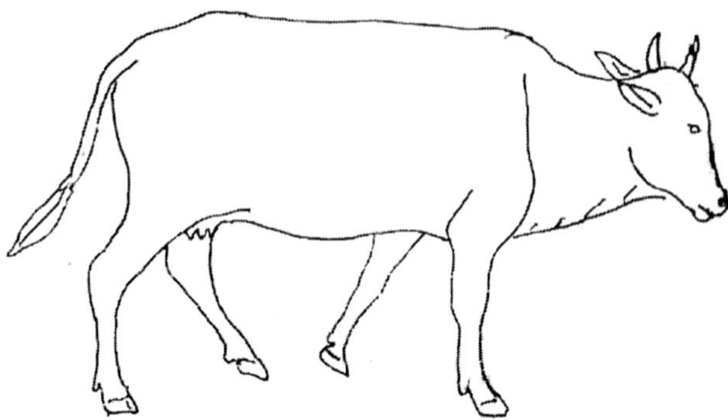

Fig. 2: Gait of normal animal. Animal generally takes a lift to full extent in each step

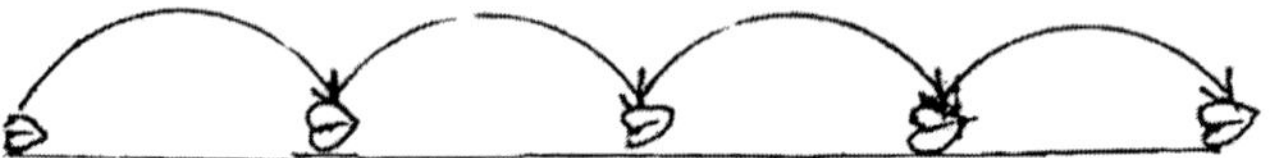

Fig. 3: Gait of normal animal (full lifting of foot)

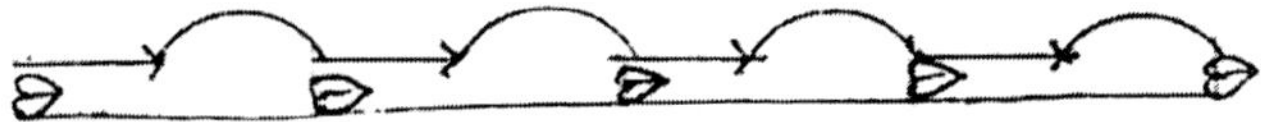

Fig. 4: Gait of a fractured patient (more dragging and less lifting of foot).

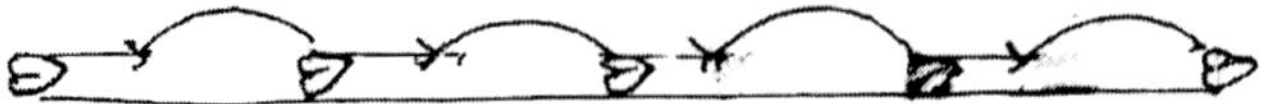

Fig. 5: Gait of animal with light Thomas splint (less dragging and more lifting of foots)

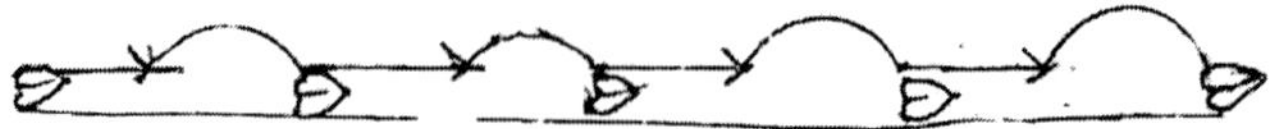

Fig. 6: Gait of animal with heavy Thomas splint (more dragging and less lifting of foot)

139

Prosthetic Fitting

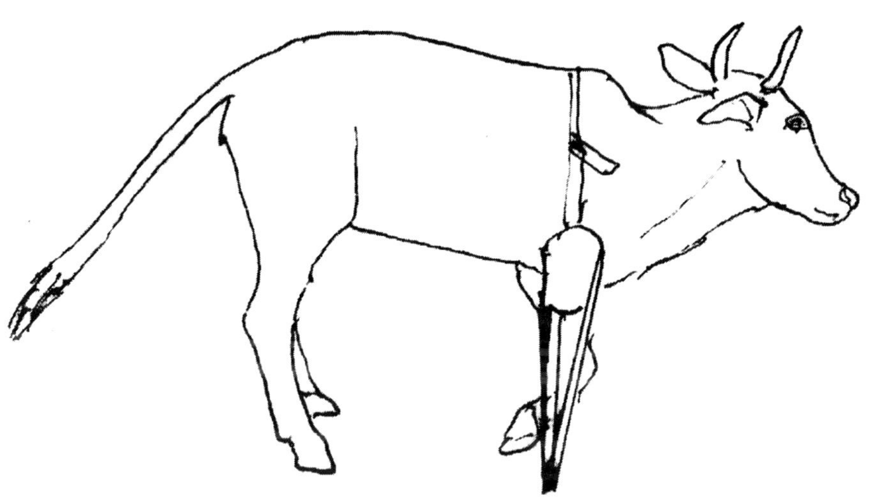

Forelimb Amputees

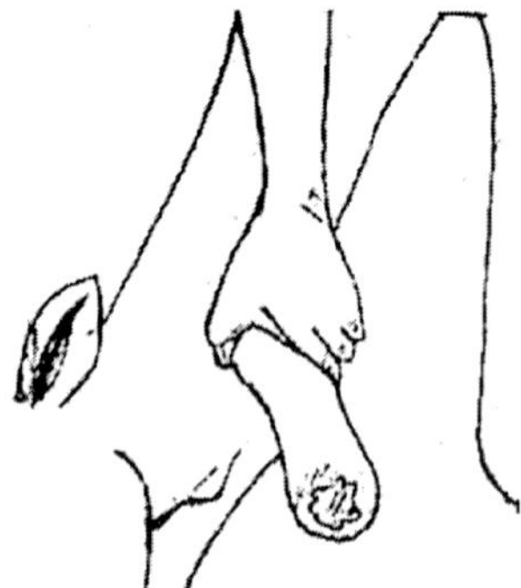

Fig. 1a: Fetlock disarticulation.

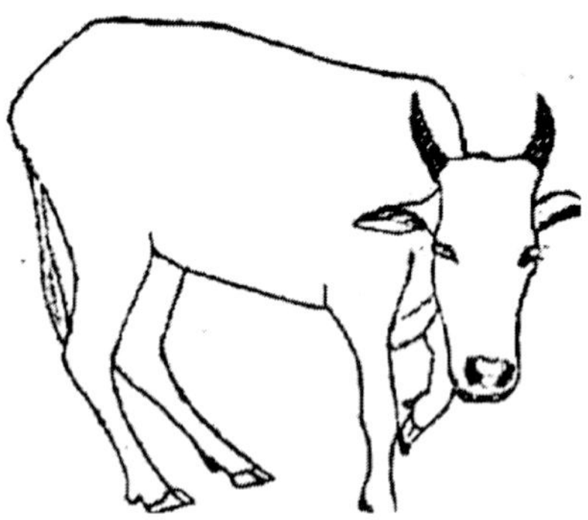

Fig. 1b: Fetlock disarticulation.

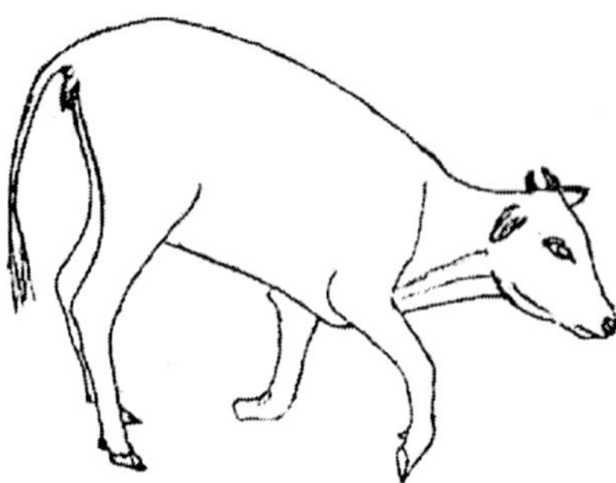

Fig. 2a: Meta carpal amputation

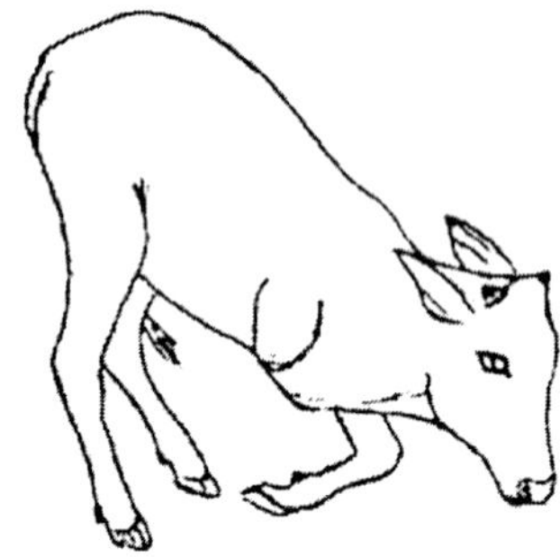

Fig. 2b: Carpo-metacarpal disarticulation

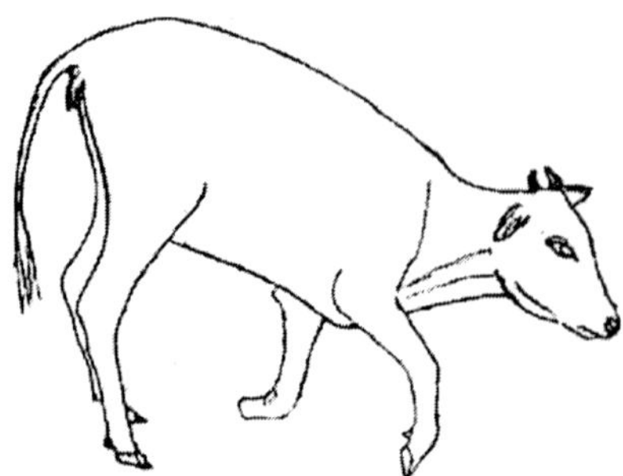

Fig. 3a: Radius ulna amputation

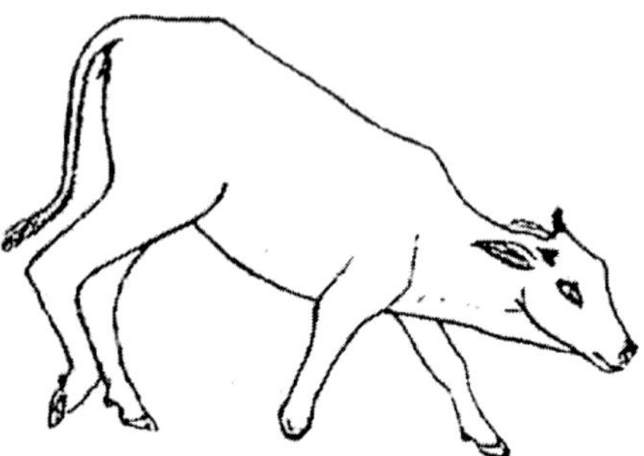

Fig. 3b: Elbow disarticulation

Hind Limb Amputees

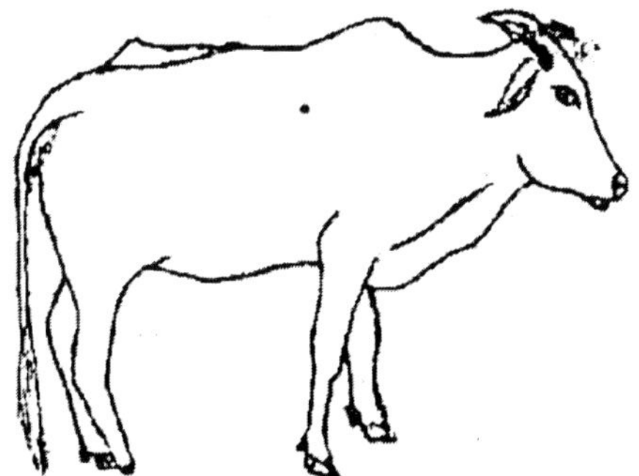

Fig. 4a: Fetlock disarticulation

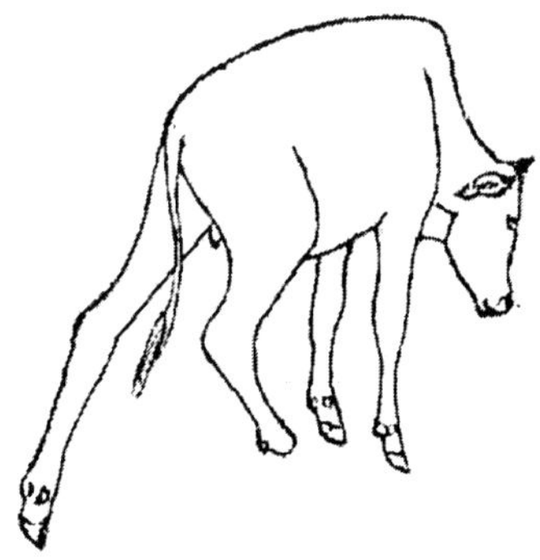

Fig. 4b: Fetlock disarticulation

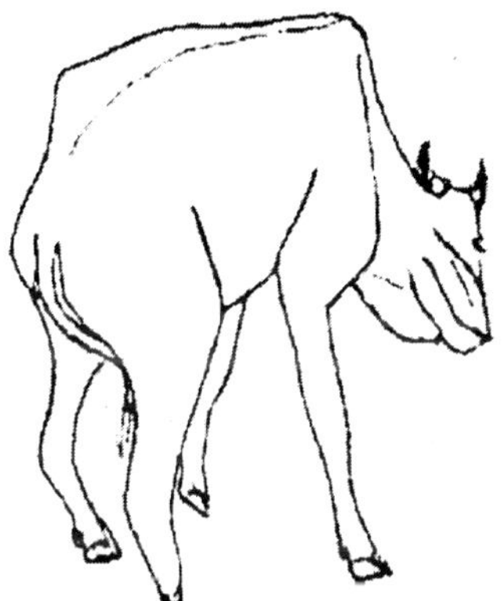

Fig. 5a: Meta tarsal amputation.

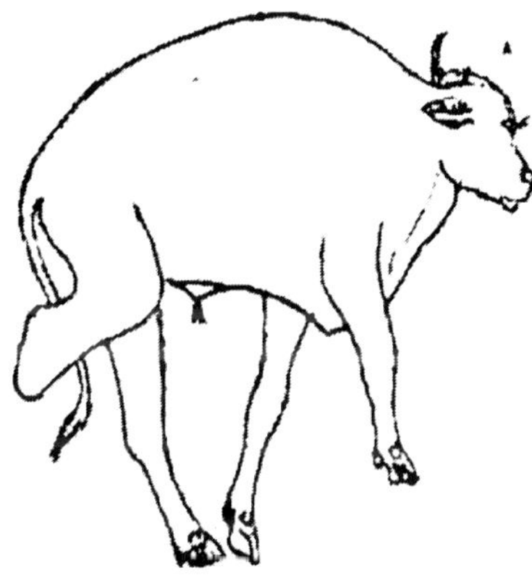

Fig. 5b: Transometa tarsal disarticulation

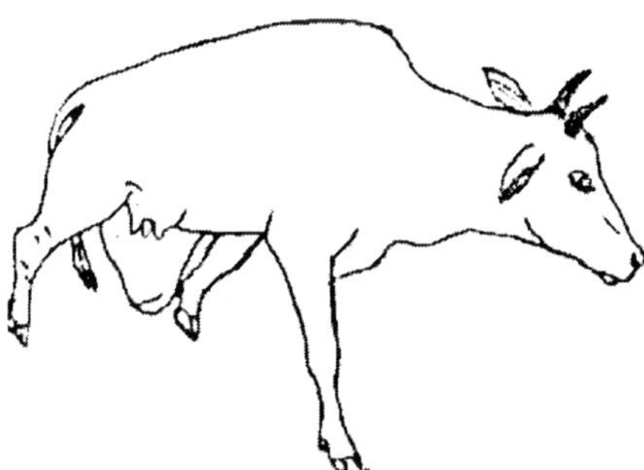

Fig. 6a: Tibiofibula

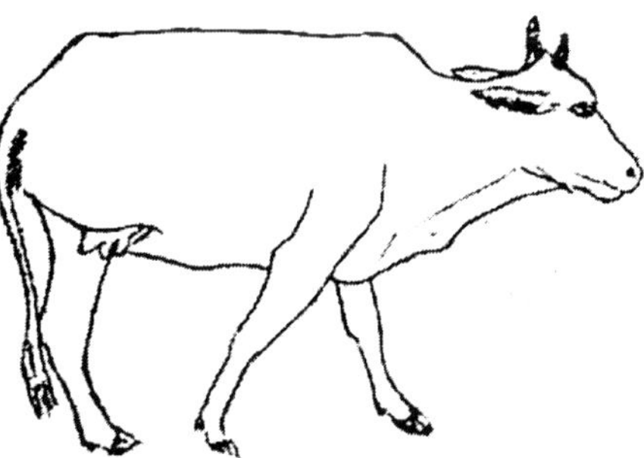

Fig. 6b: Stifle disarticulation